Anatomical Kinesiology

Barbara E. Gench, Ed.D.
Professor
Department of Kinesiology
Texas Woman's University
Denton, Texas

Marilyn M. Hinson, Ph.D.
Professor Emeritus
Department of Kinesiology
Texas Woman's University
Denton, Texas

Patricia T. Harvey, M.A., O.T.R., C.H.T.
Assistant Chief of Occupational Therapy
William Beaumont Army Medical Center
El Paso, Texas

eddie bowers publishing, inc.
2600 Jackson Street
Dubuque, Iowa 52001-3342

eddie bowers publishing, inc.
2600 Jackson Street
Dubuque, Iowa 52001-3342

ISBN 0-945483-34-1

Printed in the United States of America.

9 8 7 6 5 4

CONTENTS

PREFACE

This book is intended as a text for undergraduate courses in kinesiology for students preparing to be therapists and exercise scientists. Its contents are based upon an underlying concept in which emphasis is placed on the importance of an anatomical basis as the pivotal point around which mechanical concepts can subsequently be formed.

Portions of this book have been published under a previous title. That book was intended as a text for undergraduate students majoring in dance and kinesiology. In the present book, applications related to dance and kinesiology have been replaced by applications that are more clinically related. Where one might wonder why only selected clinical applications are presented in this book, the rationale for doing so was based on the fact that this book is written to be used as a text in a first-level kinesiology course. Professional preparation programs frequently require a second-level course of students; it is in that course that more in-depth application to the clinical setting should occur.

It should be pointed out that the selection of terminology was made in order to agree, as much as possible, with the current literature. Two problems were encountered, however, which deserve mention. The first relates to the use of singular and plural suffixes. The suffix **ae** indicates the plural; as, for example, one **vertebra**, two **vertebrae**. Certain muscles carry this suffix in their names (levator scapulae, erector spinae, tensor fasciae latae), but are commonly used with a singular verb. It was decided to parallel that usage in this text, even though it is grammatically incorrect, because to do otherwise would be confusing. The **ae** suffix has been used to indicate the plural, when appropriate, only where muscle names are not concerned.

A second problem of contradiction arose from the lack of agreement in the literature as to whether the bones or the joints flex, extend, rotate, and so on. Certain authors state that a muscle flexes the forearm; others stipulate that the muscle flexes the elbow joint; still others submit that it flexes the forearm at the elbow. The terminology selected for use in this text is that which indicates movement of the joint. Such phrases as "abduction of the hip joint" and "extension of the wrist joint" are typical of the phraseology employed.

Finally, it has been noted that pronunciations of muscle names are quite valuable and sometimes confusing. To meet this problem, a pronunciation model has been included after the name of each muscle. The pronunciations are taken from **Dorland's Illustrated Medical Dictionary**, 27th edition, W. B. Saunders, 1988. In the case where traditional spellings have been preempted by more current terminology (i.e., **deltoid** instead of **deltoideus**), the pronunciation suggested is that of current usage.

Whereas the anatomical considerations are presented in a somewhat traditional manner, including origins, insertions, innervations, and actions, it will be noted that the many related discussions focus upon muscle location and angle of insertion as indicators of muscle action. The student is thereby invited to become acquainted with the logic of movement rather than the tedium of memorization.

The chapters of the text conclude with summary remarks that are intended to help the student apply anatomical considerations to daily activities as well as in the clinical setting rather than to consider them a nonintegrated, meaningless part of the kinesiology course. Suggested laboratory experiences are included in each chapter which have, in the authors' experience, proved to be of value in the achieving of a full understanding of the materials. Quizzes have been included which relate to the topics covered in each chapter. These are provided to give the student an opportunity to evaluate progress toward understanding kinesiology.

A comprehensive bibliography has been provided. The inquiring student should find it useful in the search for related and in-depth information.

At the time that this book was written, one of the authors was serving in the United States Army. It should be noted that the views stated in this book are not the views of the United States Army.

The authors are indebted to many individuals for their valuable help during the writing of the book. Particular acknowledgment is extended to Mary Johnson for her excellent illustrations. Appreciation is expressed to Dr. Grace Gilkeson, Dr. Jean Pyfer and Dr. Ann Uhlir for their continued encouragement and support. Finally, we would like to express our gratitude to ***eddie bowers publishing, inc.*** for their aid in all phases of this manuscript's preparation.

Barbara Gench
Marilyn Hinson
Patricia Harvey

HISTORY AND NOMENCLATURE

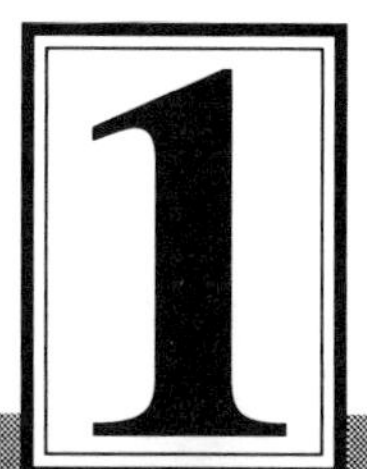

INTRODUCTION

Kinesiology has been widely accepted as an integral course in the undergraduate curriculum of those who will specialize in human movement. It is puzzling, therefore, that the meaning of the word **kinesiology** is not more commonly known. Taken literally, the word can be separated into its roots of **ology** (science of) and **kinein** (to move). Unfortunately, the resulting definition, "science of movement," is too broad to be useful, for to say that one is studying the science of movement could indicate anything from human anatomy to the development of human reflexes. Certainly these disciplines are related to kinesiology -- each shares a common object of study, the human being. Kinesiology is, however, uniquely different from all other movement sciences in that its focus is upon knowledge of the mechanics of movement which emerge from the blending of the knowledge of human anatomy with that knowledge basic to the study of physics. For example, in kinesiology, one learns to relate the facts of muscular origin and insertion of anatomy to mechanics such as joint axis and angle of insertion in order to explain the actions of a given muscle. One learns, also, to relate muscle actions and joint positions to the demands of successful performance in daily activities.

Kinesiology - Knowledge of the Mechanics of Movement

Kinesiology is seen, then, to be comprised of two sub-areas: the first is concerned with the production of movement, or lack of movement, by the muscles of the body -- the second with events which result from the application of muscular force. The first sub-area is known as **anatomy of human motion**, and is so oriented as to answer such questions as "at what angle should the elbow be held to allow surrounding muscles to exert greatest strength?" or "why are the muscles of the thigh so important to the integrity of the knee joint?" The second sub-area is referred to as **mechanics of human motion**, and includes concepts designed to answer questions such as "in what position should one's center of gravity be placed in order to be most stable?" or "how might the principles of leverage be used for the most effective transfer of a patient from a bed to a wheelchair?"

A BRIEF HISTORY

Trace the History of Kinesiology

from

Aristotle

to

Archimedes

to

Galen

to

da Vinci

to

Galilie

to

Newton

to

Galvani

to

Duchenne

The division of kinesiological materials into anatomical and mechanical sub-areas is not without some historical basis. Certainly Aristotle, who has been titled the Father of Kinesiology, was concerned not only with muscle actions but also with the influence of muscular activity upon the generation of force. It is remarkable and exciting that there was such keen interest in movement as was demonstrated by this Greek philosopher who lived more than 2000 years ago.

It was only some 100 years after Aristotle that Archimedes developed the principles of buoyancy that continue to be received as valid. It is unusual to find a kinesiology text that does not include his principles in its treatment of the mechanics of swimming.

Perhaps it was inevitable that man's curiosity about the basics of muscle contraction led Galen, a Roman who lived during the second century after Christ, to consider contractile properties of muscle. Although his explanation of the workings of nerves was more spiritual than scientific, he was nevertheless able to define agonism and antagonism with accuracy. He also coined the still-used terms of **diarthrosis** and **synarthrosis**, which relate to joint mobility.

Not until more than ten centuries after Galen did the works of Leonardo da Vinci begin. Best known as an artist, da Vinci was intrigued with the human body and its movement characteristics. Mechanics of posture, gait, and jumping all came under his careful scrutiny. His mechanical and engineering drawings are often seen today as logos of kinesiological societies, as cover designs of textbooks, and even on T-shirts.

What schoolchild has not heard of Galileo Galilie and the Leaning Tower of Pisa? Almost fairy-tale-like in the minds of many is the story of Galileo dropping various objects from the tower in the seventeenth century so he could prove that the pull of gravity is not selective: it exerts its influence to accelerate a falling body at the same rate regardless of the weight of the body. This important principle is used in many classrooms to explain the phenomena related to such things as skydiving, projectile trajectory, and force absorption.

Sir Isaac Newton (1642-1727) is fondly associated with apples, for many would have it that he was observing apples fall from an apple tree when he discovered the laws of gravity, inertia, acceleration, and action-reaction. Be that as it may, his laws are considered basic to the study of the mechanics of movement, and are used universally to explain force resolution and composition, centripetal force, angle of projection, and virtually any other problem that confronts the movement specialist.

Approximately 140 years after Newton's death, Guillaume Duchenne returned the focus of interest to the basic study of muscle function. His work was based, to some extent, on that done previously by Luigi Galvani, who verified the presence of electrical potentials in muscle and nerve. Galvani's name is remembered often by those who study Galvanic Skin Response (GSR) in lie detector tests, tests of like and dislike, etc.

Duchenne built upon Galvani's work by developing a technique of stimulating the contraction of a muscle of the body and observing the reaction of the associated body parts. Even though Duchenne admitted that the contraction of a single muscle was not representative of the complicated interchange of muscle activity in movement, his work gave the kinesiologist a firmer base for analysis than did simple palpation.

During the same time period in which Duchenne was involved in his early electromyographic studies, Eadweard Muybridge (later known as Ed Weard) became interested in studying movement in a temporal manner. There are many legends about Muybridge. One of the most interesting has it that he visited a tavern that exhibited a painting of Napoleon on a galloping horse. The painting, as did all paintings of that era, depicted the horse with one hoof on the ground. Some discussion ensued and, as a result, Muybridge wagered a considerable sum that the artist was in error; that, in fact, horses at gallop did not always have one leg in contact with the ground. There was, rather, a period in each stride during which the horse was airborne. After considerable effort, expense, and consultation, Muybridge set several cameras along a race track. As the horse passed each camera, a device was triggered so that each camera recorded the action in front of it. Muybridge won his bet! The photographic evidence proved that the horse was, in deed, airborne during part of the gallop stride. So dawned the era of motion photography as a tool for collection of movement data. Whether the many legends about Eadweard Muybridge are true or not, credit must be given to him for his applications of photography to human movement. They remain classic to the sciences of kinesiology and biomechanics.

At approximately the same point in time, C. W. Braune and Otto Fisher, to be followed somewhat later by Rudolph Fick, completed basic research related to body segment weights, centers of gravity, and other parameters of importance to assessment of strength and center of gravity. Their works are classic in the sciences of kinesiology and biomechanics, and have been augmented by the findings of Dempster in his more current efforts.

In the middle 1900s, Arthur Steindler authored what has become a classic text in kinesiology entitled **Kinesiology of the Human Body under Normal and Pathological Conditions**. Because of the importance, past and present, of his manuscript, every serious student of kinesiology is urged to add it to his or her library at the earliest possible time.

to

Muybridge

to

Braune

to

Fisher

to

Fick

to

Steindler

to

Dempster

NOMENCLATURE

We are now brought to the current day in our exploration of the historical events that have undergirded what we know as the science of kinesiology and/or biomechanics. It is of interest to note, at this point, that as our ability to analyze motion has progressed, so has our terminology. It is recognized that the many words used in conjunction with the study of human movement may be confusing to the student of the science -- perhaps they are equally confusing to the professional. What is the difference between **kinesiology** and **biomechanics**? How do **statics, dynamics, kinetics**, and **kinematics** relate to the study of human movement? What are **electromyography** and **cinematography**? How does the study of **forces** relate to the science of movement? Let us answer these questions in order.

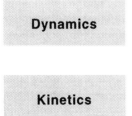

Kinesiology vs. Biomechanics

Regarding the difference between kinesiology and biomechanics, it was noted above that kinesiology can be defined broadly as the science of movement. It takes its base in a thorough knowledge of the anatomical and muscular structures of the human body. It is only when these have been mastered that mechanics of motion are introduced. Biomechanics, on the other hand, would appear to assume that its devotees already have a sound grasp of an anatomical and muscular knowledge and can proceed with an in-depth study of movement mechanics. There is, obviously, some overlap in the materials embodied by the titles of the two sciences. Whereas the kinesiologist is attentive to the mechanics of movement, he treats it somewhat superficially and only after anatomical considerations have been mastered. The biomechanist enters at this point, and with the kinesiologist's background, focuses upon the mechanics of movement and explores with all depth possible.

Statics

The terms **statics**, **dynamics**, **kinetics**, and **kinematics** have appeared since we began to use biomechanics as a scientific descriptor. Statics refers to that branch of biomechanics that is concerned with equilibrium -- that is, the **sum of all moments must equal zero**. Such a concept may seem foreign to the uninitiated; it need not be so. That basic formula of statics translates simply that with a seesaw situation in which two children of equal weight are sitting at equal distances from the axis of the seesaw, no movement will occur. The seesaw is balanced. Equivalently, if the force of buoyancy equals the force of gravity, a body will neither sink nor rise. Also, any pull or push that is matched by one of the same force will yield no movement. In each of these examples, the sum of the moments of force is equal to zero. Said another way, each moment of force is neutralized by an equal and opposite moment. So it is with the subscience of statics.

Dynamics

Dynamics is the name of the biomechanical branch of interest that is concerned with movement and its velocity, acceleration, and associated forces. Subheadings of biomechanics are kinetics and kinematics. Kinetics includes that portion of dynamics that is concerned with body mass and with muscular forces that are applied to move that mass. To determine the center of mass of a long jumper or to analyze the arm action of a high jumper is to study kinetics.

Kinetics

Students of kinematics do not concern themselves with the causes of motion but rather with the results of the causes. Projection paths of sports implements as well as of the body itself come under their close scrutiny. Spin and rebound are also of interest, as are the principles of aerodynamics.

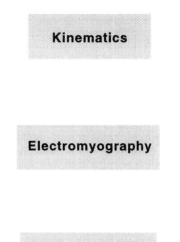

Kinematics

Electromyography and cinematography are tools for the gathering of kinesiological and biomechanical data. Electromyographic records are taken, through special electrodes, of contracting or resting muscles. Determinations can be made regarding the strength of a muscle's contraction, the beginning and duration of contraction and, indeed, whether contraction is occurring at all.

Electromyography

Cinematographic data are film records made with motion picture or video cameras. The films are usually exposed at high speeds in order to yield a slow-motion quality when they are projected. Analysis of sports movement is obviously enhanced because of the slowing of motion and also because the films provide a discrete and permanent record that can be restudied at will.

Cinematography

The study of forces is basic to the analysis of human movement. The gathering of force data is done through the use of special instrumentation that is sensitive to pushing or pulling. Peak forces as well as force profiles over time can be recorded to determine, for example, whether there is a difference in the grip strength of the right and left hands of highly skilled golfers, or to specify the amounts of force applied to the ground by an amputee between heel-down and toe-off of the normal and orthotic foot.

It is hoped that this brief discussion of nomenclature has been clarifying and has dispelled any confusion. The definitions and explanations offered are sound and appear to reflect the thinking of the current leaders in the field.

TERMINOLOGY AND BASIC CONCEPTS

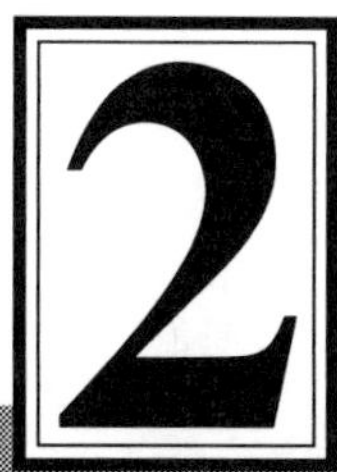

The concepts presented in this chapter are considered to be basic to a study of the anatomical aspects of kinesiology. They are developed around a terminology that has been agreed upon by kinesiologists and that appears in most of the literature.

REFERENCE POSITIONS

Two positions have been universally accepted as reference positions for joint movement (Fig. 2.1). One, called the **fundamental position**, prescribes that the subject stand in upright posture with feet parallel and close, with the arms at the sides and the palms of the hands facing the body. The second reference position, the **anatomical position**, varies from the fundamental position only in that the arms are away from the body with the palms facing forward. Either position may be used as a basis around which to describe all joint movements of the body except those of the forearm. When the palm of the hand is turned inwardly and outwardly, the anatomical reference position must be used.

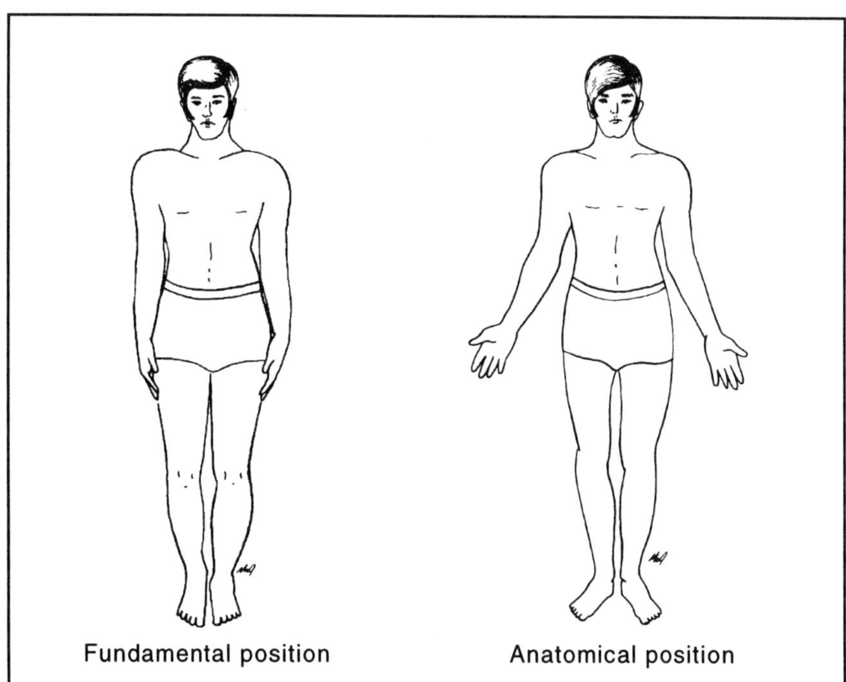

Fig. 2.1

Reference Positions

The purpose of the reference position is to supply a starting point from which movement in any direction can be described. For example, a forward swing of the arm involves flexion of the shoulder joint; extension is defined as the joint movement which allows a downward and backward swing of the arm but only until the arm has returned to the reference position. Additional backward swing of the arm requires hyperextension of the shoulder joint. Since the muscles of the shoulder which cause extension may not necessarily be the ones which cause hyperextension, the kinesiologist must be precise in describing the action of the arm in order to differentiate among the attendant activities of the surrounding muscles. The use of a reference position which has been universally accepted can provide for the required precision.

TYPES OF MOTION

The two types of motion referred to most frequently are **linear** or **rectilinear**, and **angular**. During **linear motion**, an object progresses in a straight line from one position to another with all of its parts moving in the same direction and at the same velocity. A boat, gliding through the water, is undergoing linear motion. The elevation and depression of the shoulder girdle when one shrugs the shoulders involves movement of the scapula which is linear in nature.

Linear Motion

Angular motion, also called **rotary** or **rotatory** motion, is defined as motion in which all parts of an object move along the arc of a circle around a center or axis of rotation. A propeller exhibits angular motion with all of its parts moving along the arc of a complete circle, the center or axis of which is the hub. The forearm undergoes angular motion, also, when the elbow is bent and straightened as its parts follow the arc of a partial circle around an axis at the joint.

Angular Motion

The varied movements of the human body as a whole are usually comprised of both angular and linear components. Walking, running, and jumping all combine the linear movement of the trunk with the angular movements of the limbs, and are referred to as **combination movements** involving both types of motion. When movements of only a portion of the body are described, however, they are referred to as being either linear or angular in nature, and small discrepancies are ignored. Even though the action of the scapula noted during shoulder shrugging is actually accompanied by a certain amount of angular motion, it is mainly linear and is described as such. Bending and straightening the elbow involves some gliding between the bones of that joint; however, the motion of the forearm is primarily angular and is so designated.

Combination Movements

PLANES OF ACTION

In order to facilitate the description and analysis of movements, kinesiologists have adopted the use of three anatomical reference planes. These planes, called **cardinal planes**, can be conceptualized as three large panes of glass. Each pane is oriented at right angles to the two remaining planes as they pass through the body.

Cardinal Plane

The cardinal sagittal plane (Fig. 2.2) progresses from the front to the back of the body, dividing it, by weight, into right and left halves. Movements are said to be occurring in the **sagittal plane** either when they are in the cardinal plane -- nodding the head *yes* -- or when they are in a plane parallel to the cardinal plane -- a forward and backward swing of the arms. Joint actions which result in sagittal movements are called **flexion**, **extension**, and **hyperextension**.

Sagittal Plane

Sagittal Plane and Movements

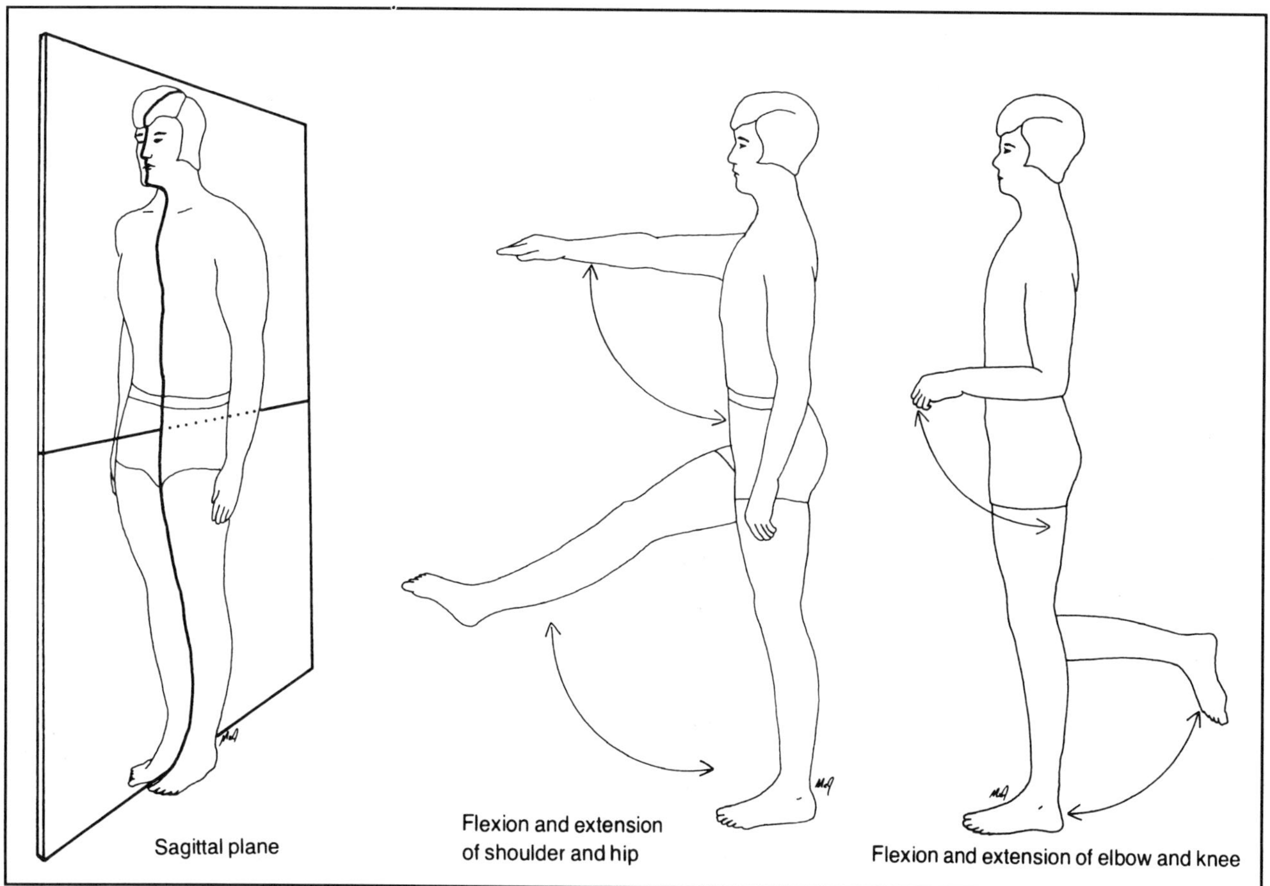

Fig 2.2

Frontal Plane

The cardinal frontal plane (Fig. 2.3) passes through the body from side to side, dividing it, by weight, into front and back halves. Almost all movements which occur in the **frontal plane** are in that cardinal plane and are exemplified by the sideward swings of the arms during the "jumping jack" exercise. Joint actions, which allow for angular movements in the frontal plane, are called **abduction** and **adduction** where the limbs are concerned and **lateral flexion** if the spine is involved.

Frontal Plane and Movements

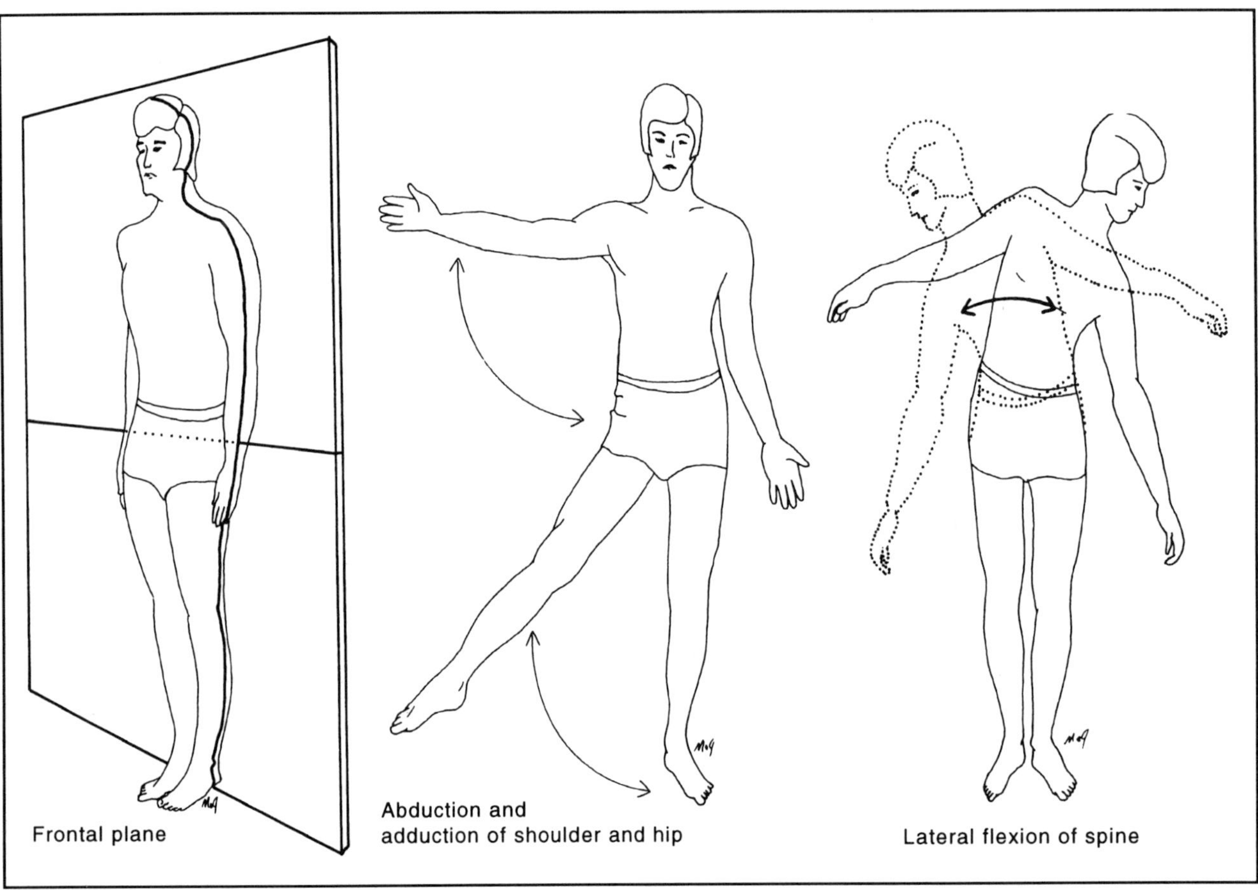

Fig. 2.3

Transverse Plane

The cardinal transverse or horizontal plane (Fig. 2.4) divides the body, by weight, into a top half and a bottom half. It would be difficult to execute a movement in this cardinal plane since all motion would have to be localized in the hip region. The many movements of the body which are said to occur in the **transverse plane** actually are in a plane parallel to the cardinal one. Turning the head to look from side to side, or turning the palms inwardly and outwardly are examples of movements in the transverse plane. Joint actions which result in such movements are called **rotation**, and, where the limbs are concerned, are further described as being either internal or external.

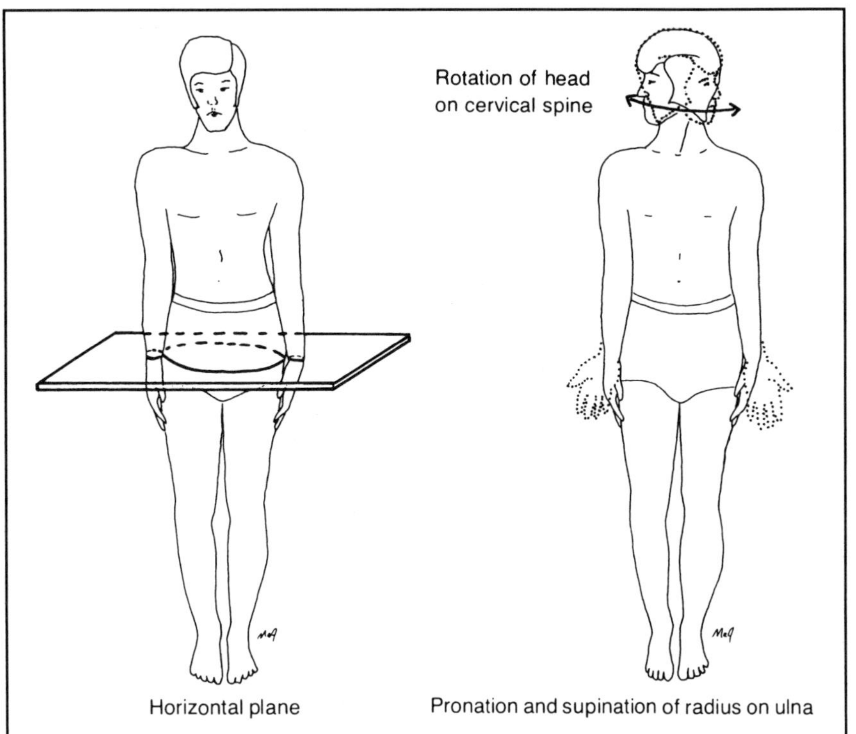

Fig. 2.4

Horizontal Plane and Movements

When the three cardinal planes are visualized as passing through the body simultaneously, it will be noted that there is a common point of intersection which is taken to be the center of gravity, or as it is also called, the center of mass.

AXES

Movements occur in a plane and, if they are angular in nature, around an axis. Each of the three cardinal planes is conceptualized with an axis which is at right angles to it (Fig. 2.5). An axis at right angles to the sagittal plane would be a horizontal one which is oriented from side to side. Because its orientation is the same as that of the frontal plane, this axis is called the **frontal axis.** An axis at right angles to the frontal plane is oriented from front to back as is the sagittal plane, and is called, therefore, the **sagittal axis.** The axis at right angles to the transverse plane is known as the **long axis** or **vertical axis** and passes downwardly through the top of the head.

Axes of Rotation

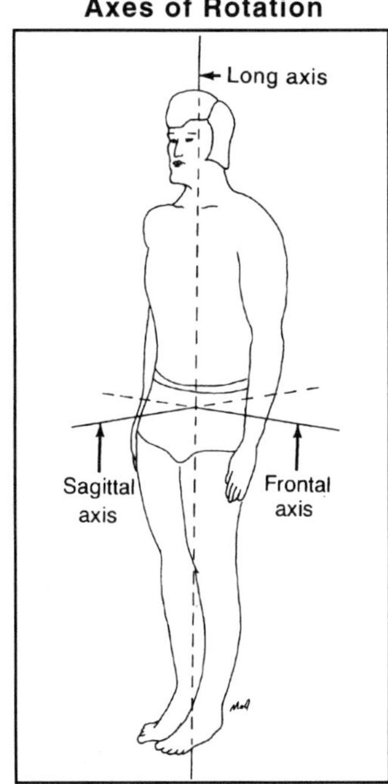

Fig. 2.5

Just as the three cardinal planes intersect at the center of gravity, so do the three cardinal axes; however, since most angular movements of the skeleton occur in planes parallel to the cardinal planes, they consequently occur around axes parallel to the cardinal axes. The forward and backward swinging of the arm is said to occur around the frontal axis even though this particular axis passes through the body from side to side at shoulder level rather than at

Frontal Axis

the level of the center of gravity. Abduction and adduction of the leg is performed around a sagittal axis which passes through the hip; inward and outward rotation of the arm occurs around a vertical axis which passes through the top of the shoulder.

Planes and their axes are inseparable. Angular movements in the sagittal plane must occur around the frontal axis, just as angular movements in the frontal and transverse planes must occur around the sagittal and vertical axes, respectively.

Sagittal Axis

It is common for a kinesiologist to refer to the **long** or **longitudinal axis** of the body. This item of terminology appears to have stemmed from some confusion regarding those joints which provide for rotation in the transverse plane. Inward and outward twisting of the arm while in anatomical position is occurring in the transverse plane around a long axis; however, when exactly the same twisting motion is performed with the arm held in front of the body and at shoulder level, the plane is frontal and the axis is sagittal. To clarify any confusion, it has become practice to describe rotational movements of the spine and limbs as occurring around their long axes if these movements are not in the transverse plane.

Long Axis

The use of both an axis and a plane is appropriate only if angular motions are being described. Since linear motion is defined as motion during which all parts of the object move in the same direction and at the same velocity, there can be no axis of rotation. Linear motion is described, then as occurring simply in a plane; angular motion is described as occurring both in a plane and around an axis.

JOINT MECHANICS

When two bones form a connection, the resulting articulation is called a **joint**. The purpose of most joints is to provide for movement of the bones of the skeleton; however, some joints are structured to yield strength or form to the skeleton.

Fibrous Joints of the Skull

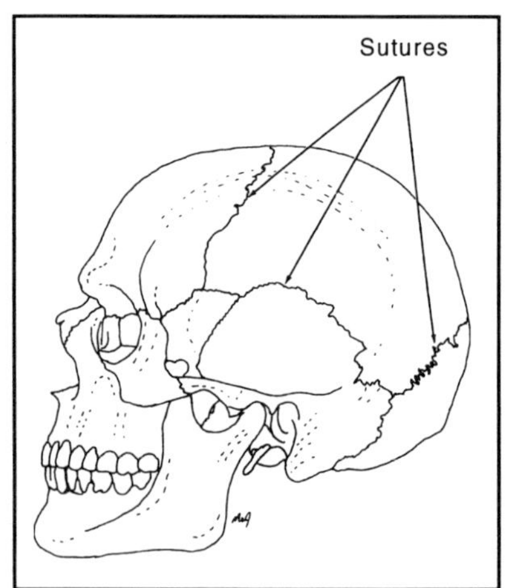

Fig. 2.6

FIBROUS JOINTS

In fibrous joints (Fig. 2.6), the connecting bones are held in almost direct contact with each other, with only a thin layer of connective tissue separating them. These joints, exemplified in the human body only by the sutures of the skull, are immovable and are designed to give form and strength to the skull.

CARTILAGINOUS JOINTS

The cartilaginous joint (Fig. 2.7) is formed by the union of bones with intervening discs of fibrocartilage which permit slight movement but great strength. The articulation between the two pubic bones as well as those between the vertebrae are examples.

Cartilaginous Joint between Pubic Bones

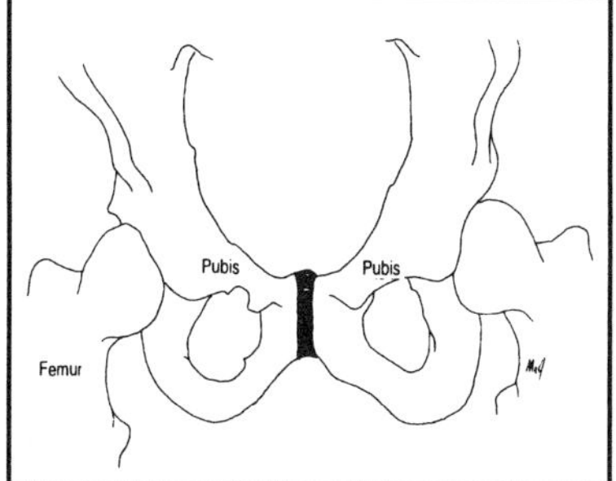

Fig. 2.7

SYNOVIAL JOINTS

Synovial or diarthrodial joints are freely movable and are characterized by the presence of a space between the articulating surfaces of the bones (Fig. 2.8). The ends of the bones which make up the joint are typically flared and are covered with cartilage. The entire joint is wrapped with fibrous tissue -- the synovial membrane -- from which is secreted the lubricant, synovial fluid. Ligaments course between the bones to provide strength.

The synovial joint, because of its freedom of movement, is of utmost importance to the study of kinesiology. Such joints are categorized according to the number of axes around which the articulating bones can rotate. The anatomical reference position will be assumed for the discussion that follows.

A Synovial Joint

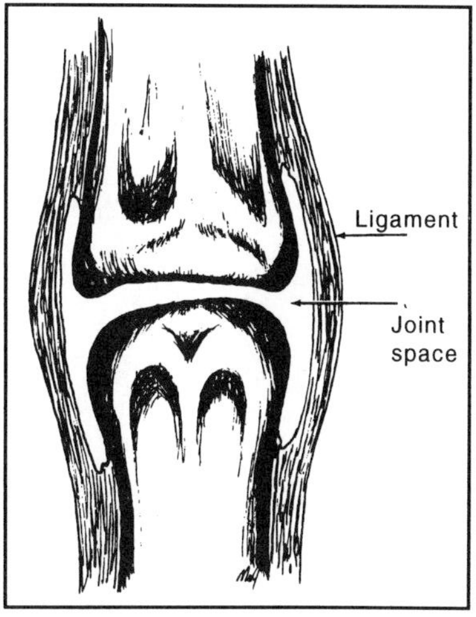

Fig. 2.8

NONAXIAL JOINT

If the movement of articulating bones is linear rather than angular, the joint is nonaxial and displays gliding rather than angular motion. The amount of motion between the bones is limited either by ligaments or bony processes which surround the articulation. Examples of gliding joints can be found between most of the carpal bones (Fig. 2.9).

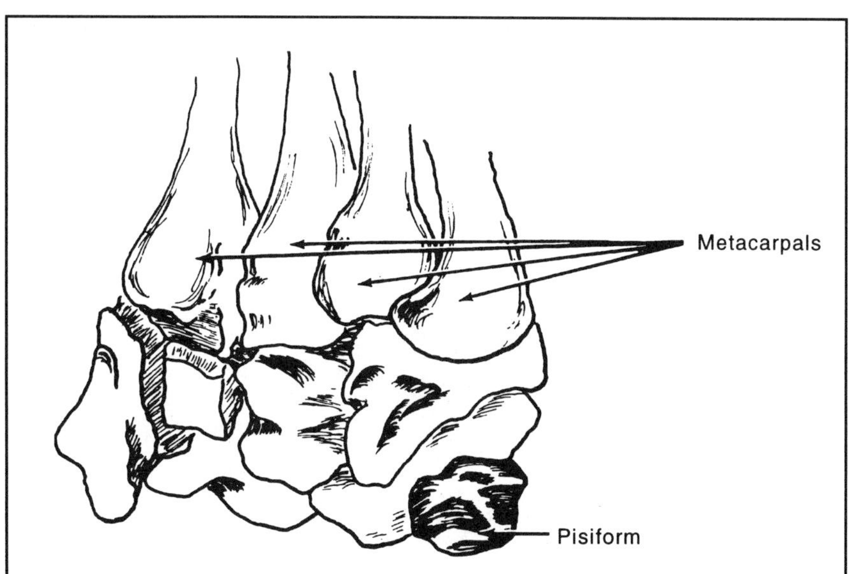

Fig. 2.9

Gliding Joints of Carpal Bones

Palpation of one of these gliding joints is shown in Fig. 2.10, wherein the pisiform bone is shown as a fist is made. The hand is then relaxed and pressure is applied with the fingers of the other hand to move the pisiform from side to side. Perhaps an easier nonaxial joint to examine is the patellofemoral joint. If the knee is extended with the heel on the floor, the patella can easily be moved along the distal end of the femur.

Palpation of Pisiform Bone

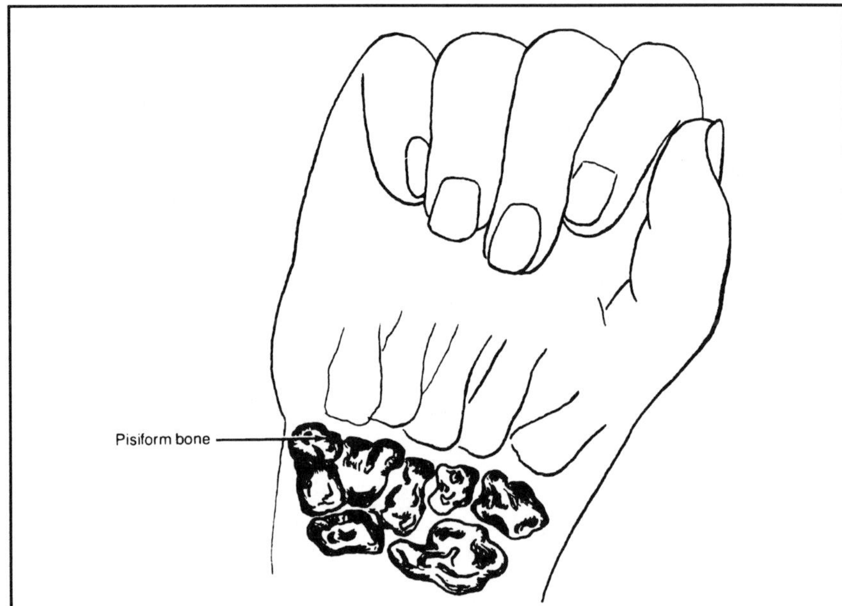

Fig. 2.10

UNIAXIAL JOINT

A joint which permits angular motion around a single axis is called a **uniaxial joint**. The elbow joint, a hinge joint, allows rotation only around a frontal axis as the elbow is flexed and extended (Fig. 2.11).

Hinge Joint of the Elbow

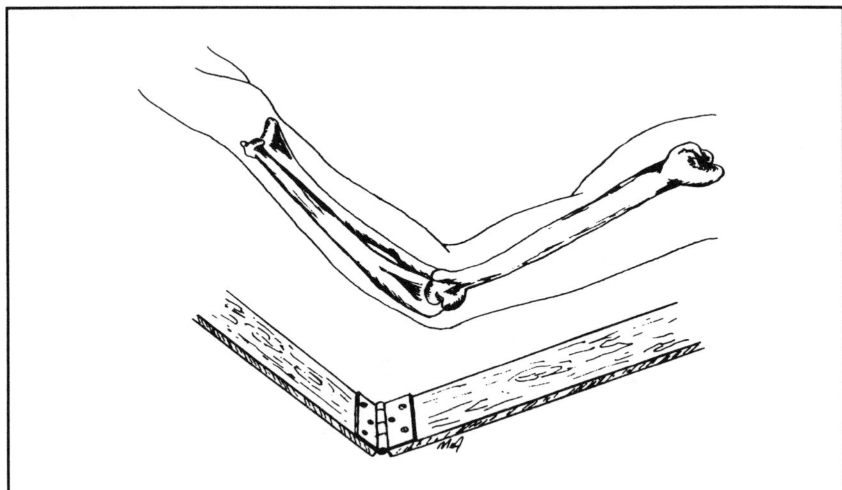

Fig. 2.11

The proximal radioulnar joint, a pivot joint (Fig. 2.12), allows rotation only around a long axis as the forearm is pronated and supinated (inwardly and outwardly rotated).

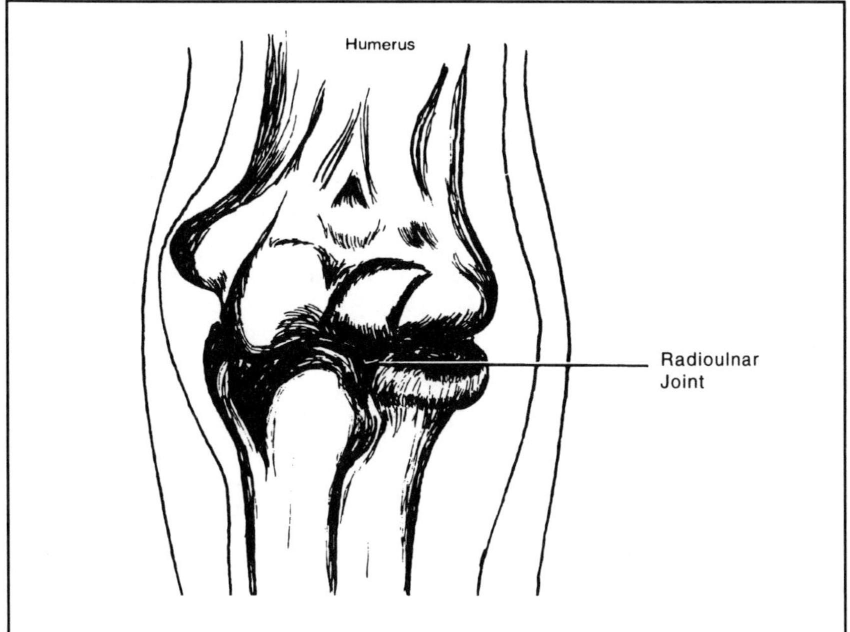

Fig. 2.12

Pivot Joint between Radius and Ulna

BIAXIAL JOINT

If a bone is permitted, by the articulation it forms with another bone, to rotate around two perpendicular axes, its articulation is biaxial. The wrist joint, a condyloid joint, is formed by the oval surface of the lunate and navicular bones of the wrist and the elliptical cavity of the radius and articular disc (Fig. 2.13).

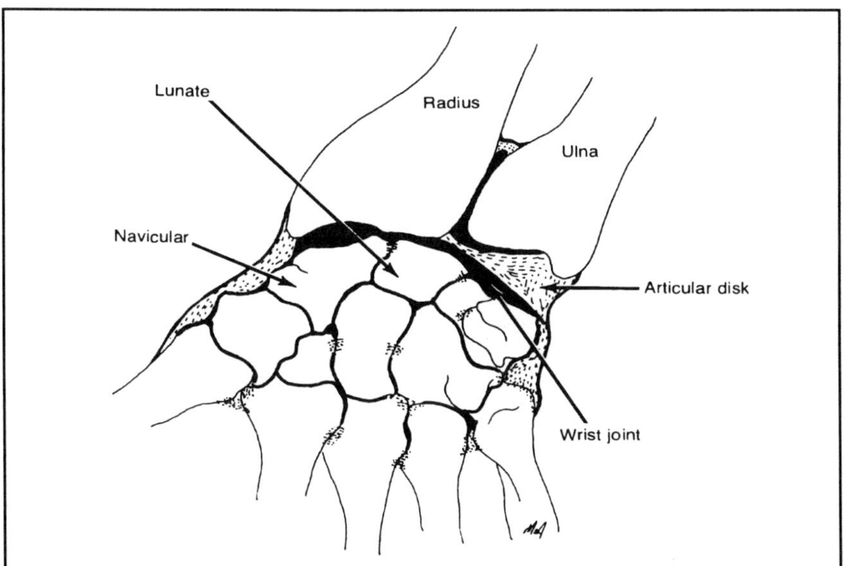

Fig 2.13

Condyloid Joint of the Wrist

This arrangement provides for rotation of the hand around a frontal axis as the wrist is flexed and extended, and around a sagittal axis as the wrist is radially and ulnarly deviated (abducted and adducted). Because the joint is elongated rather than round, no motion is allowed around a long axis.

Saddle Joint of Thumb

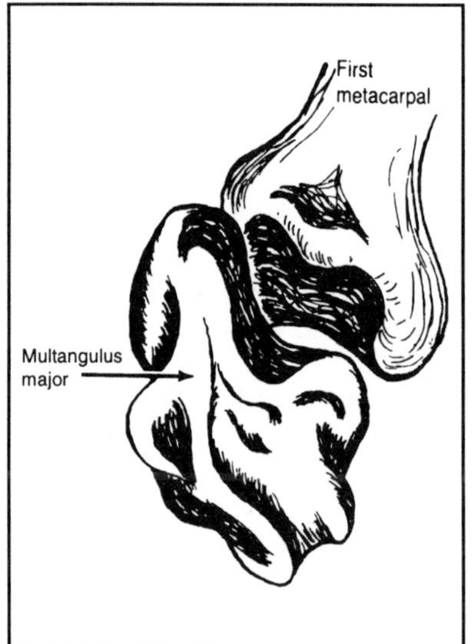

Fig 2.14

Condyloid joints, by allowing for both flexion-extension and abduction-adduction movements, are capable, also, of permitting circumduction. Using the wrist joint again as an example, it will be noted that the hand can be made to circumscribe a cone, the apex of which is at the wrist. The base of the cone is traced by the fingertips. Circumduction is a combination movement and can be performed at any joint which comprises both flexion-extension and abduction-adduction capabilities. Other examples of these joints are the metacarpophalangeal joints of the fingers.

A second variety of the biaxial joint is the saddle joint in which the opposing surfaces of the bones are shaped reciprocally in a concave and convex manner. The joint resembles a rider in a saddle and is exemplified by the carpometacarpal joint of the thumb (Fig. 2.14). The metacarpal of the thumb is the rider and the multangulus major is the saddle. The saddle joint allows for a flexion-extension type of motion (the rider rocking forward and backward in saddle), for an abduction-adduction type of motion (the rider slipping from side to side in the saddle), and for circumduction.

TRIAXIAL JOINT

The triaxial joint permits freedom of movement around the sagittal, frontal, and long axes. These joints, known as ball-and-socket joints, are formed by the reception of the globe-shaped head of one bone into the round concavity of the second bone. The best examples of the ball-and-socket joints are those of the hip and shoulder in which the three rotational axes can be easily imagined as the limb is flexed, extended, abducted, adducted, rotated, and circumducted (Fig. 2.15).

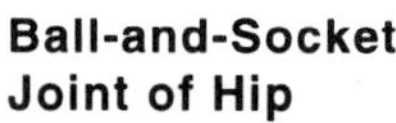

Ball-and-Socket Joint of Hip

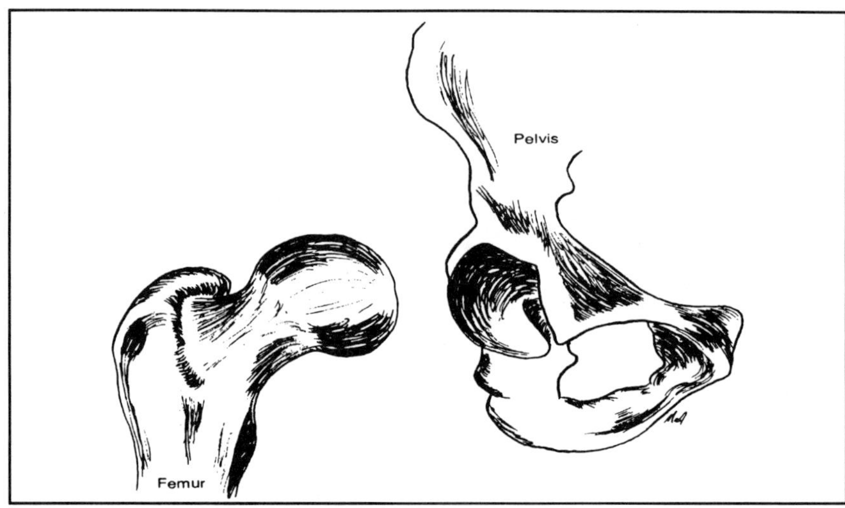

Fig 2.15

One may wonder, at this point, why such importance is attached to the axial nature of the respective synovial joints. In order to fully appreciate, rather than simply memorize, the actions of muscles, the muscles must be envisioned with respect to the axes of rotation of the joint they surround. For example, the axis of rotation of the hinge joint at the elbow passes through the two bony prominences at the distal end of the humerus (Fig. 2.16).

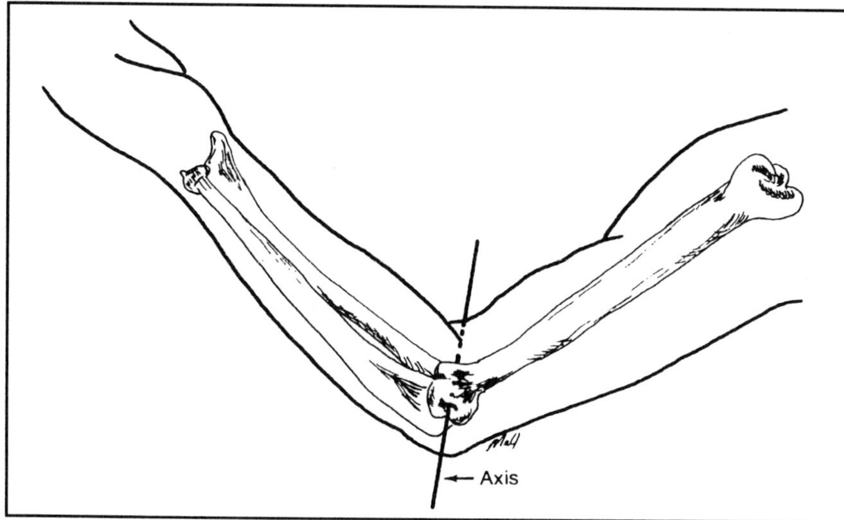

Axis of Rotation of Elbow Joint

Fig. 2.16

Any muscle which crosses the elbow joint and is anterior to the axis will flex the joint and move the lower arm forward and upward in the sagittal plane. Conversely, any muscle crossing the joint posterior to the axis will extend the joint, causing the lower arm to move downwardly and backward in the sagittal plane.

The axes of rotation of the specific joints will be discussed fully in the chapters devoted to the respective portions of the body, and the muscles will be described with regard to their locations about the axes. The tedium of memorizing muscle actions can then be replaced, in part at least, by logical deduction and palpation.

CENTER OF GRAVITY OF THE HUMAN BODY AND ITS SEGMENTS

The point in the human body at which its mass is concentrated is the total body center of gravity. The location of this point depends upon the posture of the body -- standing, sitting, arms raised, trunk flexed -- as well as upon the build of the body -- narrow shoulders, wide hips, heavy thighs -- but for purposes of this discussion, it will suffice to assume the standing position, and locate the total center of gravity in the middle of the pelvis, at or about the level of the upper sacrum.

Total and Segmental Centers of Gravity

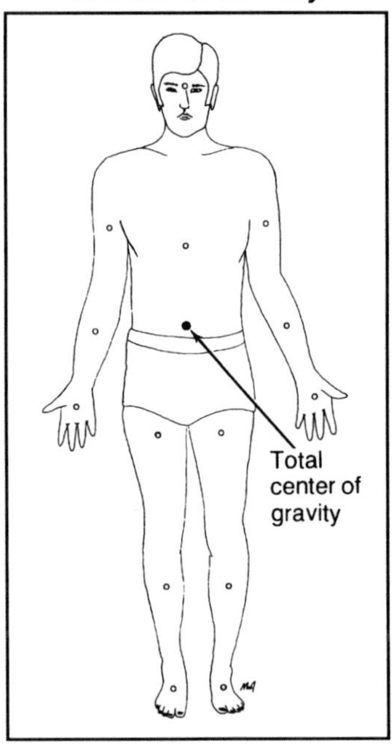

Fig. 2.17

The point in a segment of the human body at which its mass is concentrated is the segmental center of gravity. Figure 2.17 illustrates the approximate locations of these centers, as well as that of the total body center of gravity.

The importance of the various centers of gravity to kinesiology lies primarily in the fact that as segments of the body are moved against the force of gravity, their weights are considered to be localized at their centers of gravity. As will be seen in the following discussion on leverage, the location of the weight of a segment can dictate whether that segment will be capable to generating speed or force.

STABILITY

A body is stable only when its center of gravity is over its base of support. In a position of stability the line of gravity, a perpendicular line dropped from the center of gravity, must intersect the supportive base (Fig. 2.18). If the body is tilted sufficiently to cause the line of gravity to fall outside the base of support, the body will seek another base (Fig. 2.19).

An Object with Stability

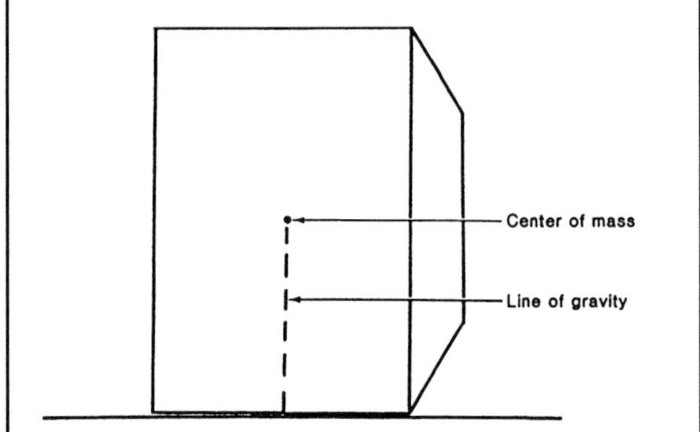

Fig. 2.18

An Unstable Object

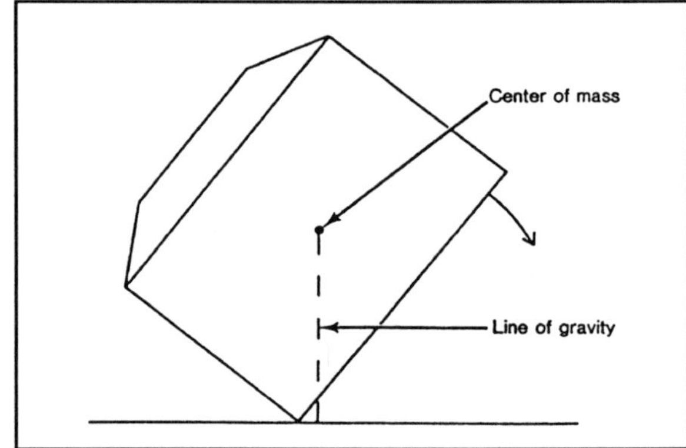

Fig. 2.19

The statements above describe, in the manner of a definition, the concept of stability or static equilibrium. The importance of this concept is far reaching both in sports and dance because of the frequent necessity to maintain stability and also to destroy it for the sake of mobility. The ballerina on pointe is faced with a difficult problem as she seeks to control her center so that the line of gravity continues to pass through the exceedingly small base of support afforded by the toe of her shoe. Conversely, the sprinter in track, who must take a position of stability for the start, aligns body parts to assure that the line of gravity intersects the base of support but falls precariously close to its front edge. The slightest forward lean will cause the line to fall ahead of the base and stability is sacrificed for mobility to begin the race.

The sprinter affords us also with a third condition; that is, the maintenance of instability. Here, the criterion of success is not to regain stability but rather to control the running lean of the body so that each successive step is an attempt to "catch up" with the center of gravity. The more the lean, the faster must be the steps taken; similarly, the slower one wishes to run -- or walk -- the less the lean required to keep the line of gravity moving ahead of the supporting foot. But lean we must, even though in slow locomotion it may be imperceptible.

Maintenance of Instability

Stability is perhaps most complicated for those who must begin a skill in the stable posture, then lose it in order to cover space, and finally regain it for the conclusion of the skill. Such would be the case for the vaulter in gymnastics. Having begun the vault in an erect posture, the approach run is initiated by the lean. Instability then becomes the condition and is maintained until the vault is completed and the ending pose is to be taken. At this point, the body alignment must be adjusted to a backward lean which allows the feet to pass under and ahead of the center. The center must then play "catch up" with the base of support and when it does, stability is regained. It is obvious that the timing required must be precise; it is small wonder that so often an additional side or forward step must be taken to gain control of the center's momentum.

Stability

Several principles present themselves in the study of stability. One of these can be identified through the examination of the various bases of support employed in sports and dance activities. When the stances of the archer, golfer, and baseball batter are considered, two points of commonality will be noted. In each case the feet are spread, and they are placed side-to-side. Comparison of the stances, at the moment of ball release, of the bowler, softball pitcher, and the basketball player performing a chest pass illustrates again that the feet are spread, but in a front-to-back direction. In all of these activities, the base of support has been enlarged to provide additional stability to the performer in that the line of gravity must travel farther before it falls outside the base. A principle emerges: the larger the base of support of an object, the more stable it is. Effective use can be made of this principle regardless of whether the criterion of success in a skill is stability or instability. The beginning tumbler can more easily achieve the balanced position of a headstand when reminded to form a triangle with the head and two hands rather than to place the head between and in line with the hands. The badminton player can profit also from the knowledge of this principle which instructs the individual, conversely, to maintain a small base of support to allow for quick reaction to the flight of the shuttlecock.

First Principle of Stability

Mention has been made of the sprinter in track who must be stable during the starting position but who must be able, in the shortest amount of time possible, to become mobile. This position of stability dictates that the line of gravity will intersect the base, but near the edge over which the line will subsequently be directed to achieve mobility. Identical problems of stance are met by competitive swimmers who affect their starts from blocks and by football players just before the ball is snapped. The opposite problem confronts the anchor person in a gymnastic pyramid. The person seeks to maintain the stability of the starting position and thus centers the line of gravity over the base so necessary adjustments can be made before the line can fall outside the edge. This **second principle** of stability states that the more nearly the line of gravity falls at the center of the base, the more stable the body.

Second Principle of Stability

A brief look at a fencer and a backpacker will afford insight to a third principle (Fig. 2.20). When on guard, the classical stance of the fencer provides that the foil is held in front of and well away from the body in the preferred hand. The nonpreferred arm is held to the rear with the shoulder in abduction and the elbow and wrist in flexion. The position of the nonpreferred arm is one of compensation for the weight of the foil. Were it not for this compensation, the center of gravity and its line would be "pulled" by the foil to a point close to the forward edge of the base, and the fencer would find difficulty in controlling the advance as well as in initiating a retreat. So it is with the backpacker who must lean forward at the hips to compensate for the backward shift of the center caused by the weight of the pack.

A Fencer and Backpacker Illustrating Compensatory Actions to Improve Stability

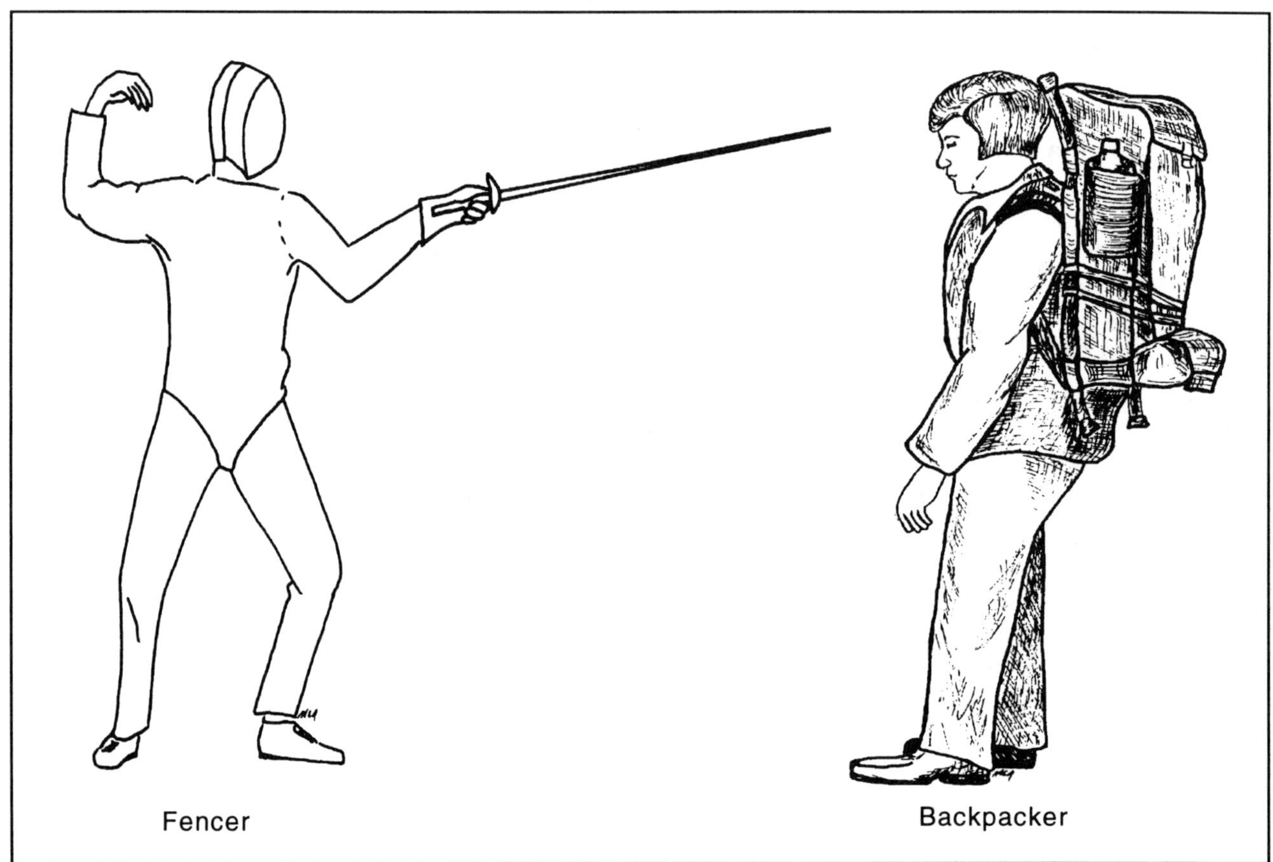

Fig. 2.20

The **third principle** becomes: when an external weight is added anywhere to the body, except directly above or below the center of gravity, the line of gravity shifts toward the weight, and compensatory movements are required to re-establish its alignment over the center of the base. Movement of a body part away from the midline causes the same effect as the addition of an external weight. This principle is important also to therapists when they work with amputees. Amputation of a limb causes the center to migrate to the opposite or "heavier" side. The amputee is unaccustomed to the new position of the center and must relearn the feeling of stability. Those who sustain the loss of both legs present a center of gravity at about the xiphoid process, and when they are placed in wheelchairs, must exercise caution when reaching for or picking up items so that they do not overlean the chair's base of support.

Third Principle of Stability

Returning to the archer, golfer, baseball batter, bowler, softball pitcher, and the basketball player with whom this discussion originated; the question of the shape of the supportive base can now be explored. These performers select a base in accordance with the direction in which they must apply force. The center of gravity fluctuates in a direction parallel to that of force application; the base is widened, therefore, in that direction to prevent the line of gravity from falling outside and causing a loss of balance. A **fourth principle** of stability instructs, then, that the base of support should be widened in the direction of force application. This principle can be broadened to include, also, force absorption. If one is expecting to be pushed from the side, the feet are placed in a side-to-side stance; expectation of a shove from the front or rear leads to a front-to-back stance. In each case, the base is broadened to make it more difficult for the line of gravity to fall outside the base.

Fourth Principle of Stability

A **fifth principle** of stability concerns the height of the center of gravity. Figure 2.21 illustrates two objects, A and B, which are identical except for the heights of their centers of gravity. Object A must be tilted farther than Object B in order to move its line of gravity outside its base; thus, the lower the center of mass, the more

Fifth Principle of Stability

Relationship of Height of Center of Gravity to Stability

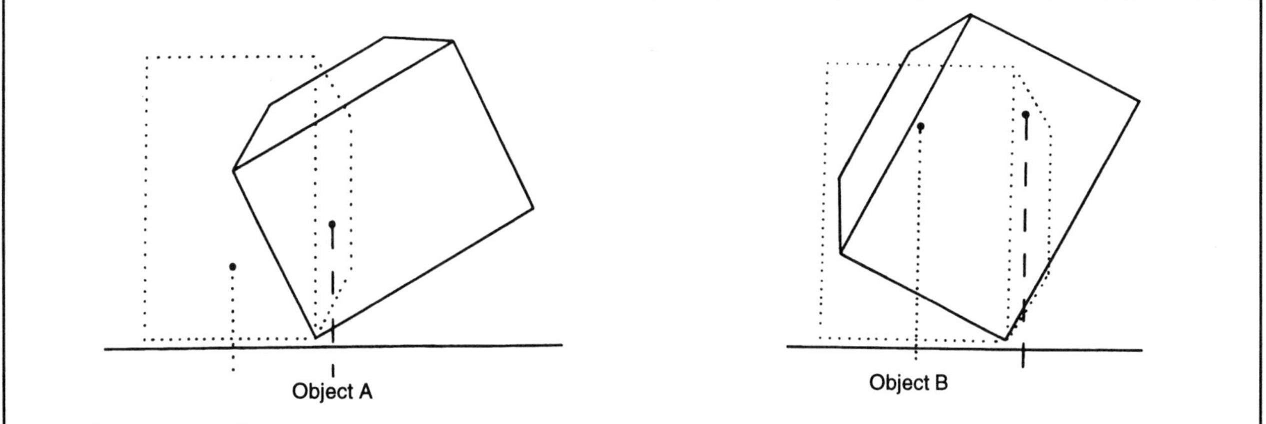

Fig. 2.21

stable the object. The short gymnast will tend to excel in balance beam; women, by virtue of their broad pelvic girdles and comparatively narrow shoulder girdles, will be more stable than men; a young child is quite unstable since the relatively heavy head causes an upward displacement of the center. Acrobats who balance two, three, or even four performers with each one standing on the shoulders of the other perform a difficult feat indeed, for as each additional performer is balanced, their collective center moves higher. Badminton, tennis, and softball players elevate their centers by extending the knees and hips slightly just before the opponent makes contact with the implement. The tennis player elevates the center by actually jumping slightly from the ground before the opponent hits the ball. In each case, the performer becomes less stable and more able to become mobile quickly without committing to any direction of progress which may either place him in an unfavorable position to affect the interception, or "tip" the opponent.

The Sum of the Moments is Equal to Zero

Discussion of stability or static equilibrium often comprises the statement, "the sum of the moments is equal to zero." The terminology may seem confusing at first glance; however, when it is remembered that a moment of force is equal to a force arm multiplied by the force applied (F x FA), a glimmer of clarification may be seen. Return, briefly, to consideration of the first class lever known as a seesaw. If the seesaw is balanced, the sum of its moments must be equal to zero; i.e., the product of its force arm and their respective forces are equivalent. Two forces of 10 kg each applied at 5 meters on either side of the axis will cause the seesaw to balance.

$$F \times FA = R \times RA \quad \textit{or} \quad F_1 \times FA_1 = F_2 \times FA_2$$

$$10kg \times 5m = 10kg \times 5m$$

and

$$moment_1 = moment_2$$

therefore

$$moment_1 - moment_2 = 0$$

In other words, the sum of the moments equals zero.

Use of the concept of sums of moments is frequent in static equilibrium, for it entails the very basis of stability. Only when all moments on one side of the body equal those on the other will the body be stable with its line of gravity passing through the center of its base of support. To hold an arm at shoulder level rather than at the side increases its moment because the force arm is increased. The increased moment must be neutralized by the other side of the body if stability is to be retained. Perhaps the other arm could be abducted, also, or the head could be tilted sufficiently so its weight multiplied by its force arm could equal the moment of the extended arm on the opposite side.

All of this is by way of reinforcing, mathematically, principles set forth above. To retain static equilibrium requires that compensation be made above and below, on either side of, and forward and back of the center of gravity to ensure that the sumof the moments is equal to zero.

The Five Major Principles of Stability

1. The size of the base of support is proportional to stability; that is, the larger the base, the more stable the body; the smaller the base, the less stable the body but the more easily mobility can be achieved.

2. Intersection of the line of gravity at the center of the base of support yields greatest stability for that base; intersection of the line near the edge of the base lessens stability but makes mobility easier to achieve.

3. The addition of weights to the body anywhere but directly above or below the center of gravity causes the center to move in a sideward direction toward the weight. Realignment of the center is achieved through compensatory movements in the opposite direction. Movement of a body part away from the midline has the same effect as the addition of a weight.

4. To maintain stability as force is being applied or absorbed, widen the base of support in the direction of the force.

5. The lower the center of gravity of a given base of support the more stable the body; the more the center is raised, the less stable the body becomes.

DETERMINATION OF THE CENTER OF GRAVITY

The center of gravity of the body is probably the parameter most frequently used to describe movement of the body through space. Because position of the center of gravity is so influential to stability or mobility of the body, and because it is also a prime factor in the calculation of the amount of work done by an individual, the procedures for its location can be of utmost importance.

The mathematical determination of the location of the center of gravity is not a complex calculation, but it is somewhat laborious if done by hand. The data needed for making the calculation include total body weight, individual body segment weight, location of the center of gravity of each segment, and horizontal and vertical coordinates of these centers. The coordinates can be obtained by projecting film of the subject on graph paper that has been labeled in arbitrary linear units. The origin of the graphic system is placed so the projected image is in the first quadrant; i.e., the coordinates X = 0, Y = 0 (0,0) are placed in the lower left-hand corner of the graph paper. A stick figure of the subject's position is then completed (Fig. 2.22). A millimeter ruler can be used to locate the centers of gravity of the various segments by using the segmental data presented in Fig. 2.23.

Stick Figure on Graph Paper

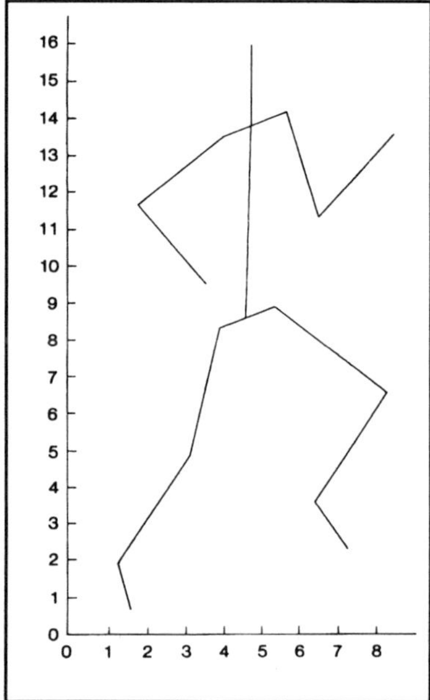

Fig. 2.22

Location of Centers of Gravity of Body Segments

Segment	Center-of-Gravity Location Expressed as Percentage of Total Distance between Reference Points
Head	46.4% to vertex; 53.6% to chin-neck intersect
Trunk	38.0% to suprasternal notch; 62.0% to hip axis
Upper arm	51.3% to shoulder axis; 48.7% to elbow axis
Forearm	39.0% to elbow axis; 61.0% to wrist axis
Hand	82.0% to wrist axis; 18.0% to knuckle III
Thigh	37.2% to hip axis; 62.8% to knee axis
Calf	37.1% to knee axis; 62.9% to ankle axis
Foot	44.9% to heel; 55.1% to tip of longest toe

* AMRL Technical Report 69-70, Wright Patterson Air Force Base, Ohio, 1969

Fig. 2.23

Location of Center of Gravity of Right Upper Leg

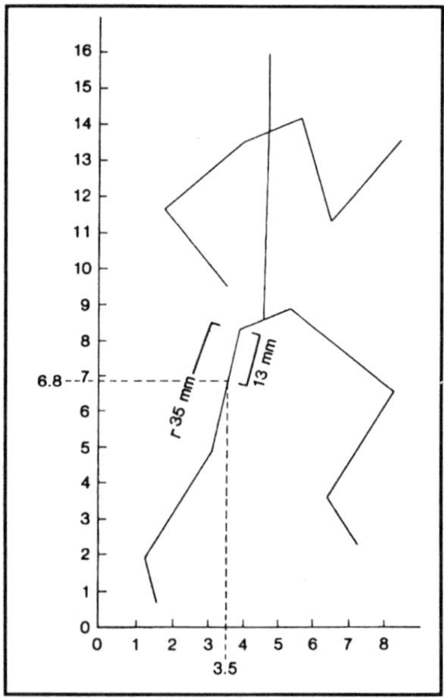

Fig. 2.24

Having marked all segments, their respective X and Y coordinates are found on the graph paper. The procedure is illustrated in Figure 2.24 for the left upper leg, which measures 35 millimeters in length. From Figure 2.23, it is found that the center of gravity of the upper leg islocated 37.2 percent of the segment length from the hip axis. Thus, 35 millimeters x .372 = 13.02 millimeters. When that distance is measured to the nearest millimeter from the hip, a mark is made on the segment and perpendiculars are dropped to the two axes. Their points of axis intersection (3.5, 6.8), are the coordinates of the center of gravity of the upper leg.

The only remaining step is to multiply both the X and Y coordinates by the weight of that body segment. These data are found in Figure 2.25. Results of multiplication are added to those of all other segments, with X coordinates kept separate from Y coordinates. The two sums are then divided by the body weight. The divisions provide X and Y coordinates of the total body center of gravity for the position analyzed.

$$X_{cg} = \frac{(X_1 \cdot Wt_1) + (X_2 \cdot Wt_2) + \ldots + (X_{16} \cdot Wt_{16})}{\text{Body Weight}}$$

$$Y_{cg} = \frac{(Y_1 \cdot Wt_1) + (Y_2 \cdot Wt_2) + \ldots + (Y_{16} \cdot Wt_{16})}{\text{Body Weight}}$$

Weights of Body Segments Relative to Total Body Weight

Segment	Percentage of Body Weight
Head	0.073
Trunk	0.507
Upper arm	0.026
Forearm	0.016
Hand	0.007
Thigh	0.103
Calf	0.043
Foot	0.015

* AMRL Technical Report 69-70, Wright Patterson Air Force Base, Ohio, 1969.

Fig. 2.25

Subscripts indicate segment number; i.e., if segment number one is the foot, its coordinates should each be multiplied by the weight of the foot, etc. It must be remembered that both the right and left arms and legs are to be considered in the calculation; however, if only one side of the body can be seen, and if bilateral symmetry of the limbs can be assumed, the calculations from the observed limb can simply be doubled.

A less mathematical solution to determining the location of the center of gravity lies in the use of a board, two 'knife-edges," and a weight scale. One end of the board is placed on the scale and the other on a block of sufficient height to level the board. The 'knife-edges" (two lengths of angle iron will do quite nicely) are placed between the ends of the board and the scale and block, respectively. Length of the board between the edges is recorded, and the scale is set to zero.

A subject whose weight is known can now lie on the board with feet toward the scale. The scale reading is recorded and the following calculation is performed.

$$\text{Center of Gravity} = \frac{\text{Scale reading X length of board between edges}}{\text{Weight of subject}}$$

Suppose our subject weighs 60 kilograms and the length of the board between knife-edges is 180 centimeters. If the scale reading is 30 kilograms, we can solve for the location of the center of gravity as follows:

$$\text{Center of Gravity} = \frac{30 \text{ kg X } 180 \text{ cm}}{60 \text{ kg}} = 90 \text{ cm}$$

The center of gravity is located 90 centimeters from the knife-edge that is on the block.

The process can be repeated if locations of the center are desired in the sagittal and frontal planes. The subject would stand on the board with his or her side to the scale and then facing the scale. Results of the calculations will yield the desired locations. It is also possible to place the subject in some other postures and determine, in the same fashion, the location of the center of gravity.

LEVERS OF THE HUMAN BODY

A lever is a rigid bar that has an axis of rotation (*A*), a point at which force is applied (*F*), and a resistance which must be balanced or overcome (*R*). The three types of levers are designated according to which of their three components, axis, force, or resistance, is between the other two components.

In a **first class lever**, the axis of rotation is located somewhere between the point of force application and the resistance (Fig. 2.26). In the **second class lever**, the resistance is between the force and the axis (Fig. 2.27). The **third class lever** is distinguished by the locations of the axis and resistance on the ends of the lever with the force application between them (Fig. 2.28).

First Class Lever

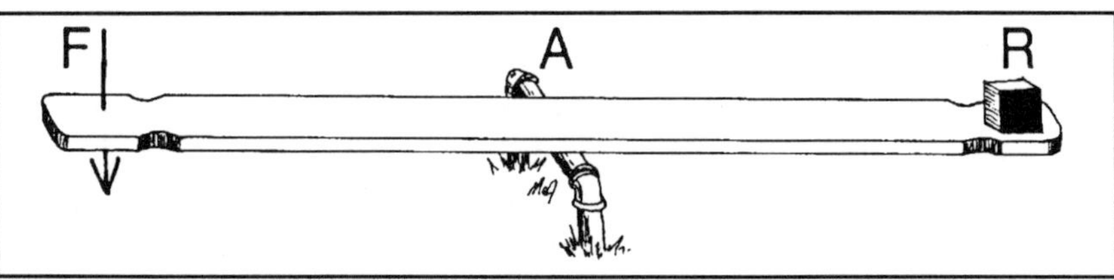

Fig. 2.26

Second Class Lever

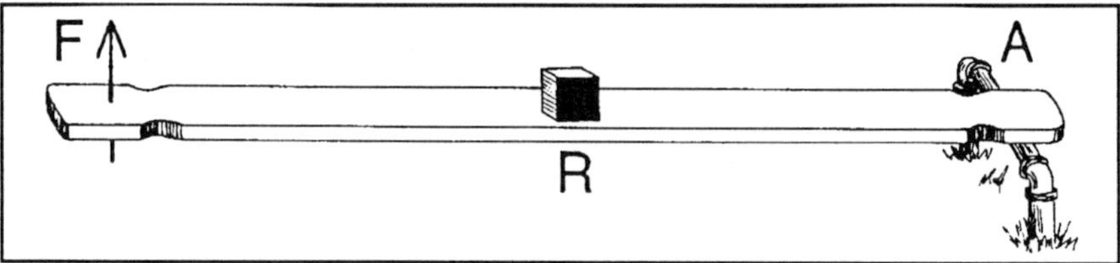

Fig. 2.27

Third Class Lever

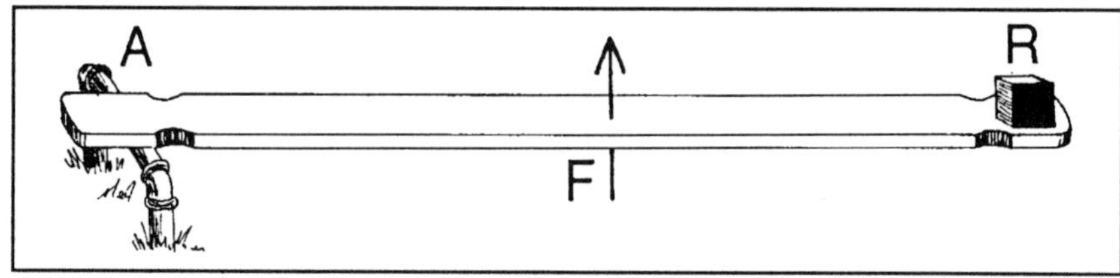

Fig. 2.28

All levers can be divided into two segments known as the **force arm**, which is the perpendicular distance between the line of force application and the axis, and the **resistance arm**, which is the perpendicular distance between the line of resistance and the axis. When the force arm is equal to the resistance arm, the lever has a mechanical advantage of one; that is, for every unit of weight the resistance represents, an equivalent unit of force will be required to balance the lever. In the case of the seesaw shown in Fig. 2.29, the force arm and the resistance arm are equal. If the child on the right weighs 25 kilograms, the child on the left must also weigh 25 kilograms if the seesaw is to balance.

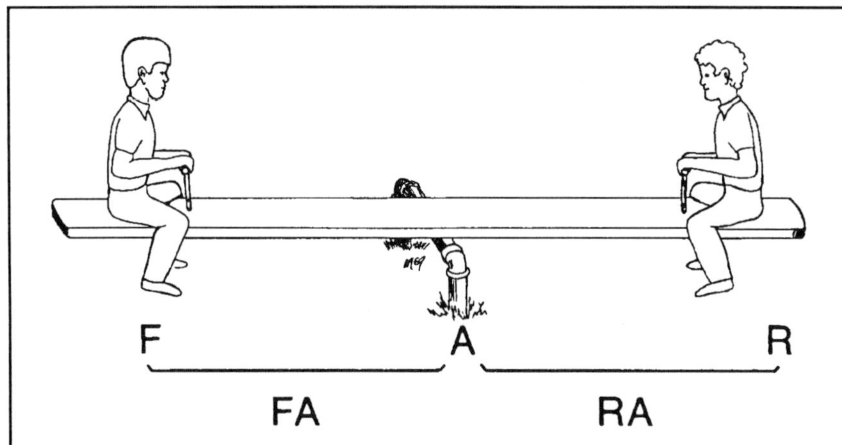

Force Arm and Resistance Arm of a First Class Lever

Fig. 2.29

The use of a screwdriver to pry open a paint can, although still a first class lever, yields a different mechanical advantage (Fig. 2.30). If the resistance arm is 2 centimeters and the force arm is 20 centimeters long, the mechanical advantage is 10. For every ten units of resistance with which the can is capped, only one unit of force is required to balance the lever.

It can be seen that mechanical advantage is equal to the force arm divided by the resistance arm -- *FA/RA*. It will be noted, also, that depending upon the location of the axis between the force application and the point of resistance, the mechanical advantage of a first class lever can range from less than one (axis located close to force point) to infinity (axis located close to resistance). The greater the mechanical advantage, the greater the resistance that can be balanced by a given force.

Application of the concept of mechanical advantage to the second class lever indicates that, regardless of the placement of the resistance along the lever, the force arm will always be longer than the resistance arm. The mechanical advantage must always be, then greater than one and can range, again, to infinity as the resistance is placed closer and closer to the axis.

First Class Level with Mechanical Advantage of Ten

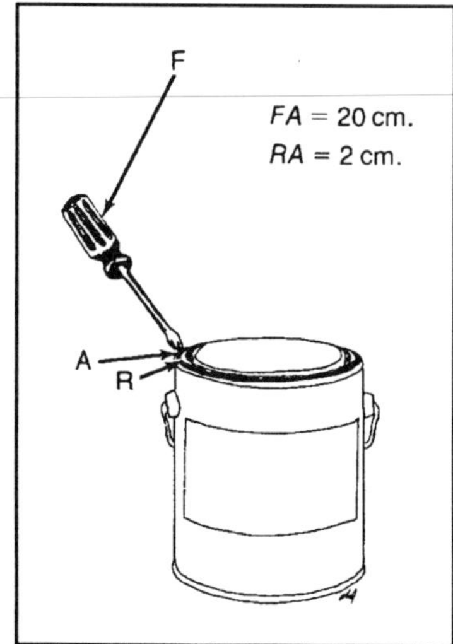

Fig. 2.30

The third class lever, conversely, yields a mechanical advantage which is always less than one. Regardless of the point at which the force is applied, the resistance arm will always be longer than the force arm.

Using mechanical advantage as the criterion, it is possible to rank the three lever types with regard to their capacity to balance and overcome resistance. The second class lever, with its mechanical advantage greater than one, has greatest capacity for strength, and the third class lever, with its mechanical advantage of less than one has the least capacity.

The student may question the phrase "**balance the lever**" used in the foregoing discussion. Levers are not usually employed to balance resistance, but rather to overcome it. All considerations regarding leverage are based upon force requirements to balance resistances. If the balancing force is known, it is known, also, that any increment in force, no matter how small, will cause the lever to move and thus overcome the resistance.

First and Second Class Levers are Seldom Found in the Human Body

The levers of the human body are the bony segments of the skeleton. Axes of the levers are the joints; points of force application are the insertions of the muscles; and the resistances are the centers of gravity of the bony segments to be moved, whether they are additionally weighted by some object to be lifted, or whether they offer only the resistance of their own weights.

In the human body, first and second class levers are seldom found. Examples of a first class lever are the triceps brachii, acting on the forearm when it is positioned above the head (see Chapter 4, Fig. 4.12), and the neck extensors pulling downwardly on the back of the head to balance its weight across the first vertebra. A second class lever is exemplified by the forearm and the brachioradialis. Since the center of gravity of the forearm is between the elbow and the insertion of the brachioradialis (see Chapter 4, Fig. 4.7), a second class system is formed.

Third class levers predominate in the human body, being found almost totally throughout the upper and lower extremities. This may seem paradoxical in view of the relatively heavy weights or resistances which we are able to lift and move. The paradox disappears, however, when we consider that our muscles are capable of exerting forces far in excess of any resistance we overcome. The quadriceps, the anterior muscles of the upper leg, are able to apply a force of 200 to 300 kilograms. A visit to the weight room will show that the maximum weight (resistance) which can be lifted by extending the knee is probably between 20 and 40 kilograms. It is clear that the human body is handicapped in its strength capability by the adverse mechanical advantage of third class levers.

One may wonder why the human body has not evolved as a system of forceful second class levers rather than weak third class levers. The reason appears to be in the fact that third class levers are capable of generating great speed. Their predominance in the human body allows us to perform throwing and kicking tasks at incredible speeds rather than having to overcome great resistances with the ponderousness of the second class lever.

Leverage calculations are relatively simple and are derived from the formula $F \cdot FA = R \cdot RA$. This is a mathematical statement of balanced levers in which F is force, FA is the force arm, R is resistance, and RA is resistance arm. Figure 2.31 illustrates a third class lever with a force arm of 4 and a resistance arm of 16. The resistance to be balanced in 5 kilograms. By rearranging the formula to $F = R \cdot RA/FA$ and substituting, force is found to be 20 kilograms. Any force in excess of 20 kilograms will overcome a resistance of 5 kilograms if the lever has a mechanical advantage of one-fourth.

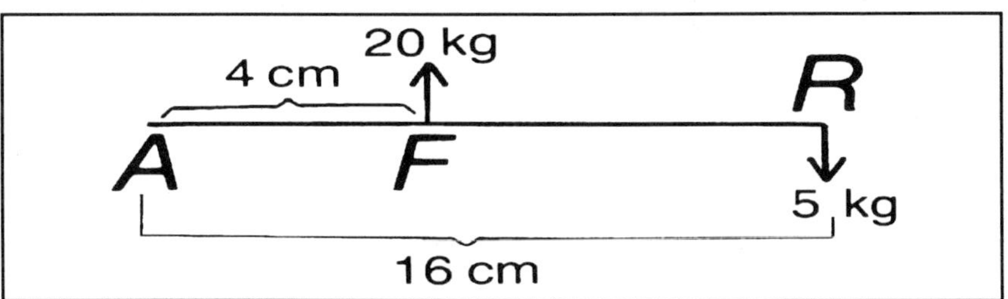

Third Class Lever with Mechanical Advantage of One-Fourth

Fig. 2.31

A second example of a leverage calculation is shown in Figure 2.32. The mechanical advantage is 7/35 or 1/5, and the force being applied is 40 kilograms. Since $R = F \cdot FA/RA$, it can be found that a resistance of 8 kilograms will be balanced. A force of 40 kilograms is required to hold a lower leg weighing 8 kilograms in full extension.

Third Class Lever with Mechanical Advantage of One-Fifth

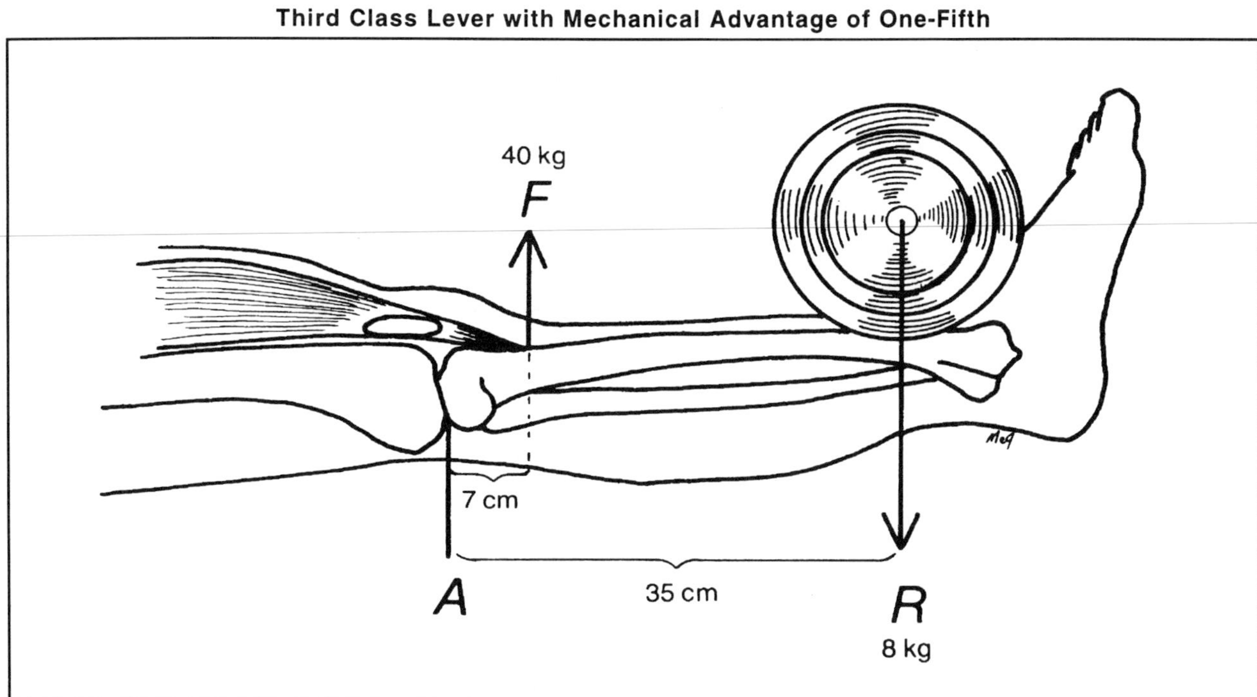

Fig. 2.32

The product of force and force arm (F x FA) is termed the **moment of force** or the **torque** of the lever. Increases either in the amount of force applied or the length ofthe force arm will increase the moment of force or torque of the lever and enable it to balance a greater resistance or the same resistance at a longer resistance arm. A statement such as, "slide backward slightly on the seesaw to improve the moment," is simply a different way of saying that leverage can be improved by increasing the length of the force arm.

COMPOSITION OF FORCES

Force is a vector quantity. It has both magnitude (kilograms, pounds, grams) and direction (horizontal, vertical, diagonal). Because it is a vector, force can be represented by a line the length of which is scaled to the units of the force, and direction of which is indicated by an arrow at the end of the line. Figure 2.33 is a horizontal force vector which is 4 centimeters long. It has been scaled so that 1 centimeter of length equals 1 kilogram of force. The vector represents, therefore, 4 kilograms of force directed horizontally and to the right.

Horizontal Force vector

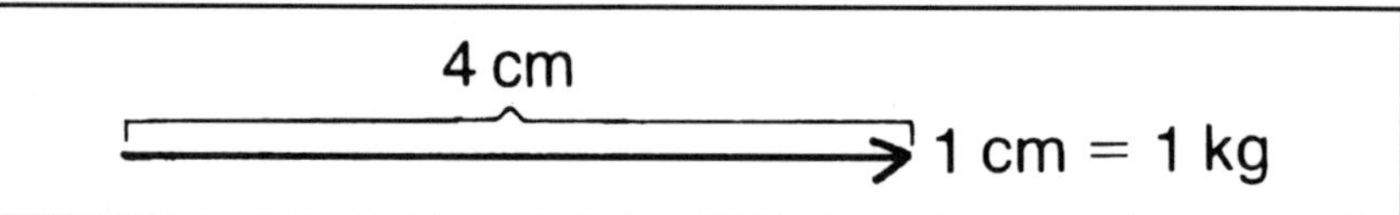

Fig. 2.33

In Figure 2.34, two forces (F_1 and F_2), each of 4 kilograms, are being applied simultaneously to an object. Their total effect, that is, their resultant (F), is 8 kilograms and is directed to the right.

Summing of Forces

1 cm = 1 kg

$F_1 = 4$ cm + $F_2 = 4$ cm = $F = 8$ kg

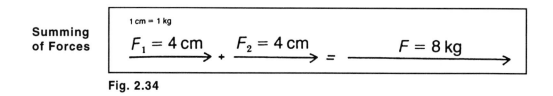

Fig. 2.34

Figure 2.35 shows two forces of different magnitudes and opposite directions being applied simultaneously to an object. The resultant of these forces is 2 kilograms directed to the left.

Subtraction of Forces

1 cm = 1 kg

$F_1 = 2$ cm + $F_2 = 4$ cm = $F = 2$ kg

Fig. 2.35

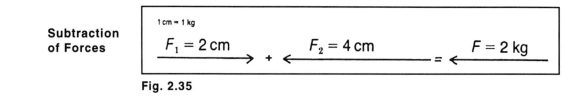

Figure 2.36 depicts several forces being applied to the scapula by the simultaneous contraction of surrounding musculature. The resultant of these forces is two units in magnitude and is directed vertically. Under the conditions shown in the illustration, the scapula will be elevated with two units of force.

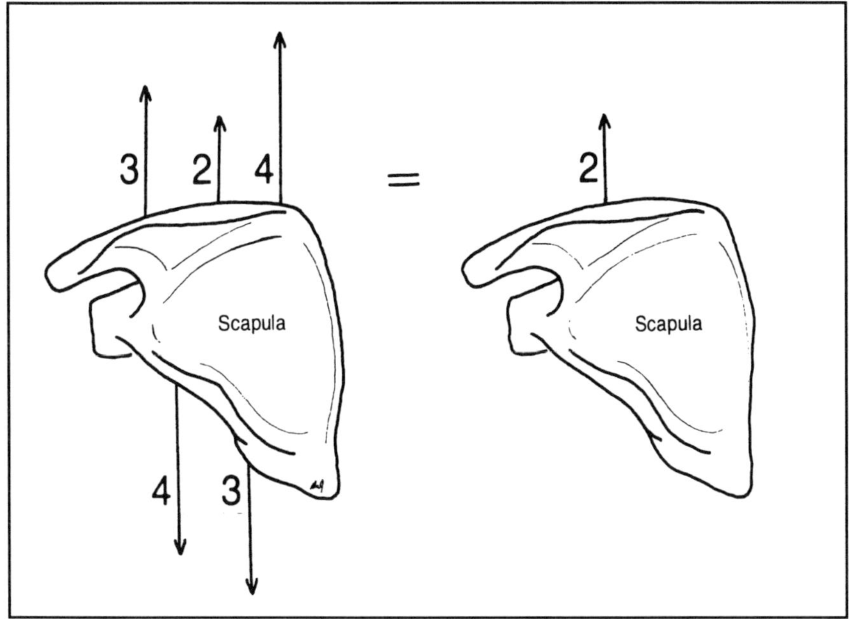

Fig. 2.36

Summation of Forces

From the above discussion, a general statement can be made: If two or more forces are applied simultaneously and along a common direction, their resultant is the algebraic sum of the forces. The direction of the resultant will be that of the remaining algebraic sign.

When forces act at an angle to each other rather than along a directional line, their resultant must be found by other means. If F_1 and F_2 (Fig. 2.37) are acting at right angles to each other, their resultant, F, will be the diagonal of a parallelogram constructed around them. The magnitude of the resultant is calculated as shown in the figure. The direction of the resultant is traditionally reported as the angle it makes, in a counterclockwise direction, with the horizontal. This angle can be found easily through the use of trigonometric functions.

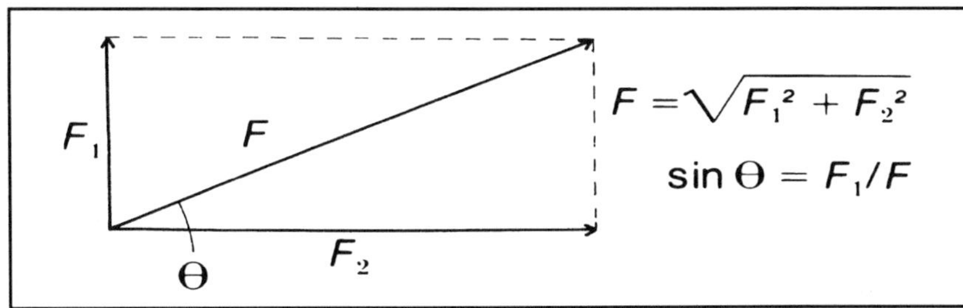

Fig. 2.37

Determination of the Resultant Force, *F*

If F_1 and F_2 are not at right angles to each other (Fig. 2.38), their resultant will still be the diagonal of a parallelogram; however, the magnitude and direction of the resultant must be calculated by use of the trigonometric law of cosines.

Determination of the Resultant, *F*, from the Two Forces F_1 and F_2

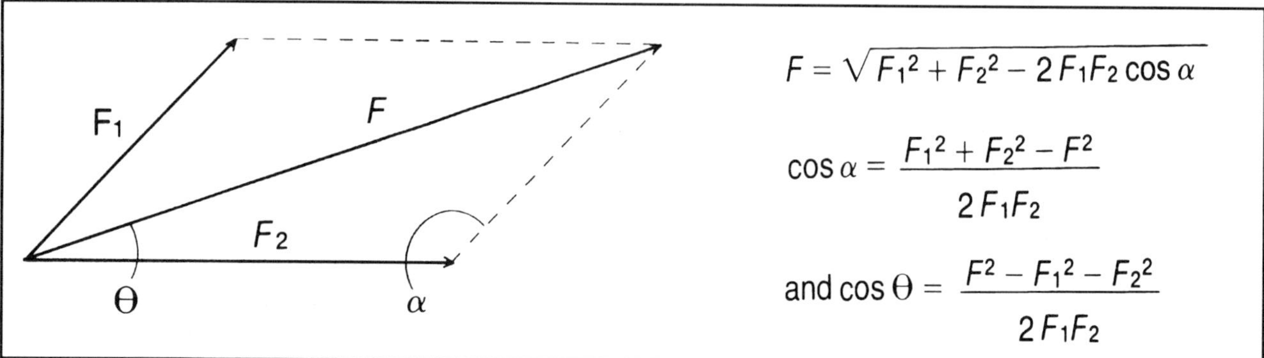

$$F = \sqrt{F_1^2 + F_2^2 - 2F_1F_2 \cos \alpha}$$

$$\cos \alpha = \frac{F_1^2 + F_2^2 - F^2}{2F_1F_2}$$

$$\text{and } \cos \theta = \frac{F^2 - F_1^2 - F_2^2}{2F_1F_2}$$

Fig. 2.38

For the purposes of this text, resultants will be incorporated in the narrative in a conceptual rather than mathematical way. The student who is interested in exploring further the mathematics of force composition is urged to refer to the several biomechanics texts which are currently available.

RESOLUTION OF FORCES

Force resolution is the converse of force composition. To resolve a force is to separate it into two forces, the directions of which are known. Only diagonal forces such as those illustrated in Figure 2.39 will be considered; such forces will be resolved into two component forces which are at right angles to each other.

Resolution of the Force, F, into its Vertical and Horizontal Components

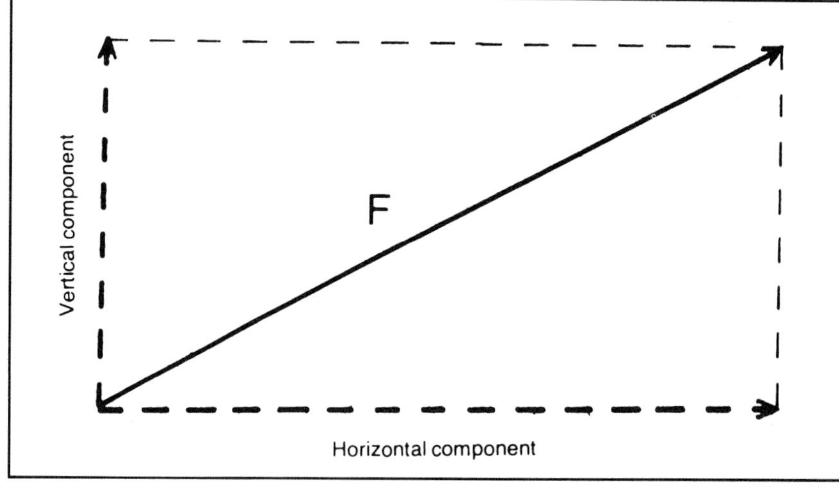

Fig. 2.39

Rules for Resolution of Forces

Rule 1. The two components of a diagonal force will be at right angles to each other and will include the diagonal force vector between them.	**Rule 2.** The lengths of the two component force vectors will be such that when the tips of the two component vectors are connected to tip of the diagonal vector, a rectangle will result.

Figure 2.39 illustrates the procedure of force resolution. From the end of the diagonal force vector *F*, two vectors are drawn at right angles and on either side of *F*. When the tips of the three arrows are connected, a rectangle is formed.

Figure 2.40 shows the application of force resolution to a problem in kinesiology. A diagonal force representing a muscle is seen to attach to the scapula. By resolving the diagonal vector, it can be observed that the muscle in question moves the scapula diagonally because of its tendency to pull the scapula toward the spine and toward the head.

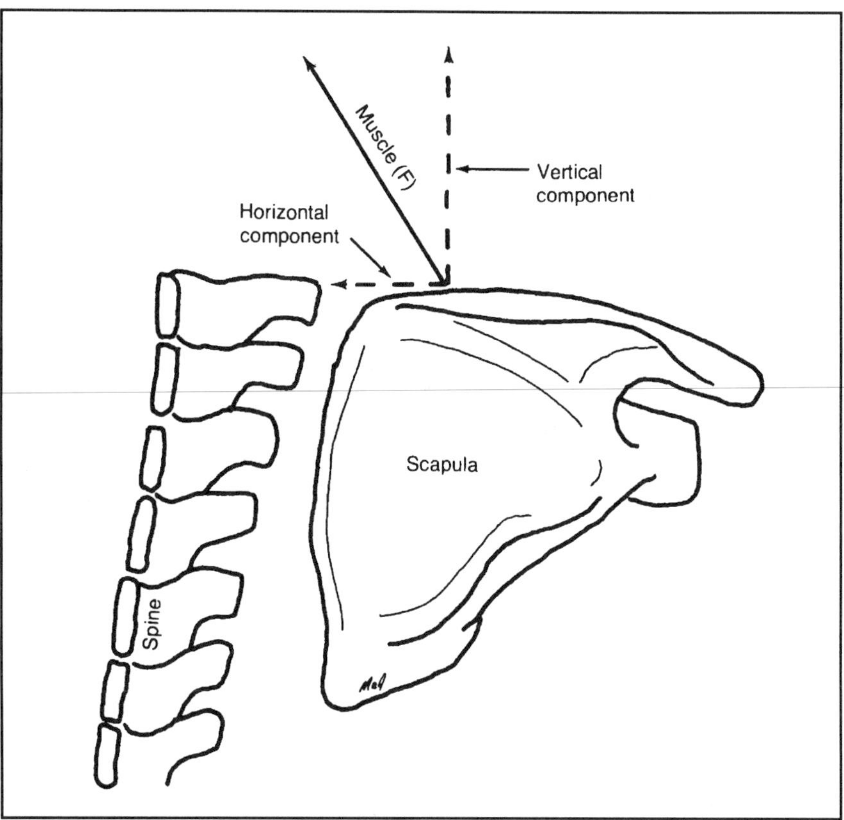

Fig. 2.40

Resolution of a Diagonal Force, *F*

Force resolution is exemplified again in Figure 2.41, in which the biceps brachii is illustrated as attached diagonally to the forearm. Resolution of the force vector of the biceps brachii is accomplished by drawing, from the end of the diagonal force vector, an arrow along the forearm and one at right angles to the forearm. The appropriate length of the two component vectors has been achieved when a rectangle results from the connection of the three arrow tips.

Force Resolution of the Pull of the Biceps Brachii

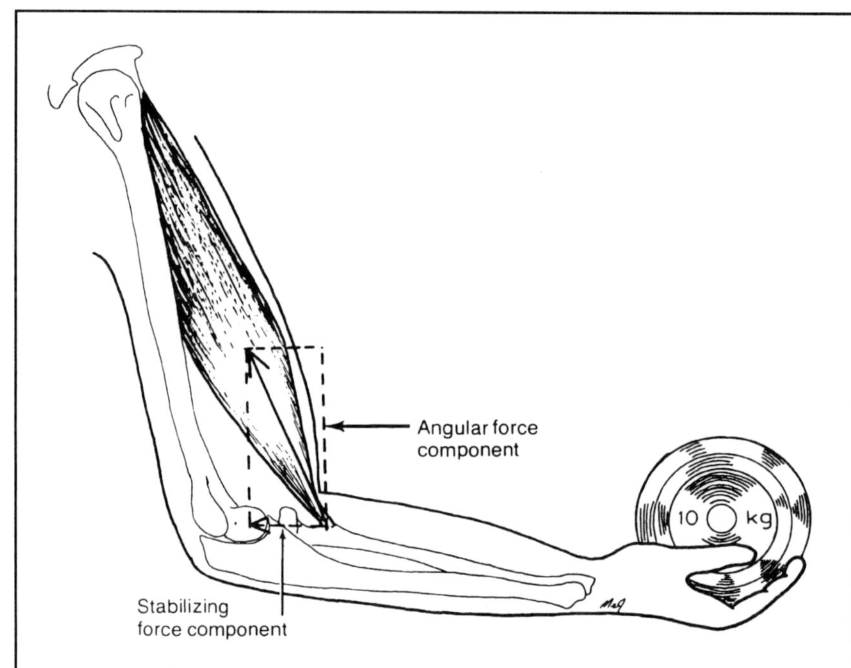

Fig. 2.41

The case of force resolution of a diagonal muscle pull against bony levers such as the forearm is a special one. The two component vectors are always envisioned as being along or parallel to the bone and perpendicular to the bone. The vector which is directed along the bone and toward the joint acts to press the articulating surfaces of the bones together; this component is called, therefore, the **stabilizing component**. The vector at right angles to the bone is the component which causes the bone to rotate about the joint axis and is called the **angular component**. Comparison of the relative lengths of the angular and stabilizing vectors will lead to conclusions regarding the effectiveness of a muscle to move the joint it crosses. The longer the angular component is in relationship to the stabilizing component, the more effectively the muscle can cause movement and the less effectively it can stabilize the joint.

Several joints of the body are crossed by muscles which, according to the position of the joint, have changeable angles of insertion. The elbow, knee, and hip joints are examples, and to illustrate this discussion, the elbow will be chosen as it is crossed by the biceps brachii.

If the elbow is held in full extension, the angle between the tendon of the biceps and the radius -- the angle of the biceps insertion -- is small. Resolution of the biceps' force yields a long stabilizing component and a comparatively short angular component -- the biceps is relatively ineffective as a mover of the forearm when the elbow is extended. As the elbow is flexed, however, the insertion angle of the biceps gradually becomes larger; the accompanying resolution comprises angular components which are lengthening as the stabilizing components are becoming shorter. The biceps is thus becoming more and more effective as a mover of the forearm and less and less effective as a stabilizer of the elbow.

When the elbow joint reaches a point of flexion in which the insertion angle of the biceps is 90 degrees, the only component of force is the angular one. At this joint position, the biceps will be at its peak effectiveness as a mover of the forearm but will apply no stabilizing force to the joint.

Continued flexion of the elbow causes the insertion angle of the biceps to become greater than 90 degrees. Resolution of the biceps' force will again yield two components, one the angular component, and the other a component directed along the bone but away from the joint. The latter component is acting to pull the joint apart and is called the **dislocating component**. The dislocating component of the biceps' force gradually elongates as the elbow joint flexes to full range; the angular component simultaneously shortens and indicates a decreasing effectiveness of the biceps as the elbow nears full flexion because much of the force generated is diverted to become dislocating force.

The biceps brachii, as well as any other muscle which can be made to insert through a range of angles, will be mechanically at its optimum to provide strength when it attaches at 90 degrees. The farther from the perpendicular the angle of insertion becomes, the weaker the muscle will be as a joint mover.

MUSCLE ATTACHMENTS

In its simplest form, a muscle has two bony attachments and crosses a single joint. When the muscle contracts, it shortens, causing its two attachments to become closer together as permitted by the joint. Typically, one attachment is on a bone which moves easily; the other attachment is on a bone more difficult to move. It is to be expected that contraction of the muscle will cause motion of the bone which is the freer of the two to move. When the body is in anatomical or fundamental reference position, one can predict very accurately which bone will move with contraction of an attaching muscle. For example, a muscle which attaches to the ribs and to the upper arm will cause the arm to move rather than the ribs; a muscle which courses from a bone in the forearm to a bone in the hand will cause the hand to move rather than the forearm. Because of the predictability of action, it is possible to distinguish between the two attachments according to which will be stable and which will move. The **origin** of a muscle is the attachment on the more stable of the two bones; the **insertion** is the attachment on the bone freer to move.

In the performance of some movements, the position of the body or the movement task to be performed may require the origin and insertion to alternate. The brachialis, an elbow flexor which attaches to the humerus and the ulna, usually acts to pull the forearm (insertion) toward the humerus (origin) when it contracts. If the forearm is stabilized, however, as it would be during the performance of the chinning exercise, contraction of the brachialis will flex the elbow by pulling the humerus toward the forearm. The origin and insertion have reversed themselves to satisfy the requirements of the task. A second example can be seen in the rectus abdominis. It is listed as a flexor of the spine, with its origin at the pubis and its insertion on the ribs. It is to be expected, therefore, that contraction of this muscle will cause the spine to bow and the shoulders and trunk to bend forward toward the hips. This expectation will be correct if the body is in anatomical position, because the bearing of weight precludes significant movement of the hips toward the torso. If the upper body is held stable, however, contraction of the rectus abdominis will rotate the pubic crest upwardly around the hip joints for upward tilt of the pelvis. Origin and insertion have, thus, been reversed. Reversals such as these are treated as special cases, however, because the anatomical or fundamental reference position is always assumed to pertain.

Muscle Attachments
Proximal
Distal
Medial
Lateral

One school of kinesiological thought recommends the use of **proximal** and **distal** or **medial** and **lateral** to describe muscle attachments. According to this terminology, the brachialis would be depicted as a muscle with proximal attachment on the humerus and distal attachment on the ulna. Whereas this terminology has the advantage of consistency (proximal seldom becomes distal, etc.), it does not inform the reader of the true nature of the movement to be caused. To know that a muscle that attaches to the scapula and to the back of the head is contracting with an origin on the scapula is to know that muscular effort is being spent to move the head, not the scapula. Knowing only that the muscle attaches proximally on the head and distally to the scapula does nothing to describe the type of the movement to be expected.

Physiologically, a muscle is comprised of a contractile portion and one or more cord-like structures called **tendons**. The type of muscle envisioned most frequently is that shown in Figure 2.42. The contractile portion in the center rounds smoothly to form a *belly* and then becomes tendinous on each end. The biceps brachii is an example of such a muscle. Through its tendons, it attaches to bony prominences on the scapula and radius (see Chapter 3, Fig. 3.26). Not all muscles have such typical characteristics, however. Some do not originate with a tendinous attachment, but rather make attachment through the sheaths of the contractile fibers, themselves. Examples are the muscles that attach to the scapula (see Chapter 3). The reason for the different structures would appear to stem from the size of the surface area of attachment. If the area is large, contraction force can be spread sufficiently to allow attachment via the fiber sheaths. If the area is small, the muscle must terminate in strong tendons that can transmit large amounts of force to their respective bone prominences.

EXCURSION RATIO

Muscle tissue is characterized by the properties of extensibility, elasticity, and contractility. Its extensibility property allows it to stretch; its elasticity permits it to return from stretch to its resting length; its ability to contract allows it to shorten from the resting length. In Figure 2.42, a typical muscle is depicted at its resting, stretched, and contracted length. The ratio of stretched length to contracted length is referred to as the **excursion ratio of the muscle**. For the muscle illustrated, the excursion ratio is 2:1; that is, the muscle is capable of stretching to a length twice as long as it can shorten. A ratio of 2:1 is considered average for muscles of the human body, and is, for the most part, adequate to allow joints to move through their full ranges. Where muscles cross several joints, however, their excursion ratios may be inadequate to allow either for simultaneous extension or flexion of the several joints involved. This is exemplified by the muscle which extends the fingers. It is a multiple-joint muscle, crossing some five joints between its origin above the elbow and its insertion on the third phalanx of each finger. When an attempt is made to hold the wrist and fingers in full extension, it will be noted that the wrist is limited in its range. If the fingers are allowed to curl, the wrist can extend farther -- evidence that the contractile ability of the muscle is not sufficient to move all of the joints it crosses through their full ranges of extension. Similarly, the extensibility of the muscle will not allow all the joints to flex simultaneously. It is impossible to maintain a firm fist while also flexing the wrist because the muscle is incapable of stretching to that extent.

Relative Lengths of a Typical Muscle During Stretch, Contraction, and Rest

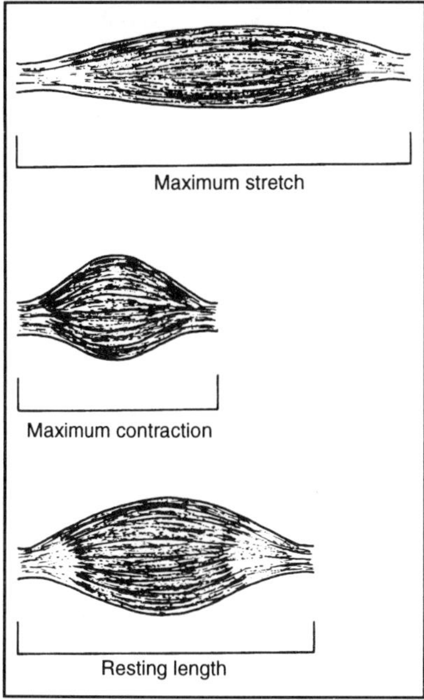

Fig. 2.42

MUSCLE FIBER ARRANGEMENT

Muscle fibers are arranged according to two basic patterns, longitudinal and penniform (Fig. 2.43). Included under the longitudinal arrangement are strap, rhomboidal, triangular, and fusiform muscles. These are exemplified in the human body by the sartorius, pronator quadratus, pectoralis major, and biceps brachii, respectively, and have in common an above average excursion ratio, but are somewhat limited, when compared to penniform muscles, in strength. Penniform muscles are subcategorized as single penniform, bipenniform, and multipenniform. The flexor digitorum longus, rectus femoris, and deltoid are examples of these penniform arrangements and, together with all other penniform muscles, offer comparatively low excursion ratios but are extremely strong.

Fiber Structure of Human Muscles

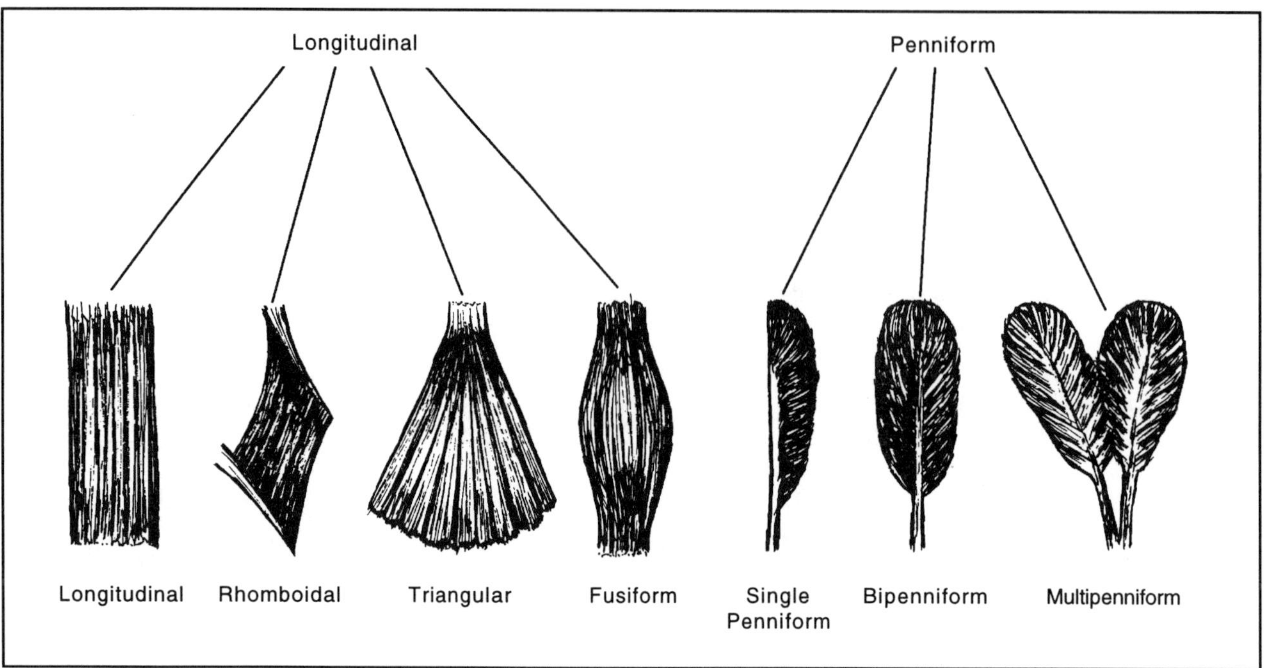

Fig. 2.43

Knowledge of the fiber arrangements of the many muscles of the body can be of help to kinesiologists as they seek to explain a specific muscle's contribution to movement. Muscles which are required for strength of movement are, in general, penniform; it is not surprising that many of the muscles of the lower limb are of that arrangement. Muscles of the upper limb are more of the longitudinal type demanded for range of movement.

THE ANATOMY OF CONTRACTION: AN OVERVIEW

Whereas an intense treatment of neuroanatomy is beyond the scope of this book, it may be helpful to provide a brief overview of the structure of the nervous system and the physiology of muscle contraction. Remarks will be limited to the central and peripheral nervous systems and to contraction mechanics of striated muscle; they should be considered only as a review of more basic material.

The structural unit of the nervous system is a neuron. It is composed of a cell body and processes called axons and dendrites. Nerve impulses are conducted to the cell body by dendrites and away from it by axons. Through this basic structure and its combination with other neurons, impulses are passed from the central nervous system to the peripheral nervous system and also returned to it. It is the combination of many axon fibers, which makes up the nerve.

The majority of axon fibers are surrounded by a myelin sheath, which is laid down to Schwann cells. These cells engulf the axon and rotate around it several times, adding a layer of myelin with each rotation, until the sheath is complete. The purpose of the sheath is to prevent significant flow of ions between the extracellular spaces and the axon. The sheath acts, therefore, much as an electrical insulation.

At intervals along the axon, the sheath is interrupted, exposing uninsulated areas called the nodes of Ranvier. Ions flow with ease through the nodes and allow a nerve impulse to jump from node to node rather than to be conducted continuously through the fiber. Such **saltatory** progress of the impulse is thought to contribute to the higher velocities of nerve transmission of myelinated fibers as compared to their unmyelinated counterparts.

Nerves - Simple or Complex Structure

It can be seen that a nerve is a complex structure comprised of myelinated and unmyelinated axons, which carry nerve impulses throughout the body. Axons vary considerably in length, some are less than a centimeter long, whereas others extend for over a meter. Even with such variation, however, it is necessary for axons to junction or synapse either with the cell body at their origination and/or with dendrites at their ends.

In its simplest form, a synapse is a narrow gap between the flared end of an axon and the cell body or a dendrite of another cell body. At the flared termination of the axon are vesicles containing an excitatory substance that is secreted by the arrival of a stimulus and increases the permeability of the postsynaptic membrane to sodium ions. Sodium ions, carrying their electropositive charge, rush through the membrane and reverse the normal negative charge that is characteristic of the resting state of the membrane. Depolarization is now complete and the impulse has been transmitted across the synapse.

Almost immediately after depolarization occurs, the membrane once again becomes impermeable to sodium ions. Not only is further inward movement blocked but also is any outward flow. The membrane is, however, permeable to potassium ions, which are attracted from inside the membrane to the outside because of the electronegative state created there by depolarization. This rapid diffusion of the potassium ions returns the membrane to its resting voltage and repolarization has begun. It cannot be complete, however, until the sodium and potassium ions are returned to their original locations outside and inside the membrane. This process is accomplished by the sodium and potassium pumps -- a relatively slow and energy consuming process. When the ions have been returned, repolarization is complete and the membrane has reestablished its true resting state.

Depolarization and repolarization do not occur only in the area of the synapse, as might be supposed from the foregoing discussion. Rather, depolarization, followed closely by repolarization, travels in wavelike fashion along the length of an axon. It will be recalled that the wave of movement along myelinated fibers is saltatory in nature, whereas it occurs through the entire length of unmyelinated fibers. It is the wave of depolarization that is thought of as the transmission of a nerve impulse.

Any interruption in the wave of depolarization will, of course, block nerve transmission. Among such interruptions are trauma, nutritional imbalance, and local anesthetics. Local anesthetics have been developed expressly to prevent the secretion of excitatory transmitters by the vesicles of the axons. Nutritional imbalances of potassium, sodium, and calcium can impede the processes of depolarization and repolarization and can result in increased or decreased excitability of the membrane.

Nerve Trauma - First Degree to Fifth Degree

Trauma to nerve tissues ranges generally from first to fifth degree in severity. First-degree trauma is characterized by the presence of pressure extreme enough to block transmission but not cause degeneration of tissue. Numbness in the feet after sitting on hard surfaces for long periods of time may be indicative of the exertion of pressure on the sciatic nerve.

Fifth-degree trauma involves the complete severance of a nerve trunk with accompanying loss of sensation and muscular paralysis. Surgery involving the rejoining of the severed ends or of uniting them by grafts is often indicated for these types of trauma. Under satisfactory conditions, regeneration of axons can occur at the rate of 1 to 2 mm per day. Not all regenerating axons find their original paths, however. Some may find their way to the wrong end organ. Example of such misdirection can be felt when rubbing a scar causes pricks of sensation on the opposite side of the trauma.

Just as the neuron is the structural unit of the nervous system, the muscle fiber (or cell) is the basic unit of the muscular system. Muscle fibers are typically arranged in parallel fashion throughout the muscle, although they may or may not be parallel to the length of the muscle. Various arrangements are possible and are discussed later in this chapter. It should be noted, however, that when a muscle fiber contracts, it does so by applying force through its length.

The transmission of a nervous impulse to a muscle fiber is basically the same as has been discovered above regarding neural synapses. The synapse between an axon and muscle fiber is called the neuromuscular junction (also called a myoneural synapse). The appearance of the neuromuscular junction differs from that of the neural synapse in that the axon that terminates at a muscle fiber does so by branching into a rootlike structure called sole feet or endplate feet. These invaginate to the muscle fiber; however, they do not enter the fiber membrane and, therefore, require the same synaptic mechanism discussed above to transmit impulses. Excitatory transmitter is released in the presence of a stimulus and initiates the wave of depolarization over the synapse and through the muscle fiber. Perhaps the major distinction between nerve and muscle fiber depolarization is that whereas depolarization down a nerve is accomplished for the sole reason of propagating an impulse to an end organ, depolarization of the muscle fiber -- itself an end organ --

is to provide for its contraction. Accepting, therefore, that the concepts of waves of depolarization and repolarization are as viable for muscle fiber as they are for nerve fiber, we can turn to a review of the current theory of the mechanics of contraction.

Muscle Fiber Structure

It has been noted that the basic unit of a muscle is the muscle fiber. Most muscle fibers extend the length of the muscle itself and are innervated by a single neuromuscular junction located in the middle of the fiber. Within the fiber, numerous myofibrils are organized in parallel with the length of the fiber and comprise, in turn, myosin and actin filaments, which are also arranged in parallel with the fiber length. The actin (light) and myosin (dark) filaments interdigitate somewhat to give rise to the appearance of microscopic bands of color called I (light or isotropic) and A (dark or anisotropic). Z-bands attach the myofibrils together at their ends and provide the structure that requires all filaments to be side by side. Since actin filaments are shorter than myosin filaments, they are capable of closing and opening on each other in a sliding sort of way to provide for shortening and lengthening of the myofibril, the muscle fiber, and, therefore, the muscle itself.

Myofibrils form an intracellular matrix called the sarcoplasm, which provides a special organization of tubules that communicate to extracellular spaces and, therefore, to extracellular fluids. This so-called T-system allows the action potential of depolarization to reach the interior of the fiber.

It is important to recall that a single axon may, at its termination, branch to innervate as many as 1000 muscle fibers and as few as 10. Regardless of the number of fibers with which an axon communicates, all of them (a motor unit) will respond to a nerve impulse transmitted along the axon. Their simultaneous response is called a twitch and will differ from other twitches within the muscle in terms of speed of contraction, the frequency of contraction, and the strength of contraction.

Fast-Twitch and Slow-Twitch Fibers

Speed of contraction is related both to the diameter of the axon, the thickness of the myelin sheath and to the physiologic properties of the innervated fibers. Large, well-myelinated axons can transmit impulses at speeds exceeding 100 meters per second. Small, unmyelinated fibers are capable of transmitting at the considerably slower speeds of only centimeters per second. These axon characteristics, coupled with **fast-twitch** and **slow-twitch** muscle fibers, provide for almost infinite possibilities within the range of contraction speeds.

Frequency of contraction is related to the refractory period of both the transmitting axon and the contracting fibers. Long refractory periods slow contraction frequency, just as short refractory periods increase contraction frequency. Another aspect that may relate to contraction frequency is that of endurance of motor units. It could be postulated that refractory periods in concert with ability of the fibers to resist fatigue may further contribute to our ability to perform motor skills with coordination and efficiency.

Contraction strength is related to the size of the fiber and the innervating axon. The larger these are, the stronger will be the contraction. In contrast to popular belief, the strength of the nerve impulse has no effect; if the stimulus is strong enough to cause transmission, it will produce maximum contraction of the motor unit -- the **all-or-nothing law**.

All or Nothing Law

In summary, the design of the neural and muscular systems of the human body can be likened to a multiwire cable linking the central nervous system to the musculature of the skeleton. Within the cable are myelinated wires capable of transmitting to the muscle (motor) as well as wires that can transmit back to the central nervous system (sensory). Speed of transmission within the cable varies according to thickness and myelination of the wires. The wires branch as they approach the muscle and invaginate, randomly, a number of fibers. Through the process of depolarization and repolarization, the fiber and its subparts -- the myofibril and actin and myosin filaments -- provide for shortening and lengthening of the muscle as a whole.

TYPES OF MUSCULAR FORCE

The two general modes of contraction of muscle are static and dynamic. During static contraction, a muscle does not change in length. There is, therefore, no observable motion in the joint over which the muscle crosses. Such contractions may or may not be maximal depending upon the requirements of the task. When a firm fist is made, both the extensors and flexors contract statically, each to neutralize the tendency of the other to move the wrist joint. The firmer the fist, the more the contraction approaches maximum. When static contractions are embodied in strength-gaining programs, they are referred to as **isometric contractions** and are usually characterized by maximum effort. Forceful pressing of the hands together in front of the chest is an example of an isometric exercise involving static contraction.

Isometric Contractions are Static Contractions

Dynamic contractions are accompanied by changes in muscle length. When the muscle shortens, the contraction is said to be concentric and the joint crossed by the muscle will be made to move according to action with which the muscle is credited. For example, the biceps brachii is an elbow flexor; when it contracts concentrically it shortens, causing the elbow to flex. The contraction may be partial or maximal; however, when such contractions are performed for the purpose of strength gain, they are typically of a maximal level. Concentric contractions can be of two types, isotonic or isokinetic. Isotonic contractions are those required when a given weight is moved through a range of joint motion. Bench presses, and arm curls with barbells are common weight-lifting examples of isotonic contractions against the resistance of weights, whereas pushups, sit-ups, and chin-ups exemplify isotonic contractions during which the body is the resistance.

Isokinetic contractions differ from their isotonic counterparts in that the muscle must shorten at a certain rate of velocity to ensure a constant rate of limb movement. Specially geared isokinetic exercisers are used to ensure not only appropriate contraction rates but also that the muscle can contract maximally, if desired, through the complete range of motion.

Eccentric vs. Concentric

Dynamic contractions need not always involve shortening of the muscle. Suppose the right elbow is flexed to a 90-degree angle and in the hand has been placed a five-kilogram weight. If the musculature of the elbow is of sufficient strength, the weight can be held in position (static contraction of the elbow flexors), or even brought toward the shoulder by flexing the elbow farther (concentric contraction). If the musculature is weak, however, the weight in the hand will gradually extend the elbow regardless of voluntary effort to resist. The elbow flexors are vigorously active, but are being forced to lengthen by the "**too-heavy**" weight. Such contractions are eccentric contractions and are as much a part of human movement as are concentric contractions. Without the muscle's ability to lengthen as it contracts, we would not be able to lower resistances after we have lifted them. A forward elevation of the arm is accomplished by concentric contraction of the flexor muscles of the shoulder. Lowering of the arm to the side of the body is accomplished by eccentric contraction of the same muscles; otherwise the arm would fall, uncontrolled, in response to the pull of gravity. It may seem surprising that the opposite muscles, the shoulder extensors, are not involved in returning the arm to the side; however, when it is remembered that the function of a muscle is to pull against a bone, it will follow that the extensors will be recruited only if it be desired that the arm be returned to the side with a force greater than that naturally afforded by gravity.

ROLES OF THE MUSCULAR SYSTEM

The muscles of the human body can assume various responsibilities as they carry out movement tasks. These responsibilities, or roles, are those of agonist, antagonist, stabilizer, and neutralizer.

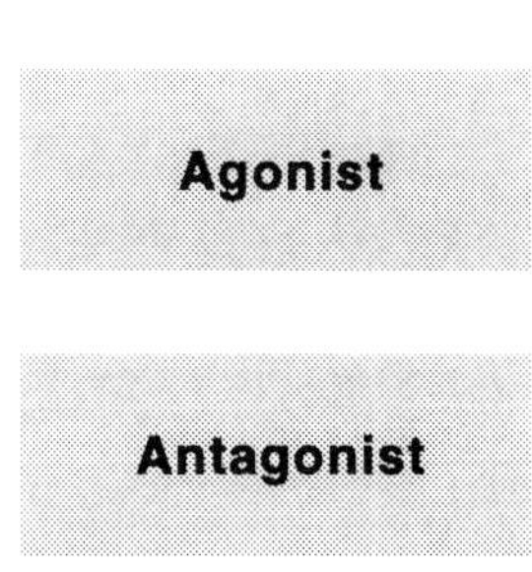

A muscle acts as an agonist when it is directly involved in causing a given joint action. The influence of an agonist upon a joint action may be either a primary one or an assistive one, depending upon the size, angle of insertion, and force arm to the joint's axis of rotation.

An antagonist is a muscle on the opposite side of the joint axis from the agonist and, as such, causes the opposite joint action. Antagonists can also be primary or assistive in their involvement, and are important to muscular control in two ways: (1) antagonists must relax to some degree in order to allow agonists to move the joint of concern; (2) antagonists must function to protect the joint structure from injury during powerful movement patterns. During knee extension against resistance, for example, the quadriceps are the agonists and hamstrings are the antagonists; however, the quadriceps can affect extension only if the hamstrings relax and allow the knee joint to move. If knee extension is performed powerfully, the hamstrings, after their initial relaxation, must contract against the momentum of the lower leg to prevent a tearing of the ligaments and other soft tissues of the joint. Since contraction of the antagonists typically applies stabilizing force, the centrifugal force developed by the lower leg is neutralized. It should be noted, at this point, that when the knee is flexed against resistance, the quadriceps reverse roles to become antagonists while the hamstrings become the agonists.

Stabilizers

Stabilizers are muscles which act, during a particular movement task, to support a body part or to make that body part firm against the influence of some force. Part 4 of the trapezius and pectoralis minor stabilize the scapula so that a firm base of support exists when a person is using crutches.

Neutralizers

Neutralizers are muscles which contract to prevent unwanted actions which occur as a result of the contraction of other muscles. Several examples of neutralizers can be found among the muscles which move the scapula. For example, the rhomboids lie between the spine and the scapula. Their line of pull dictates that when they contract, they will pull the scapula both upwardly (elevation) and toward the spine (adduction). Suppose the movement pattern being attempted requires the scapula to elevate only; some other muscle (an abductor) must be recruited which will, when it contracts, neutralize the adducting force of the rhomboids.

SPURT AND SHUNT MUSCLES

The terms **spurt** and **shunt** occurred originally in engineering terminology; however, they are used occasionally in kinesiology to describe the relationship of muscular origins and insertions to the joints these muscles cross. A shunt muscle is one which originates closer to a joint it crosses than it inserts. The brachioradialis is an excellent example of a shunt muscle at the elbow joint. A spurt muscle is one which originates farther from the joint than it inserts and is exemplified at the elbow joint by the brachialis.

Several muscles of the human body cross more than one joint and, as they do so, have characteristics of both shunt and spurt muscles depending upon the joint being regarded. The biceps brachii, hamstrings, and quadriceps are all examples of such muscles and display shunt characteristics at the shoulder or hip joint but are spurt muscles at the elbow or knee.

Shunt muscles are notable in that resolution of their lines of pull result in longer stabilizing vectors than angular vectors. Spurt muscles, on the other hand, provide for longer angular vectors than stabilizing vectors. The hamstrings and quadriceps, then, are mainly effective as stabilizers of the hip joint and movers of the knee joint.

Similarly, the gastrocnemius is a stabilizer of the knee joint and a mover of the ankle joint.

There is some controversy among kinesiologists regarding the validity of the spurt-shunt theory. Some researchers insist that the qualities of spurt and shunt muscles are due simply to the fact that their respective force arms have different lengths. Others offer that any differences noted are caused by the ratios of length of contractile tissue to length of tendinous material of the various muscles. Regardless of the viewpoint, however, the concept appears to be much the same.

NEWTON'S LAWS

Sir Isaac Newton is the discoverer of three laws, or truths, which form the basis for the mechanical analysis of all motion. As motion is analyzed, therefore, the laws must present the front line of defense, and when the questions "why?' or "why not?" perplex one, those questions should be examined initially from the viewpoint of the laws. More often than not, the answer will be found thereby.

THE FIRST LAW: INERTIA

An object will remain in its state of motion until it is acted upon by an external force sufficiently large to disturb that state.

Law of Inertia

It must be remembered, when exploring the ramifications of the first law, that objects which are at rest are in a state of motion -- that of no motion. The law addresses itself, therefore, both to objects which are moving and to objects which are still. Examples can be found in which either the condition of rest or of movement is prevalent over the other; frequent examples can be found also which illustrate the blending of both aspects of motion.

Application of the law of inertia to situations in which the object of concern is at rest can be made by recalling the often-heard statement, "the hardest part of lifting a weight is getting it off the floor." Certainly the statement is true, for the barbell will tend to exercise its inertia by remaining on the floor -- a good thing for those who frequent the weight room! Similarly, it can be said that the most demanding part of using a wheelchair is in overcoming of inertia of the chair and weight of the body as one attempts to start the chair moving.

It would be remiss not to point out that the law of inertia can place excessive demands on the muscular systems of the body. Consideration must be given to the choice of muscles to be used when lifting, pushing, and pulling. Heavy, difficult tasks must be matched with large, powerful muscles if injury is to be avoided. This is particularly important during lifting, when the tendency is to lift with the small muscles of the back rather than the large muscles of the hip and thigh.

Application of Newton's first law to situations in which inertia of movement predominates is seen particularly well in bowling. It is typical to teach beginning bowlers to deliver a "straight" ball -- one that has no sidespin. Once the ball has been released, it will tend to continue its state of motion by rolling in a straight line down the alley. There is no external force being applied, except the friction of the ball against the wood, and friction will not cause the ball to veer to the side. The bowler has only to concentrate on directing the ball toward the pocket. As the bowler becomes more skilled, however, the straight ball delivery may be changed to that of a hook in which a counterclockwise spin (or clockwise, if the bowler is lefthanded) is imparted to the ball. Upon release, the ball will again yield to its inertia and travel in a straight line down the alley. As friction slows the ball, the external force of the spin imparted is allowed to manifest itself and when it exceeds the inertia of the ball, will cause the ball to veer, or hook, into the pocket. Obviously, the timing must be quite precise; if the ball is rolled with a great deal of force, the spin will not be able to overcome the inertia and the hook will not occur. If the ball is rolled with too little force, the hook will be premature.

Inertia of the moving body has no doubt been appreciated also by the beginning snow skier who often complains that although lessons are quite adequate in their treatment of initiating movement on skis, they are dismally lacking in methods of stopping. Unless friction between the skis and snow can be increased by proper edging or waxing techniques, the skier is likely to become an inertia casualty.

Law of Acceleration

THE SECOND LAW: ACCELERATION

The acceleration of a body is proportional to the force imparted to it and inversely proportional to its mass. In symbols,

$$A = \frac{F}{M}, \text{ or } \text{Acceleration} = \frac{\text{Force}}{\text{Mass}}$$

By rearranging the terms of the formula the law can be stated differently; for example: the force which can be generated by a body is directly proportional both to its acceleration and to its mass.

$$F = MA, \text{ or } \text{Force} = \text{Mass X Acceleration}$$

Conceptualization of the second law is simplified by examining it through both of its forms. The first form instructs us, for instance, that application of the same amount of force to a golf ball and a 12-pound shot will cause the golf ball to accelerate more than the shot because of its smaller mass. The second form indicates, however, that if these two objects are made to accelerate equally, the shot, because of its greater mass, will make the larger dent when they land. Certainly neither of these two statements is surprising, but when the forms of the law are extended to other events, they become of great importance to the analysis of technique.

When the human body is considered as the object of acceleration in such situations as jumping or leaping, the force applied is that which results from the strength of the contracting muscles, and the mass is that of the body itself. If increased acceleration is demanded to increase the height of a jump, the performer must either apply more force by strengthening the muscles and/or reduce the mass of the body.

When force is to be applied to implements or other human beings, attention must be given to increasing both acceleration and mass. An archery arrow is a more lethal projectile over short distances than a bullet because, even though its acceleration is less than that of the bullet, its mass is considerably greater. At long distances, the bullet can be more damaging since air resistance so slows the arrow that even its greater mass cannot compensate.

The second law is of particular importance in the selection of sports implements. Certainly it is true that the large baseball bat in the hands of a powerful hitter deserves respect, for if the ball is contacted, it will react with great force. The large bat in the hands of a weak hitter causes no concern whatsoever since the ball probably will not be hit. Unless the hitter is strong enough to accelerate the bat properly, he will swing late. Even if contact is made, it will probably result in a slow foul ball. So it is with the tennis player who consistently swings late -- the fault may not lie in technique at all, but rather with a "**too heavy**" racket. Young girls and boys learning golf will have difficulty controlling their swings if they must use their mothers' or fathers' "**hand-me-down**" clubs. Bowlers often fall into this trap by theorizing that the heavier the ball, the easier the strike. Unfortunately, loss of control and incomplete pin action is, more often than not, the result of improper ball selection.

THE THIRD LAW: ACTION-REACTION

Law of Action-Reaction

When one body exerts a force on a second, there is an equal and opposite force exerted by the second body on the first. Throwing a ball overarm, for example, involves a forceful forward action of the arm. The accompanying reaction tends to rotate the rest of the body backward. If the feet are contacting the ground securely, however, the body cannot comply and the reaction is transmitted to the ground in so subtle a manner that it is seldom observable. Verification of the presence of the law can be found, however, if one imagines the outcome of daily living activities such as pushing and pulling if they were performed on a slippery surface such as ice. Without firm foot contact, reactions of the body can manifest themselves and the feet will slip from under the body in the direction of the reaction (or in the opposite direction to the action).

An outgrowth of the law of action-reaction is a principle referred to as transfer of momentum and relates to the redistribution of angular momentum generated by the movement of body parts. For example, when one wishes to execute a vertical jump, the arms will be forcefully elevated to above the head just as the feet leave the ground. The momentum established by the arms will be transferred to the body when the arms reach the overhead position and become still.

ABSORBING AND IMPARTING FORCE

Two principles relating to absorbing force are derived from Newton's laws, and instruct us in successful and non-injurious force absorption.

Force Absorption Principles

1. The velocity of a moving object should be slowed gradually.
2. The area of force absorption should be as large as possible under the confines of proper performance.

Illustrative of the first principle are those activities in which an implement must be caught. The phrase "**give with the ball**" is meant to prevent it from bouncing off of the hands instead of being caught. Force is absorbed by elongating the time over which the velocity of the object is slowed. If objects are moving excessively fast, it may be necessary to lengthen the absorption time even more by allowing the arms to swing backwardly after the initial "give" or even by taking a backward step.

The second principle of force absorption, to the effect that the area of absorption should be enlarged as permitted by the situation, may best be illustrated from the viewpoint of winter sports. Skis and snowshoes are both pieces of equipment that have been developed because of this principle, for without the enlarged area over which the body weight is spread, locomotion through deep snow would be virtually impossible. It will be recalled also that the rescuing of individuals who have fallen through thin ice should be performed in a prone position so that the rescuer's weight will be dispersed over a large surface area, thus lessening the tendency to break through also.

Discussion to this point has involved means of **absorbing** force safely and successfully. If one were to reverse the two principles cited, descriptions of the successful **imparting** of force would be seen.

Principles of Imparting Force

1. Increase the velocity of a moving object to impart additional force.
2. Reduce the area over which force is imparted to increase the effect of force.

The recipient of an injection is hopeful that both principles will be minded by the shot giver; i.e., that the needle will be moved rapidly and that it will be sharp.

A quiz for this material can be found in the back of this book on page 281.

LABORATORY EXPERIENCES

1. Stand with your arms at your sides as you raise one foot from the ground and notice that it is relatively difficult to remain stable. Now, abduct your arms to shoulder level and use them to help stabilize your position. Explain why the arms contribute to your ability to maintain stability while standing on one foot. Extend your explanation to include the tightwire walker who uses a long balancing pole while moving along the wire.

2. What foot stance (side-to-side, front-to-back, and so on) would you use when performing the following activities?
   a. removing a heavy object from an overhead closet shelf
   b. standing, facing forward, in a moving vehicle
   c. standing, facing sideward, in a moving vehicle

3. Explain why it is more difficult to walk in sand than on a hard surface such as concrete.

4. Drop a golf ball on a hard surface and then on a pillow. Describe the difference between the two reactions of the ball in terms of the principles of force absorption.

5. Categorize each of the following activities according to whether it is linear, angular, or a combination motion.
   a. bicycling
   b. glide in the sidestroke
   c. free fall of a sky diver
   d. action of the leg during the football punt
   e. riding a sled down a hill

6. Classify each of the following tools according to whether it is a 1st, 2nd, or 3rd class lever.
   a. scissors
   b. pliers
   c. tweezers
   d. shovel
   e. furniture dolly

7. Compare and contrast the three lever types.

THE SHOULDER

3

EVOLUTION

When man became a biped, the long, slow, and purposeful journey in evolution required to meet the demands of upright posture was begun. Among the pertinent developmental changes were those of the shoulder complex. With the elimination of its weight-bearing responsibilities, the shoulder has become admirably adapted to its new purpose of providing mobility of the upper limb.

BONES OF THE SHOULDER

The bones which comprise the shoulder complex are the scapula, the clavicle, and the humerus. The scapula, a broad, long bone, acts as a platform on which movements of the humerus are based. The clavicle holds the scapula and humerus away from the body for more freedom of movement of the arm. The humerus represents the first link in the chain of bony levers of the upper limb.

Scapula
Clavicle
Humerus

The scapula, clavicle, and humerus exhibit an intricate interplay of action toward the goal of aligning the glenoid fossa in a favorable direction for movement of the humerus, as hardly any action of the humerus can take place without associated and supplementary actions of the scapula. Throughout the entire range of motion of the humerus in the frontal and sagittal planes, approximately one-third of the mobility is the contribution of scapular movement; the remaining two-thirds of the mobility occurs at the ball-and-socket joint of the shoulder. It follows, then, that without the "free swinging" nature of the scapula, the humerus would be severely limited in its range of motion. A more detailed analysis of scapulohumeral motion will be discussed later in the chapter.

BONE MARKINGS

Figures 3.1 and 3.2 are offered as reviews of the anatomical landmarks of the scapula, clavicle, and humerus. All the bone markings which will be used in the discussion of muscular attachments are noted.

Left Scapula, Clavicle, and Humerus

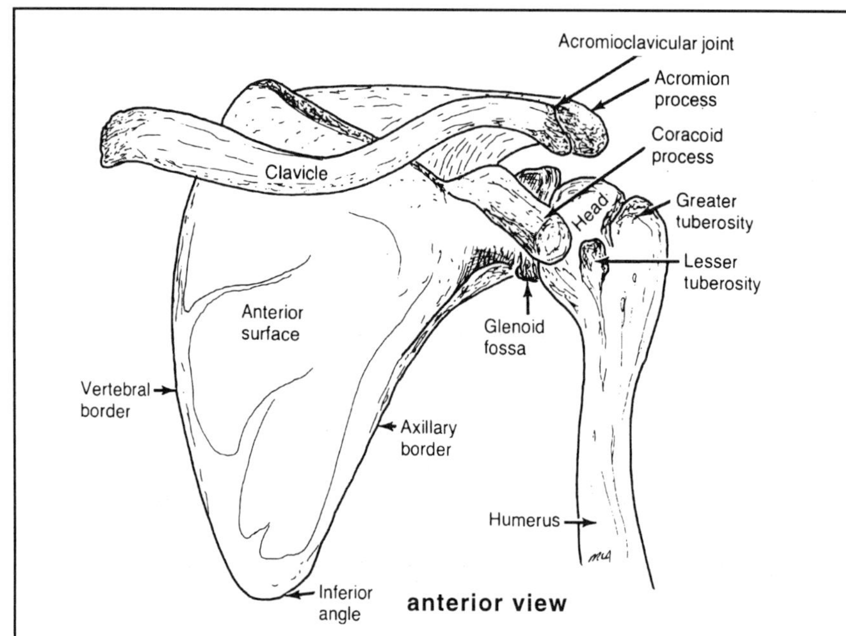

Fig. 3.1

Left Scapula, Clavicle, and Humerus

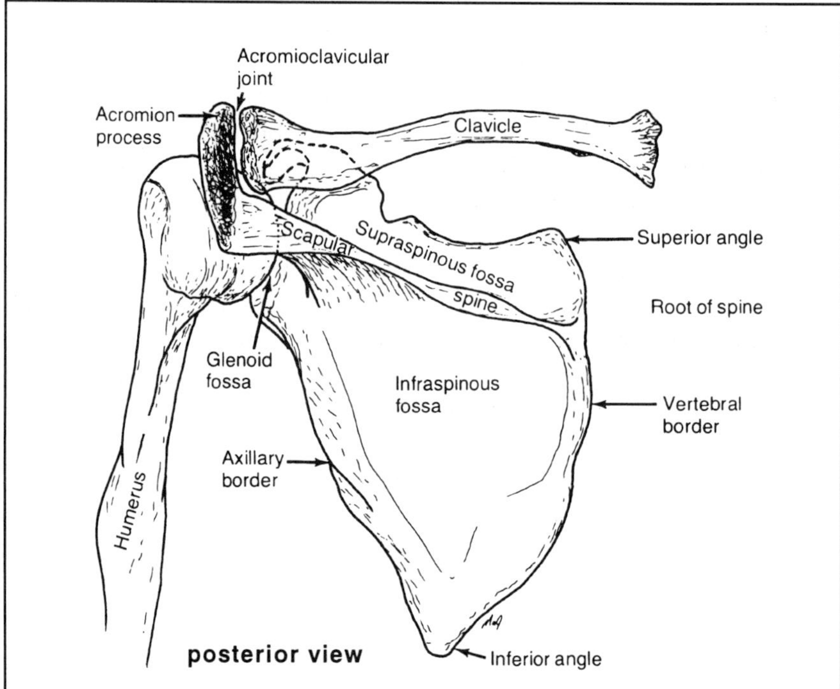

Fig. 3.2

JOINTS OF THE SHOULDER

Three joints comprise the shoulder complex. The sternoclavicular and acromioclavicular joints allow the scapula to glide along the surface of the rib cage. The glenohumeral joint is the articulation between the humerus and the scapula.

STERNOCLAVICULAR (SC) JOINT

The sternoclavicular, or SC, joint (Fig. 3.3) joins the sternum and the clavicle; it is the only bony articulation between the upper limb and the torso. The stability of this joint is dependent upon its ligamentous structures. An intra-articular disc, found between the manubrium, first costal cartilage, and the clavicle, separates the joint into two synovial compartments. This fibrocartilaginous structure is rarely affected by trauma. The intra-articular disc allows the sternoclavicular joint to function as a modified ball-and-socket joint which is responsible for rotational movements of the clavicle around three axes: elevation and depression (sagittal axis), anterior and posterior movements (vertical axis), and rotatory movements (frontal axis) (Fig. 3.4). During elevation and depression, the clavicle may be observed moving on the disc, while during other movements, the disc moves with the clavicle. The sternoclavicular joint does have a small articulation with the first rib through the attachment of its ligamentous structures and the intra-articular disc. Due to these attachments, the sternoclavicular joint has posteromedial orientation.

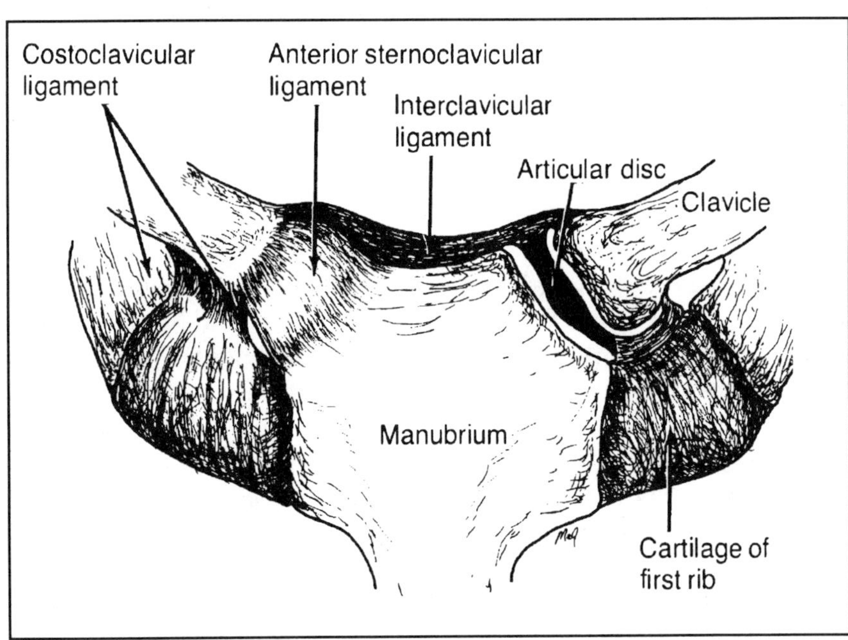

Fig. 3.3

Sternoclavicular Joints

Axes of Sternoclavicular Joint and Accompanying Scapular Actions

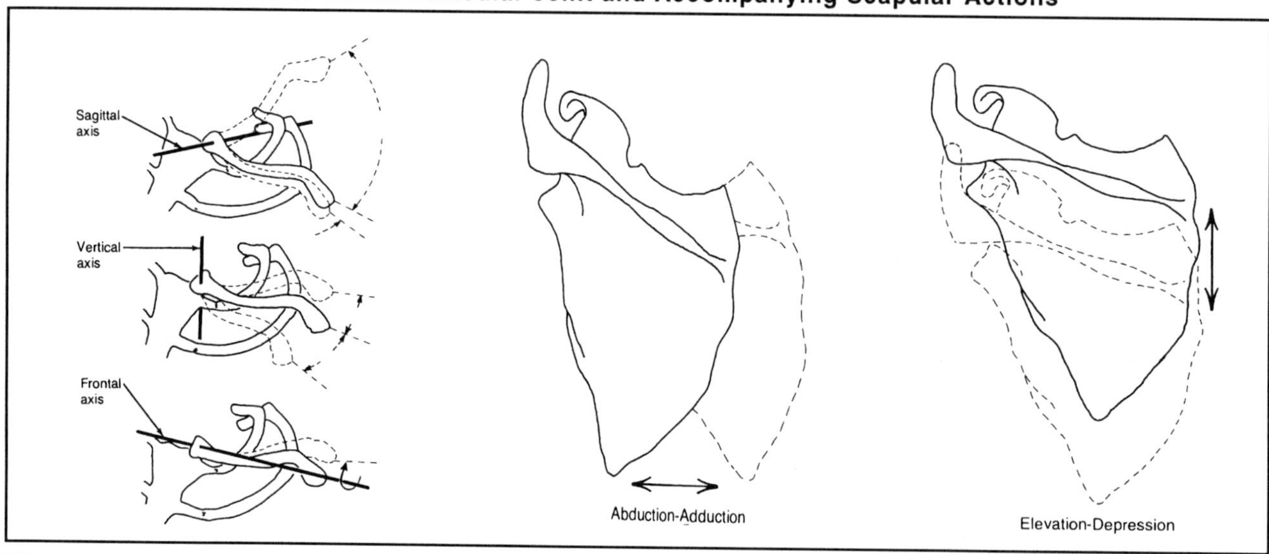

Fig. 3.4

Approximately 30 to 35 degrees of elevation is present at the sternoclavicular joint and most of this motion occurs between 30 to 90 degrees of glenohumeral elevation. Anterior/posterior motion at the sternoclavicular joint is approximately 35 degrees, and rotatory movement about the frontal axis is 45 to 50 degrees. Rotatory movements at the sternoclavicular joint occur after 70 to 80 degrees of glenohumeral elevation. The actions of the scapula which result from movement of the clavicle include abduction and adduction and elevation and depression. These movements are more linear than angular with scapular abduction/adduction accompanied by horizontal adduction and horizontal abduction of the clavicle and scapular elevation/depression accompanied by elevation and depression of the clavicle. Both pairs of actions combine to cause a gliding of the clavicle on the acromion process.

The ligaments surrounding the sternoclavicular joint are the interclavicular, costoclavicular, and anterior and posterior sternoclavicular ligaments (Fig. 3.3). The paired sternoclavicular ligaments run downward and medially from the clavicle to the sternum. These ligaments reinforce the joint capsule and limit the amount of rotation that occurs at the sternoclavicular joint during depression of the clavicle. The posterior sternoclavicular ligament is considered to be the strongest of the pair and plays a major role in preventing upward and lateral displacement of the clavicle.

The interclavicular ligament attaches itself to both clavicles and the sternum. This ligament becomes taut as the lateral end of the clavicle is depressed. The costoclavicular ligament may be found between the medial clavicle and the first rib. This ligament contains anterior and posterior fibers which assist in restricting upward displacement and downward rotation of the medial clavicle.

ACROMIOCLAVICULAR (AC) JOINT

The acromioclavicular, or AC, joint (Fig. 3.5) is the articulation of the clavicle with the acromion process of the scapula. The joint is a triaxial synovial joint which contains a meniscus between its articular surfaces that provides for surface contact and force transmission. Due to the arrangement of the ligaments around the joint, there is little motion that takes place between the acromion and the clavicle. Approximately 10° of rotational movement occurs at this joint with full glenohumeral elevation. Movements about the acromioclavicular joint are described as anteroposterior rotation of the clavicle on the scapula, superoinferior rotation, and inferior and superior axial rotation. These rotational movements occur around three axes which allow for the following scapular actions: upward and downward tilt about a frontal axis; upward and downward rotation about a sagittal axis; and "winging" of the scapula about a vertical axis (Fig. 3.6).

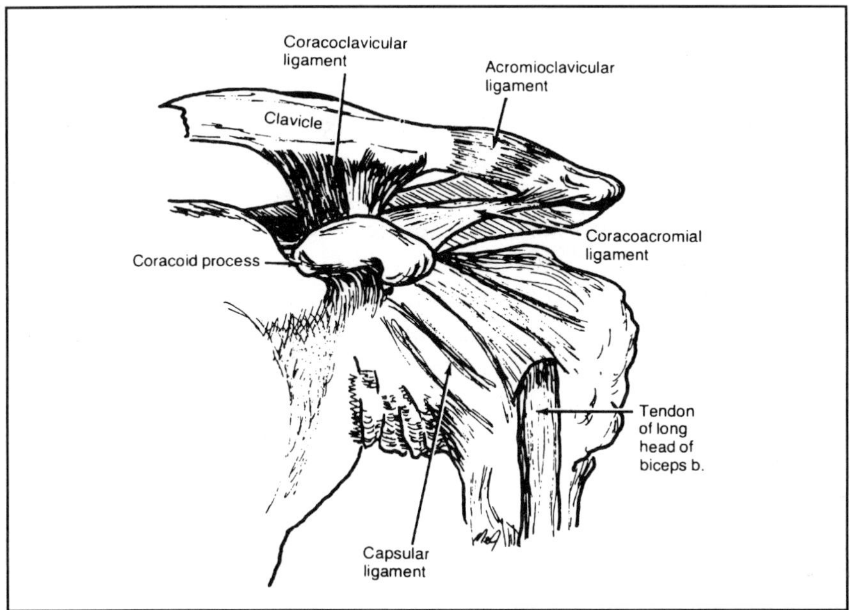

Fig. 3.5

Acromioclavicular Joint

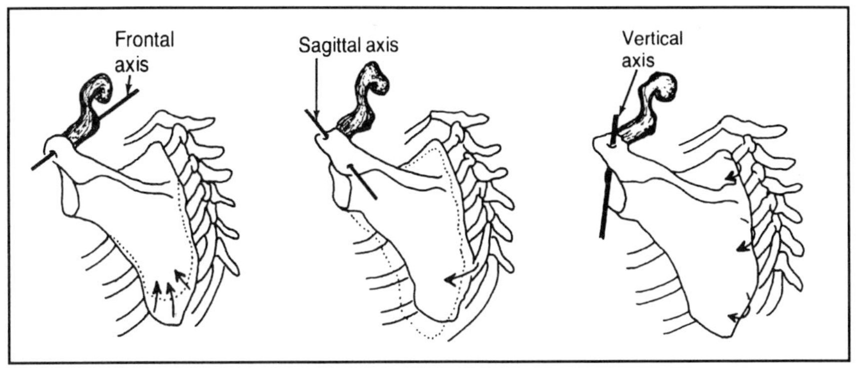

Fig. 3.6

Axes of Acromioclavicular Joint

The capsule of the acromioclavicular joint is weaker and looser than that of the sternoclavicular joint, and thus the integrity of the joint is largely dependent on the ligaments. The ligaments that surround this joint are the superior and inferior acromioclavicular ligaments and the coracoclavicular ligament. The acromioclavicular ligaments bind the clavicle to the acromion process and restrict anteroposterior movements of the joint. The coracoclavicular ligament binds the clavicle to the coracoid process to not only provide stability to the joint, but also to act as the major force in connecting the clavicle to the scapula. This ligament is made up of two components; the conoid and trapezoid ligaments. The conoid ligament restricts inferior separation of the scapula from the clavicle. When this ligament becomes taut, it produces posterior rotation of the clavicle. The trapezoid ligament restricts medial displacement of the scapula on the clavicle. When the acromioclavicular joint is dislocated, it is usually the coracoclavicular ligament that is torn.

Weakest Link: Clavicle or AC Joint

As mentioned before, the acromioclavicular joint is weaker than the sternoclavicular joint. Forces, such as those incurred by falling on the outstretched arm or on the tip of the shoulder, will be transmitted to the clavicle and will tend to either dislocate the clavicle from its two attachments or to fracture it. Since the sternoclavicular joint is the strongest link in the clavicular chain, dislocations of the medial head of the clavicle are seldom seen. In children, the clavicle itself appears to be the weakest link, for it is not unusual to see fractured "**collar bones**" after falls from trees or fences. In adulthood, however, the acromioclavicular joints tend to be the weakest link; dislocations at this joint, called shoulder separations, are all-too-common among athletes who engage in contact sports. A contributing factor to the high incidence of shoulder separations among football players may well be their pregame drill of standing slightly off-center to each other and vigorously bumping shoulders. The forceful contact can cause severe stretching of the coracoacromial ligament and thus disable it as a stabilizer of the acromioclavicular joint.

The acromion, the coracoacromial ligament, and the coracoid process forms the coracoacromial arch. Under this structure passes the proximal humerus, rotator cuff, and subacromial bursa. Glenohumeral motion depends on the integrity of these structures which are confined closely under this arch. When one of these structures is disrupted, inpingement will result, and normal glenohumeral rhythm will be lost.

GLENOHUMERAL JOINT (SHOULDER JOINT)

The glenohumeral joint (Fig. 3.7), a synovial ball-and-socket joint, is the freest joint of the body. It is formed by the large globular head of the humerus and the glenoid fossa of the scapula. The glenoid fossa is small and shallow and contacts only about one-third of the head of the humerus at a given time. The glenoid articular surface is deepened by a structure known as the glenoid labrum. The labrum contributes to the articular stability of the glenohumeral joint. This arrangement makes possible the extensive mobility of the joint; however, stability is minimal, being provided by the joint capsule and surrounding muscles rather than by the structure of the joint itself.

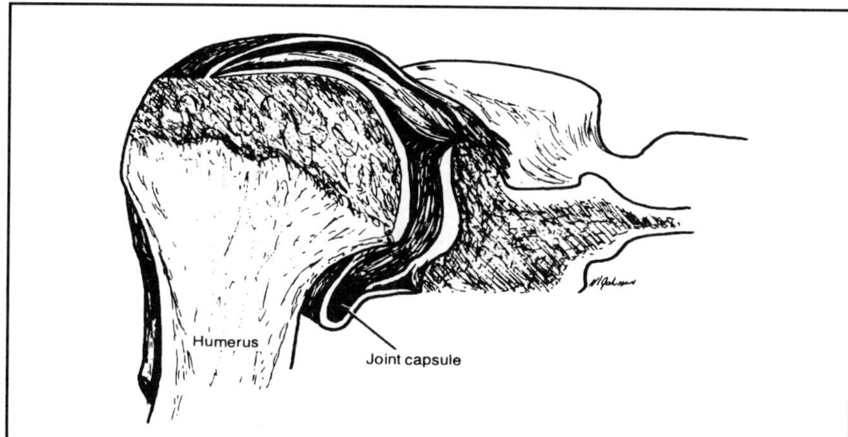

Glenohumeral (Shoulder) Joint

Fig. 3.7

The glenohumeral joint permits rotation about three axes, all three of which pass through the head of the humerus (Fig. 3.8). Flexion, extension, and hyperextension of the joint move the humerus about a frontal axis; abduction and adduction move the humerus about a sagittal axis; and internal and external rotation move the humerus about its long axis. In addition, the joint can allow horizontal

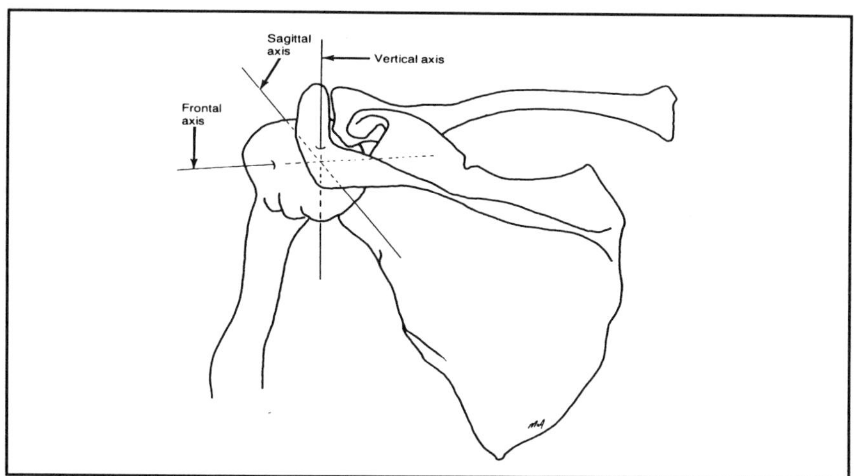

Axes of Glenohumeral (Shoulder) Joint

Fig. 3.8

adduction and abduction (Fig. 3.9) which comprise the movement of the humerus in a horizontal plane from in front of the body to the side (horizontal abduction), or from the side of the body to the front (horizontal adduction). Neither horizontal abduction nor horizontal adduction can occur from anatomical reference position. They must be preceded either by flexion or by abduction of the joint and are, therefore, regarded as combination movements. It should be noted, however, that when the actions of a given muscle include horizontal abduction or adduction, the required preliminary flexion or abduction movement is disregarded in movement analysis.

Horizontal Adduction and Abduction of Glenohumeral (Shoulder) Joint

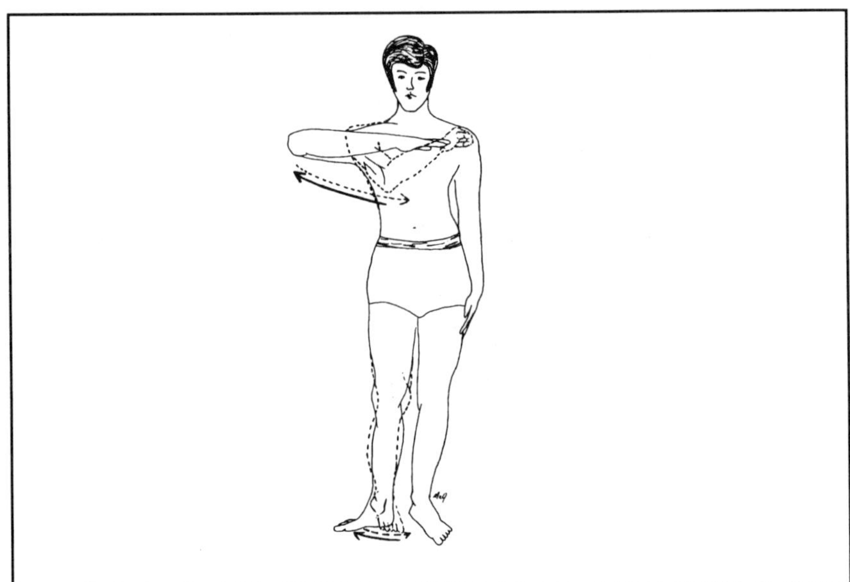

Fig. 3.9

The capsule of the glenohumeral joint is thin and weak. The glenohumeral capsule is reinforced by a ligamentous complex that is made up of the superior, middle, and inferior glenohumeral ligaments and the coracohumeral ligament. These ligaments all become functional during motion of the glenohumeral joint. The coracohumeral ligament originates from the coracoid process of the scapula, blends in with the rotator cuff and capsule, and inserts on the greater and lesser tuberosities of the humerus. It becomes taut with external rotation, flexion, and extension of the humerus and resists inferior subluxation of the joint. This ligament is considered to be the most important ligamentous structure in maintaining glenohumeral integrity and stability.

Throughout the anterior wall of the joint capsule, the glenohumeral ligaments may be found. The superior and middle glenohumeral ligaments tighten with external rotation of the humerus and provide anterior stability to the shoulder joint. The inferior glenohumeral ligament is made up of fibrous bands that stretch around the head of the humerus. This ligament becomes taut when the humerus is abducted 90 degrees or more and, thus provides anterior and posterior stability to the glenohumeral joint.

Bursae

A considerable amount of motion accompanies humeral rotation at the shoulder joint, and consequently there is a build-up of friction within the joint, between bones and tendons, between skin and bone, between muscle and bone near a tendon insertion, and between muscle layers. The synovial fluid secreted within the joint capsule minimizes the joint friction, and fibrous pockets known as **bursae** act to decrease the irritating effects of friction between the other anatomical structures. These bursae are lined with a synovial membrane similar to that of the joint, and contain a lubricating fluid which allows their inner surfaces to slip easily on each other. The overall result is much like holding a bag of water between the palms of the hands and moving them back and forth. Friction is negligible when compared to that which results from the same movement of the hands when the palms are allowed to contact each other.

Two bursae commonly recognized in the shoulder joint are the **subacromial** and **subdeltoid bursae.** These bursae allow smooth gliding motions to occur between the rotator cuff and the overlying acromion and acromioclavicular joints. Commonly, these two bursae are joined together as one and referred to anatomically as the subacromial bursa. The subacromial bursa does not communicate with the glenohumeral joint; however, if the rotator cuff is injured or ruptured, a communication between the joint and the bursa may develop.

Bursae:
Subacromial
Subdeltoid
Subscapularis

Another bursa that is important to the shoulder complex is the **subscapularis bursa**. This bursa is found between the upper portion of the subscapularis tendon and the neck of the glenoid. Its function is to protect the tendon of the subscapularis as it travels under the coracoid process and over the neck of the glenoid. In many instances, this bursa connects with the glenohumeral joint between the superior and middle glenohumeral ligaments. Several bursae are located around the shoulder complex and may be found between the capsule and the coracoid process, near the insertions of the infraspinatus and teres minor muscles; near the attachment of the trapezius to the scapular spine, between the coracoid process and the coracobrachialis; and between the tendons of the latissimus dorsi and teres major.

Normally, the membrane of the bursa is loose and thin; however, it tends to thicken with age and become filled with scar tissue from previous injuries. Inflammation and swelling frequently accompany the degeneration, and the bursa is then no longer able to separate the two muscle groups as they glide over each other. Elevation of the arm allows contact between the muscles and their adjacent structures and is, therefore, accompanied by acute pain -- a condition known as **bursitis**. The subacromial and subdeltoid bursae are commonly involved in this pathological process.

MUSCULATURE

The musculature of the shoulder is divided into two groups. Group 1 is comprised of the muscles which move or stabilize the scapula, and Group 2 is comprised of the muscles which move the humerus.

GROUP 1: SCAPULA MOVERS

The muscles which stabilize or move the scapula are the trapezius, rhomboids, levator scapulae, serratus anterior, pectoralis minor, and subclavius. All of these muscles except the subclavius have dual actions; however, only their actions on the scapula will be considered here.

Trapezius (trape'zius)

The trapezius (Fig. 3.10) is a flat triangular muscle located superficially on the upper back. It is subdivided into four parts which are easily palpated between the spine and scapula.

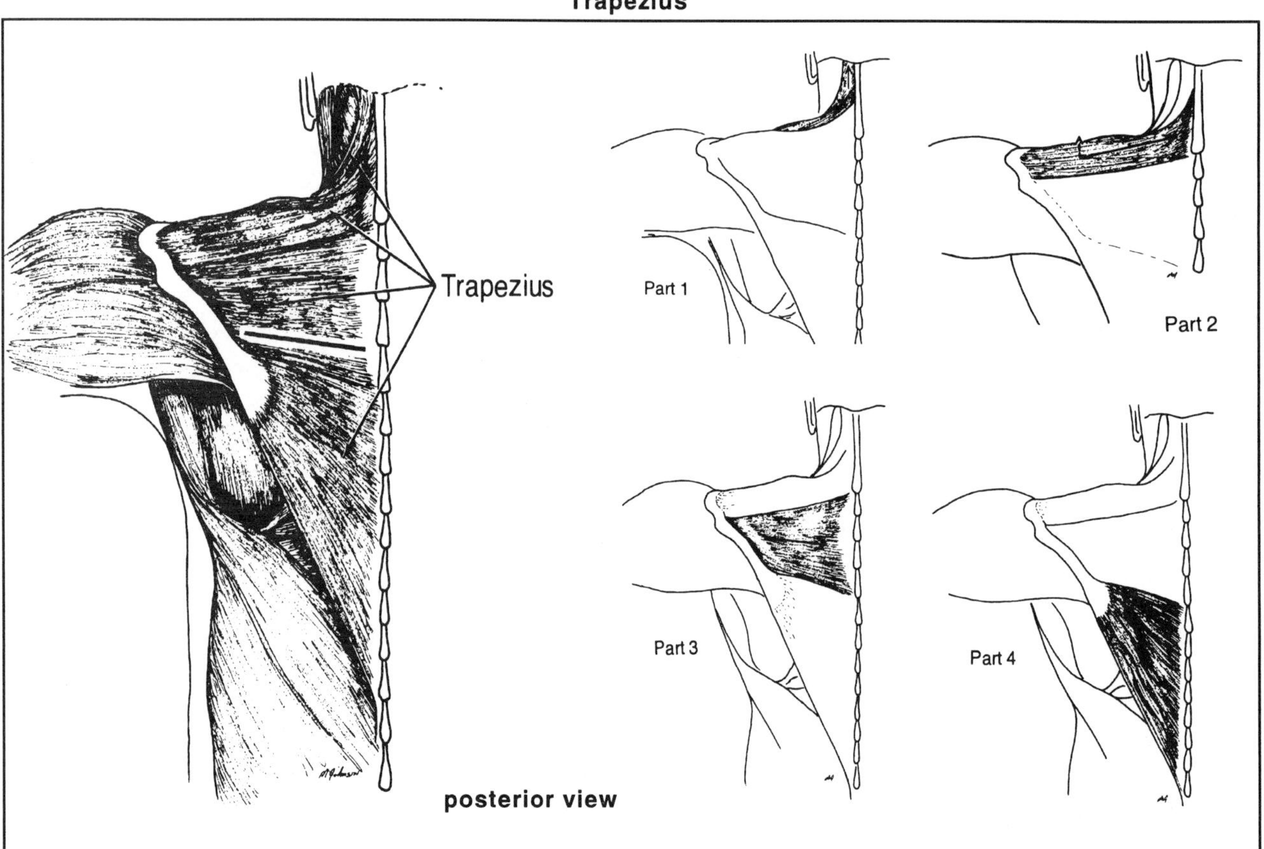

Fig. 3.10

Origin	Part 1:	Occipital bone.
	Part 2:	Ligamentum nuchae.
	Part 3:	Spinous processes of the seventh cervical and first three thoracic vertebrae.
	Part 4.	Spinous processes of the fourth through twelfth thoracic vertebrae.
Insertion	Part 1:	Outer third of clavicle.
	Part 2:	Acromion process.
	Part 3:	Scapular spine.
	Part 4:	Root of scapular spine.
Innervation	Spinal accessory nerve and third and fourth cervical nerves.	
Action	Part 1:	Elevation.
	Part 2:	Elevation, adduction, upward rotation.
	Part 3:	Adduction.
	Part 4:	Depression, adduction, upward rotation.

Since the trapezius lies primarily in the frontal plane, its contraction causes frontal plane movements of the scapula. **Part 1**, with its attachments on the base of the skull and clavicle, will pull upwardly on the clavicle when it contracts. The force on the clavicle is transferred to the scapula via the acromioclavicular joint to elevate the scapula.

Part 2 has a diagonal fiber direction -- its origin being slightly higher than its insertion. Resolution of the line of pull yields two component forces, of which one is directed toward the head (elevation) and one directed toward the spine (adduction). The third action of Part 2, upward rotation, occurs because the muscle crosses the acromioclavicular joint superior to the sagittal axis of that joint and, during contraction, pulls the acromion toward the neck by pivoting the scapula around its articulation with the clavicle.

Part 3 of the trapezius courses horizontally between the spine and scapula. Its only action is, therefore, adduction.

Part 4, like Part 2, represents a diagonal force vector; however, its origin is lower than its insertion. The two component forces for this portion of the trapezius are directed downwardly (depression) and toward the spine (adduction). Because Part 4 attaches medial to the acromioclavicular joint and approaches that attachment from below, it upwardly rotates the scapula by pulling downwardly on the root of the scapular spine.

By comparing the actions of the four parts of the trapezius, both agonism and antagonism can be seen. Parts 1 and 2 are agonistic to each other in elevation, but are antagonistic to the depressive action of Part 4. Parts 2 and 4 are agonists during upward rotation, and parts 2, 3, and 4 are agonists during adduction.

Levator Scapulae (leva'tor scap'ulae)

The levator scapulae (Fig. 3.11) is located on the lateral and posterior aspect of the neck. It lies beneath Part 1 of the trapezius and cannot be palpated except through that muscle portion.

Levator Scapulae

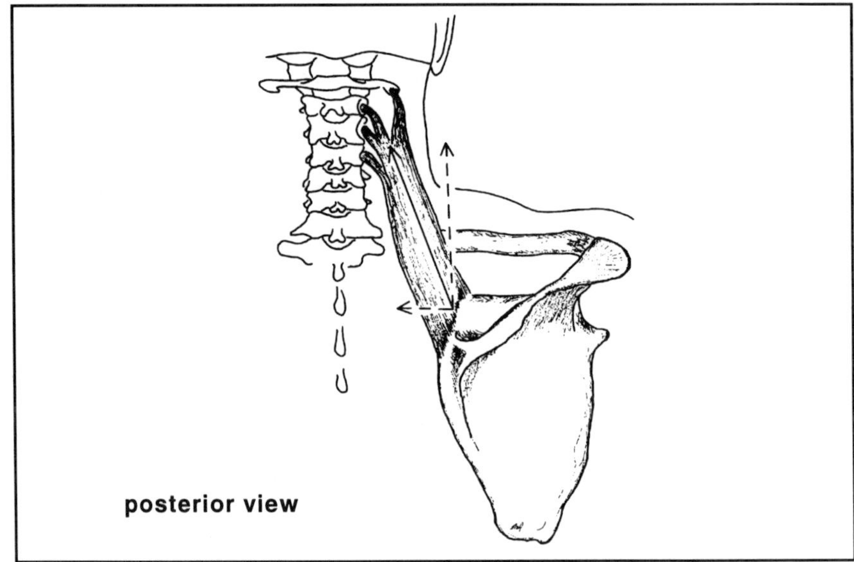

Fig. 3.11

Origin	Transverse processes of the first four cervical vertebrae.
Insertion	Vertebral border of the scapula, between the superior angle and the root of the scapular spine.
Innervation	Third and fourth cervical nerves, and a branch of the dorsal scapular nerve.
Action	Elevation, adduction, downward rotation of the scapula.

The line of pull of the levator scapulae is a diagonal one which, when resolved, yields a long vertical component and a comparatively short horizontal component. Its function as an elevator is, therefore, better than its function as an adductor. Downward rotation of the scapula is accomplished by pulling upwardly on the vertebral border of the scapula in order to lower the inferior angle. The rotation action is more easily visualized when it is remembered that downward rotation is the return from upward rotation; the levator scapulae downwardly rotates only if the scapula is already rotated upwardly to some degree.

The levator scapulae is important to the support and stability of the scapula during regular upright posture and when weights are carried on the shoulder or in the hand. Not only do weights tend to depress the shoulder, they also cause the center of gravity to shift in their direction. To compensate for both conditions, the shoulder is elevated by contracting the levator scapulae and parts 1 and 2 of the trapezius.

Rhomboids (rhom'boids)

The rhomboids (Fig. 3.12) are located beneath Part 3 and the uppermost portion of Part 4 of the trapezius. The rhomboids are divided into rhomboid major and rhomboid minor. Functionally, however, they may be considered a single muscle. The rhomboids cannot be palpated directly.

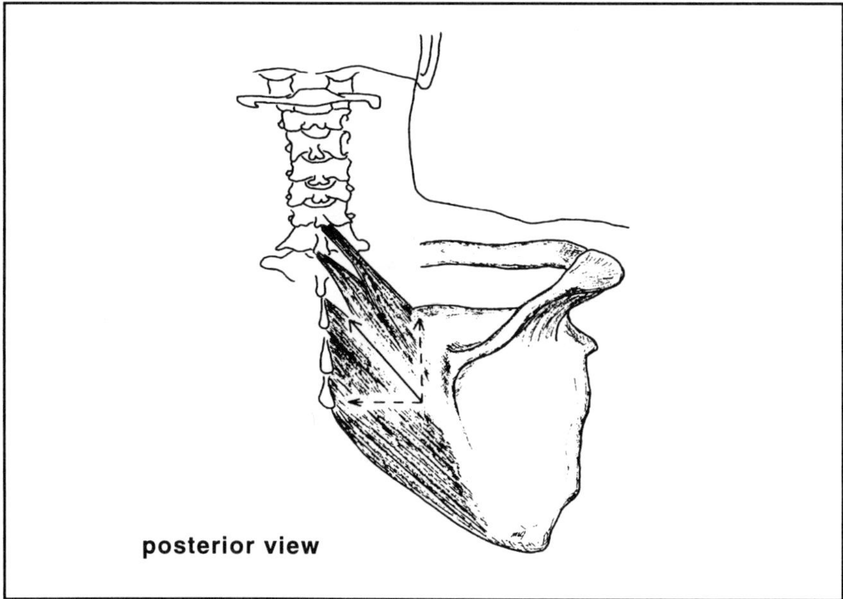

Rhomboids

Fig. 3.12

Origin —— Spinous processes of the seventh cervical and first five thoracic vertebrae.
Insertion —— Vertebral border of scapula from the vicinity of the scapular spine to the inferior angle.
Innervation — Dorsal scapular nerve.
Action —— Elevation, adduction, downward rotation of the scapula.

Resolution of the diagonal line of pull of the rhomboids produces the two components which explain the elevation and adduction action of the muscles. The downward rotation action is provided particularly by the lower fibers, which contract to pull medially and upwardly on the inferior angle of the scapula. The rhomboids are active also in maintaining normal posture as they prevent extreme upward rotation of the scapula and hold the inferior angle close to the rib cage. The latter function may be illustrated by asking a partner to place his hand against the small of his back. The examiner can easily insert a finger beneath the vertebral border of the scapula, because the trapezius and rhomboids are relaxed. When the subject is instructed to lift the hand away from the back, the rhomboids will contract strongly to pull the scapula to the ribs and will force the examiner's fingers out from underneath the scapula.

Serratus Anterior (serra'tus ante'rior)

The serratus anterior (Fig. 3.13) takes its name from the saw-toothed fashion with which it attaches to the ribs. The muscle lies beneath the scapula and courses along the surface of the ribs to attach to the front of the rib cage underneath the pectoralis major. The muscle may be palpated in the area below the axilla as the arm is raised overhead against resistance.

Serratus Anterior

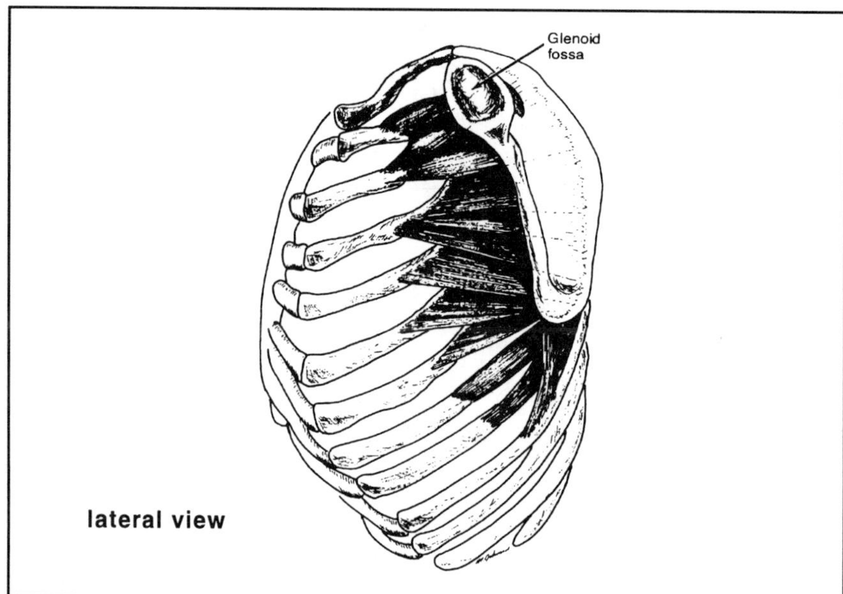

Fig. 3.13

Origin — Upper nine ribs at the side of the chest.
Insertion — Vertebral border of scapula between the superior and inferior angles.
Innervation — Long thoracic nerve.
Action — Abduction and upward rotation of the scapula.

The direction of the fibers of the serratus anterior is very nearly horizontal to make the muscle quite effective as a scapular abductor. The lower fibers are effective as upward rotators since they are in a position to exert a lateral pull on the inferior angle as Part 4 of the trapezius pulls downwardly on the root of the scapular spine. In these two actions -- scapular abduction and upward rotation -- the serratus anterior is considered to be one of the most important muscles of the shoulder. Loss of the serratus anterior seriously impairs ability to reach forward with the arm since that action must be accompanied by abduction of the scapula to align the glenoid fossa is a forward direction. Similarly, subjects who have suffered paralysis of the serratus anterior are typically unable to raise the arm overhead because of muscular insufficiency in upward rotation. The serratus anterior also acts with the rhomboids to prevent winging of the scapula by holding the scapula close to the rib cage.

Pectoralis Minor (pectora'lis mi'nor)

The pectoralis minor (Fig. 3.14) is located on the front of the chest. It is covered by the pectoralis major and, though it cannot be palpated directly, it can be examined on a subject who has placed the hand on the small of the back. If pectoralis major is relaxed, the coracoid can be located, and the proximal portion of the pectoralis minor can be felt contracting as the subject lifts the hand off the back.

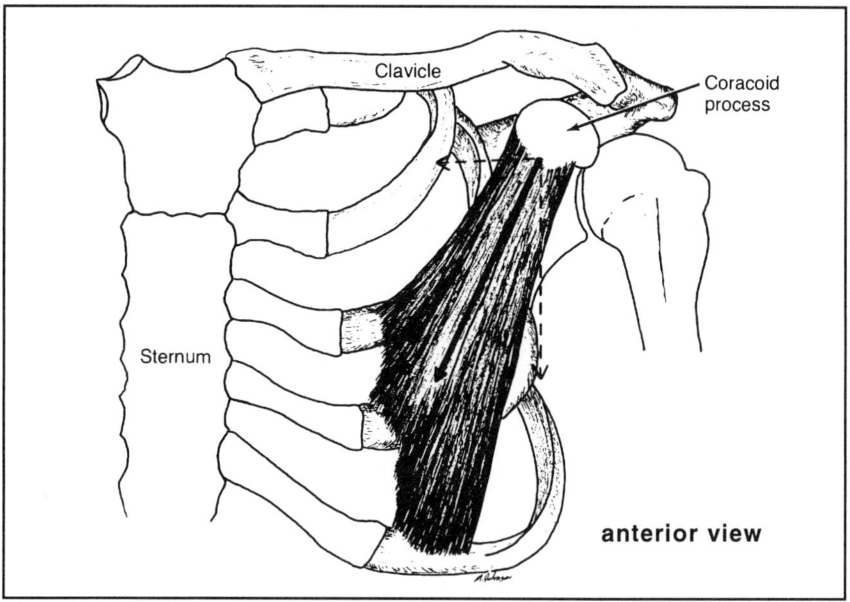

Pectoralis Minor

Fig. 3.14

Origin — Third, fourth, and fifth ribs just lateral to their costal cartilages.
Insertion — Coracoid process of the scapula.
Innervation — Medial anterior thoracic nerve.
Action — Abduction, depression, downward rotation, upward tilt of the scapula.

The fibers of the pectoralis minor are directed downward, inward, and forward from their attachment on the coracoid. The ability of the muscle to depress the scapula is easily recognized as a function of the downward direction; however, at first glance, its abduction, tilt, and downward rotation actions are not so clearly envisioned. To abduct, the pectoralis minor pulls the coracoid medially around the rigid brace supplied by the clavicle; consequently, the scapula slides laterally along the rib cage and the acromion glides forward against the distal end of the clavicle. To tilt the scapula, the pectoralis minor pulls downwardly on the coracoid to rotate the scapula around the frontal axis of the acromioclavicular joint. The downward rotation function of this muscle is a result of the downward pull on the end of the coracoid which returns the scapula to anatomical position.

Subclavius (subcla'vius)

The subclavius (Fig. 3.15) is located underneath the clavicle and is covered by the pectoralis major. It cannot be palpated directly.

Subclavius

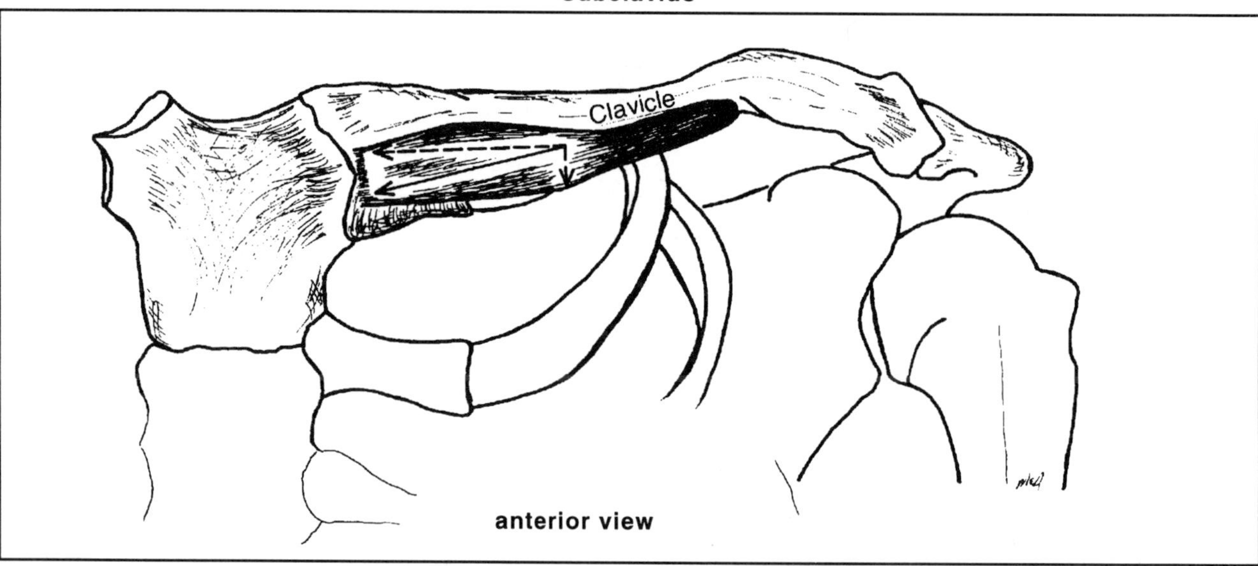

Fig. 3.15

Origin — Cartilaginous junction of the first rib.
Insertion — Inferior surface of middle half of clavicle.
Innervation — Fibers of the fifth and sixth cervical nerves.
Action — Stabilizes sternoclavicular joint; weak depressor of clavicle.

Resolution of the line of pull of the subclavius yields the two component vectors shown in Figure 3.15. The relative length of the components, when compared to each other, infers that the muscle is effective in pulling the clavicle toward the sternum to stabilize the sternoclavicular joint but is lacking in ability to depress the clavicle.

COMMENTS

Figure 3.16 illustrates direction of scapular movement in the frontal plane. The muscles which provide for the movements are noted in conjunction with the directional arrows. Thus it can be seen, for example, that the levator scapulae, parts 1 and 2 of the trapezius, and the rhomboids all have some ability to elevate the scapula. Similarly, depressors, adductors, abductors, and upward and downward rotators can be noted at a glance. Mention was made earlier that the muscles which move the scapula are also the muscles which stabilize the scapula. In general, mobility of the scapula is desired if the task to be accomplished is based upon extended range of the humerus. Reaching forward, upward, or backward with the arm is dependent upon scapular mobility. Conversely, stability of the scapula is desired when force is being applied by or to the arm. Hanging from a high bar in preparation for chinning oneself applies an upward force to the arm which is transmitted to the scapula causing it to elevate. In order to moderate the elevation, the scapular depressors contract and the scapula is made firm. In using crutches, the scapula must be stabilized as the force is applied to the handles. The scapula must be stabilized during the pushing phase as one maneuvers about in a wheelchair.

Scapula Movers

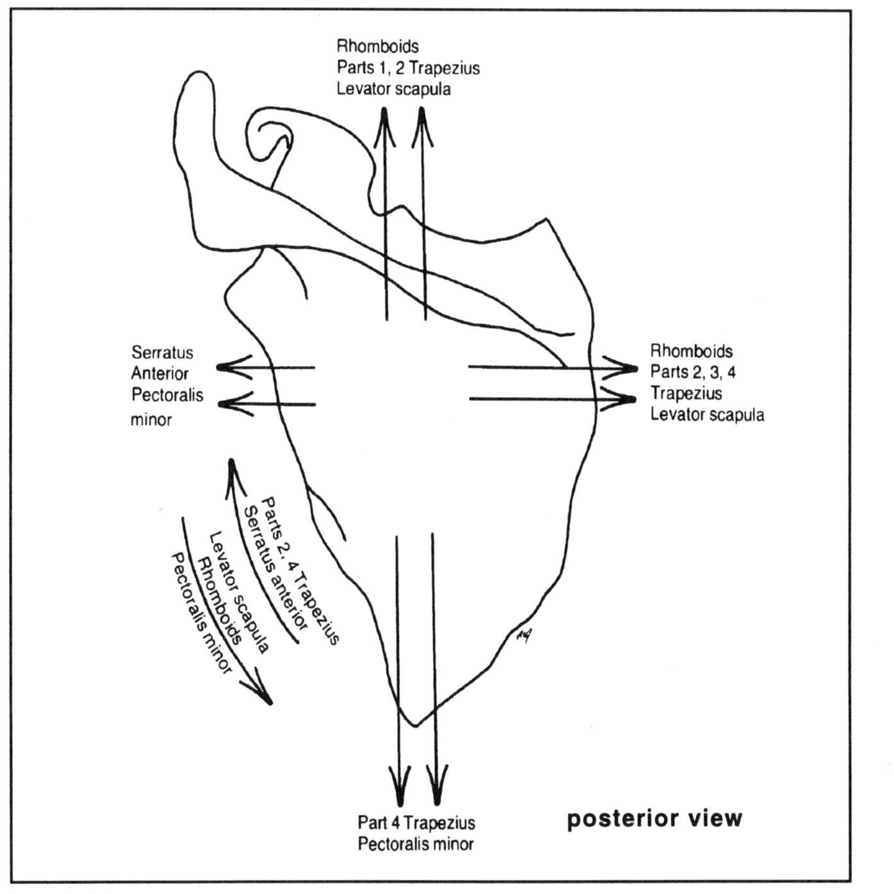

Fig. 3.16

GROUP 2: MUSCLES WHICH MOVE THE HUMERUS

Muscles of Group 2 are the deltoid, pectoralis major, latissimus dorsi, teres major, infraspinatus-teres minor, subscapularis, supraspinatus, biceps brachii, coracobrachialis, and the long head of the triceps brachii. Their actions on the humerus depend upon their relationships to the three axes of rotation of the glenohumeral joint and include flexion-extension-hyperextension, abduction-adduction, horizontal abduction-adduction, internal-external rotation, and circumduction.

Deltoid (del'toid)

The deltoid (Fig. 3.17) is a superficial muscle comprised of three portions located on the point of the shoulder and the upper arm; the muscle is comparatively large and is penniform in structure. All portions of the muscle may be directly palpated and observed.

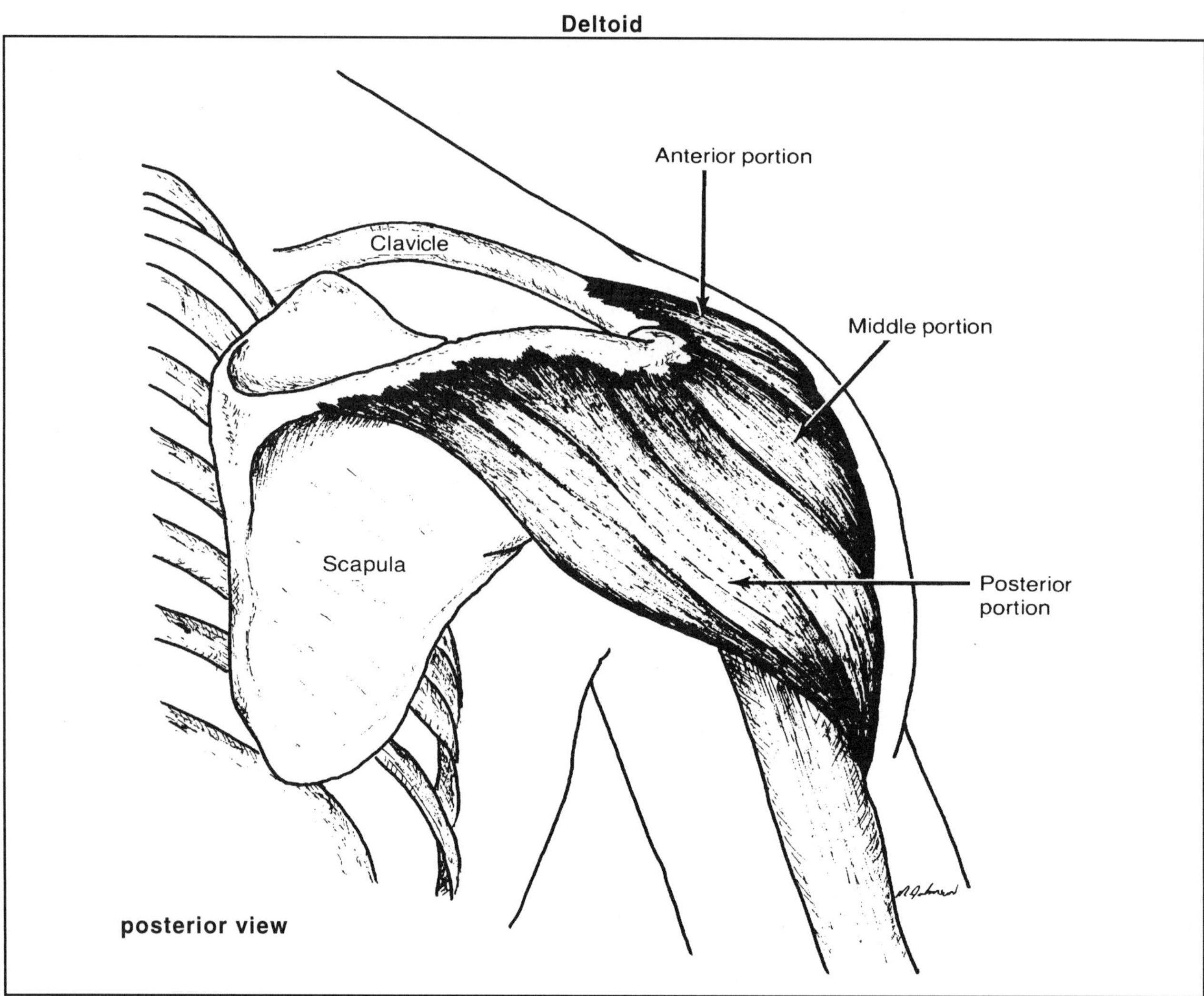

Fig. 3.17

Origin —— Outer third of the clavicle, top of the acromion process, and scapular spine.
Insertion —— Deltoid tuberosity, at the midpoint of the humerus on the lateral aspect.
Innervation — Axillary nerve.
Action —— As a whole the deltoid acts to abduct the glenohumeral joint. The fibers most important to this action are those of the middle portion. The anterior portion acts in flexion, horizontal adduction, and internal rotation of the glenohumeral joint; the posterior portion causes extension, horizontal abduction, and external rotation of that joint.

The actions of the deltoid can be clarified if they are studied with respect to the three axes of the shoulder joint. The muscle as a whole courses lateral to the sagittal axis and, therefore, performs the abduction movement. It will be seen, however, that the most anterior and posterior fibers are very close to this axis, and will have limited effectiveness in abduction. In some individuals, these fibers will be directly aligned with the axis and consequently will be inactive during any frontal plane movement. In others, these fibers may even pass medial to the axis to become weak adductors.

The location of the deltoid with respect to the frontal axis indicates that some fibers are anterior to this axis and will flex at the joint; other fibers are posterior to the axis and will extend at the joint. The fibers farthest from the axis will be most effective in these actions.

When the humerus is envisioned in the transverse plane during horizontal adduction and abduction, a portion of the deltoid is seen to be located anterior to the axis and will horizontally adduct; the portion located posterior to the axis will horizontally abduct. The effectiveness of the respective fibers increases with their distances from the long axis. Internal and external rotation are performed also by the anterior and posterior portions, respectively. Since fibers of the middle portion cross the long axis, they will have no function either in rotation or in horizontal abduction/adduction.

Supraspinatus (supraspina'tus)

The supraspinatus (Fig. 3.18) is a powerful muscle located, as the name implies, in the supraspinous fossa of the scapula. It is covered by Part 2 of the trapezius and cannot be palpated directly. The muscle is a member of the rotator cuff.

Supraspinatus

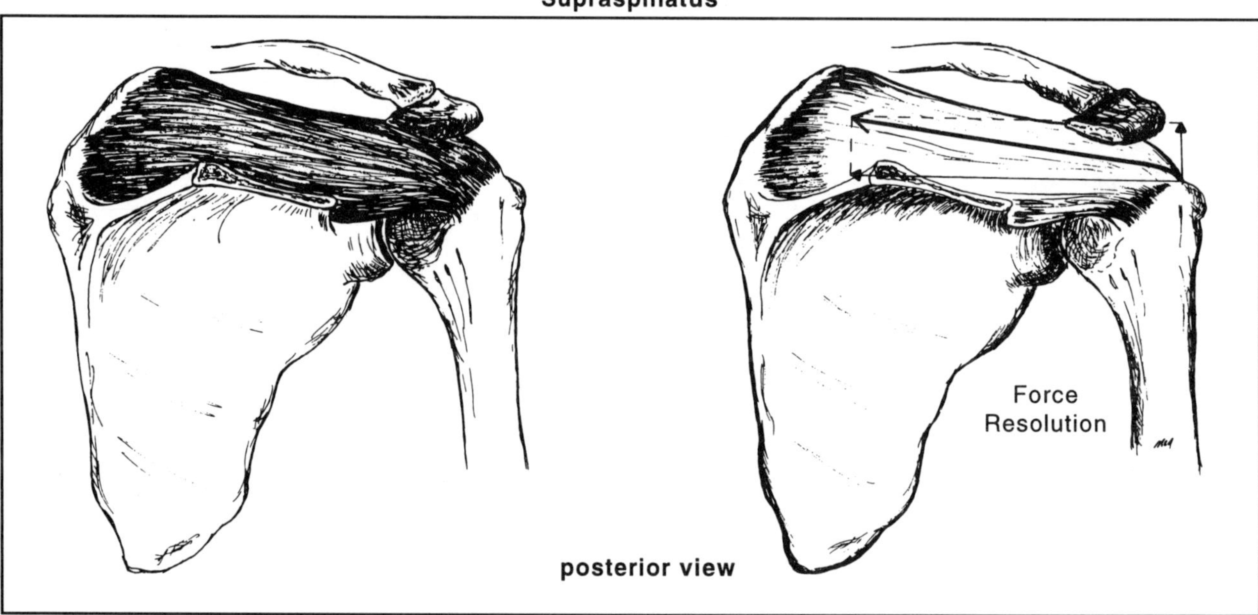

Fig. 3.18

Origin — Supraspinous fossa.
Insertion — Top of the greater tuberosity of the humerus.
Innervation — Suprascapular nerve.
Action — Abduction, external rotation of the glenohumeral joint.

The supraspinatus is primarily effective as an abductor of the shoulder joint (Fig. 3.18). Not only does it course well superior to the sagittal axis, but it is also in a position to pull the head of the humerus into the glenoid fossa. In this latter action, it complements the pull of the deltoid during abduction (see "Rotator Cuff" in this chapter).

The external rotation function of the supraspinatus is accomplished because its distal attachment is on the posterior portion of the greater tuberosity. The line of pull of the muscle is, therefore, slightly posterior to the long axis of the shoulder joint.

Pectoralis Major (pectora'lis ma'jor)

The pectoralis major (Fig. 3.19) is the large muscle on the front of the chest. It is superficial and may be palpated directly. The muscle is divided into a clavicular and a sternal portion.

Pectoralis Major

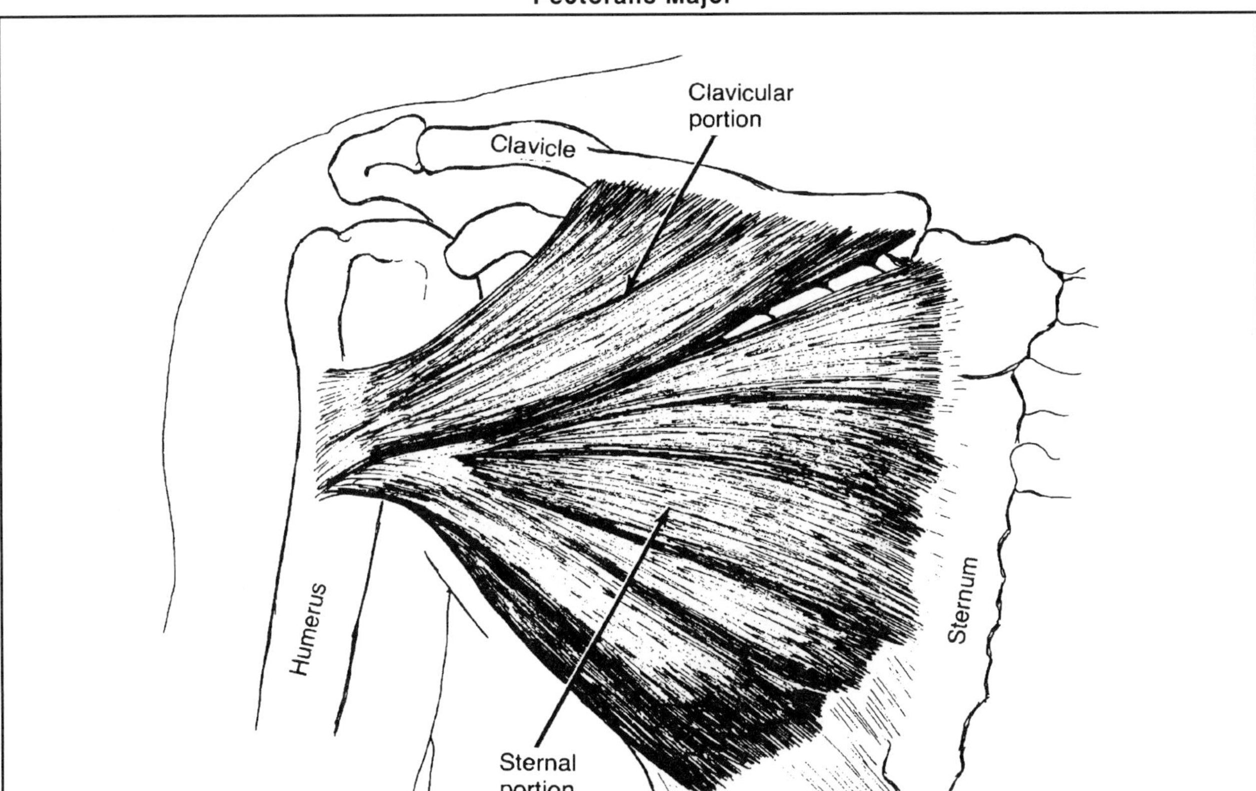

Fig. 3.19

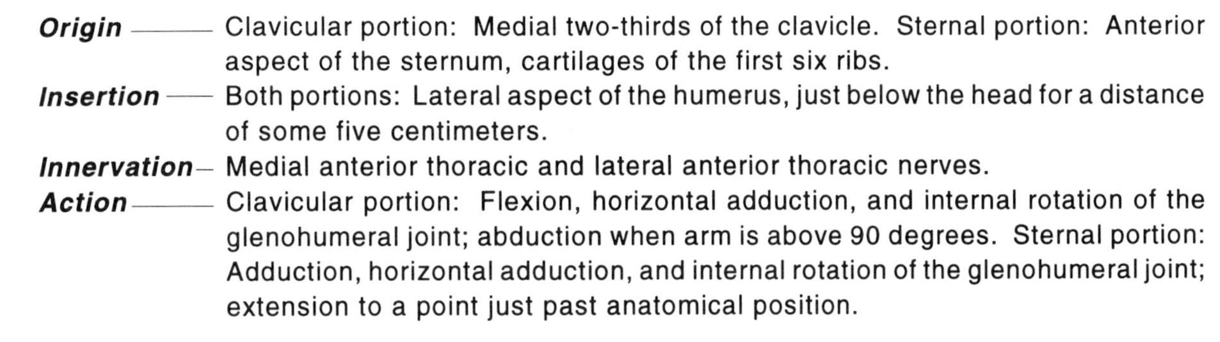

Origin — Clavicular portion: Medial two-thirds of the clavicle. Sternal portion: Anterior aspect of the sternum, cartilages of the first six ribs.

Insertion — Both portions: Lateral aspect of the humerus, just below the head for a distance of some five centimeters.

Innervation — Medial anterior thoracic and lateral anterior thoracic nerves.

Action — Clavicular portion: Flexion, horizontal adduction, and internal rotation of the glenohumeral joint; abduction when arm is above 90 degrees. Sternal portion: Adduction, horizontal adduction, and internal rotation of the glenohumeral joint; extension to a point just past anatomical position.

When the two portions of the pectoralis major are envisioned in relationship to the shoulder axes, it will be noted that regardless of the height at which the arm is held from the side, the sternal portion crosses the joint inferior to the sagittal axis and will, therefore, function as an adductor. The clavicular portion, however, crosses directly over this axis until the arm is above the horizontal, at which position it is made to cross the joint superior to the axis; the muscle will then act as an abductor.

The flexion ability of the clavicular portion is brought about because of its advantageous attachment on the clavicle. This portion crosses the shoulder joint well in front of the frontal axis to become a powerful flexor. The sternal portion is also located anterior to the frontal axis; however, since its origin is lower than its insertion, it pulls downwardly on the upper humerus to extend the shoulder joint. This extension action ceases when the arm has been moved to a position in which the axis and the two attachments are in a line with each other.

The anterior relationship of both portions to the long axis of the glenohumeral joint allows the pectoralis major to be an effective horizontal adductor and internal rotator, regardless of the position of the humerus in the transverse plane. The latter action will be enhanced when the humerus is in a position of external rotation since the distance over which the muscle pulls against the humerus will be lengthened.

Coracobrachialis (coracobrachia'lis)

The coracobrachialis (Fig. 3.20) is a small muscle located medially on the upper humerus. It may be palpated just medial to the short head of the biceps brachii when the shoulder joint is flexed and resistance is applied at the elbow.

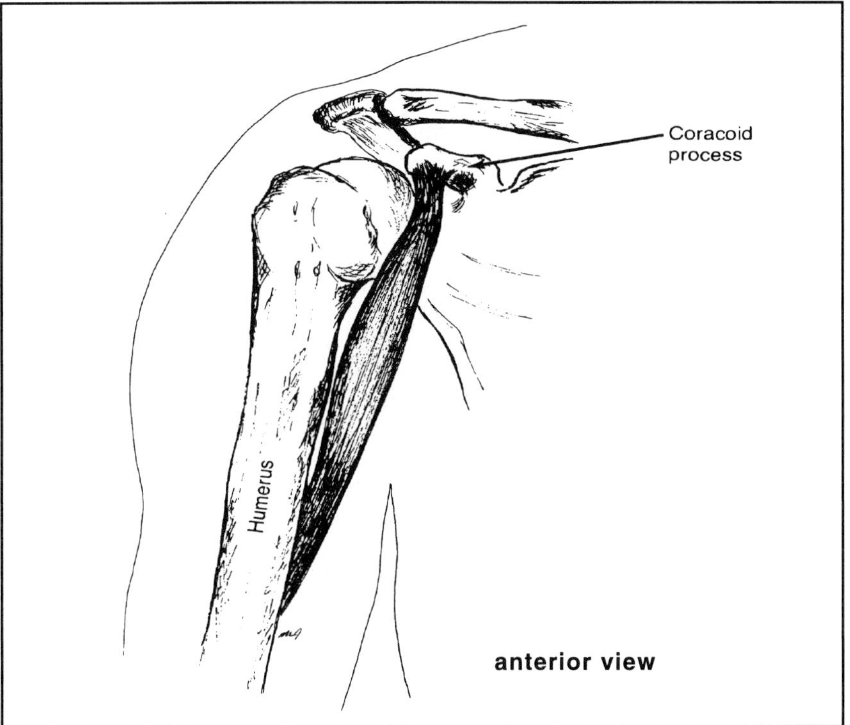

Coracobrachialis

Fig. 3.20

Origin ——	Coracoid process of the scapula.
Insertion ——	Medial and anterior aspect of the humerus opposite the distal attachment of the deltoid.
Innervation —	Musculocutaneous nerve.
Action ——	Flexion, horizontal adduction, adduction, and internal rotation of the glenohumeral joint; extension when the arm is overhead.

The coracobrachialis, because of its size and the location of its two attachments, is of limited effectiveness in its actions. The muscle crosses the shoulder joint inferior to the sagittal axis for adduction; anterior to the frontal axis for flexion; anterior to the frontal axis if origin is below insertion for extension; and anterior to the long axis for horizontal adduction and internal rotation. In all of the actions, the line of pull of the coracobrachialis is quite close to the respective axes. The muscle can act, therefore, in only an assistive manner at best, but is probably most effective as a flexor and an adductor of the shoulder joint.

Latissimus Dorsi (latis'simus dor'si)

The latissimus dorsi (Fig. 3.21), a very broad muscle, is located on the lower back. It is superficial except for a small upper portion which is covered by Part 4 of the trapezius. It can be palpated particularly well at the side of the rib cage during resisted adduction of the glenohumeral joint.

Latissimus Dorsi

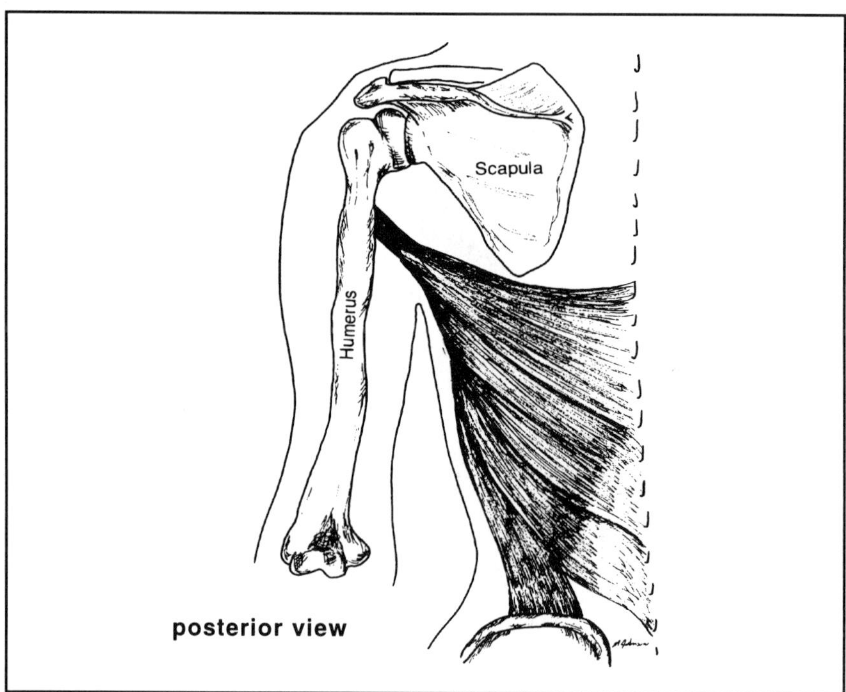

Fig. 3.21

Origin — Spinous processes of lower six thoracic vertebrae and all lumbar vertebrae; posterior surface of sacrum, iliac crest; lower three ribs.
Insertion — Anterior aspect of the humerus, parallel to the tendon of the pectoralis major.
Innervation — Thoracodorsal nerve.
Action — Adduction, extension, hyperextension, horizontal abduction, and internal rotation of the glenohumeral joint.

The latissimus dorsi is favorably located with respect to all of the shoulder joint axes. The muscle courses well inferior to the sagittal axis to be a powerful adductor; it is inferior and anterior to the frontal axis of the shoulder regardless of the position of the humerus, and, since its origin is lower than its insertion, is an excellent extensor; it crosses the shoulder joint lateral to the long axis when the humerus is in the transverse plane to act as a horizontal abductor; its line of pull is medial to the long axis when in anatomical position to function as an internal rotator.

Teres Major (te'res ma'jor)

The teres major (Fig 3.22) is a thick muscle located at the posterior edge of the axilla just above the latissimus dorsi. The muscle is superficial and may be palpated directly.

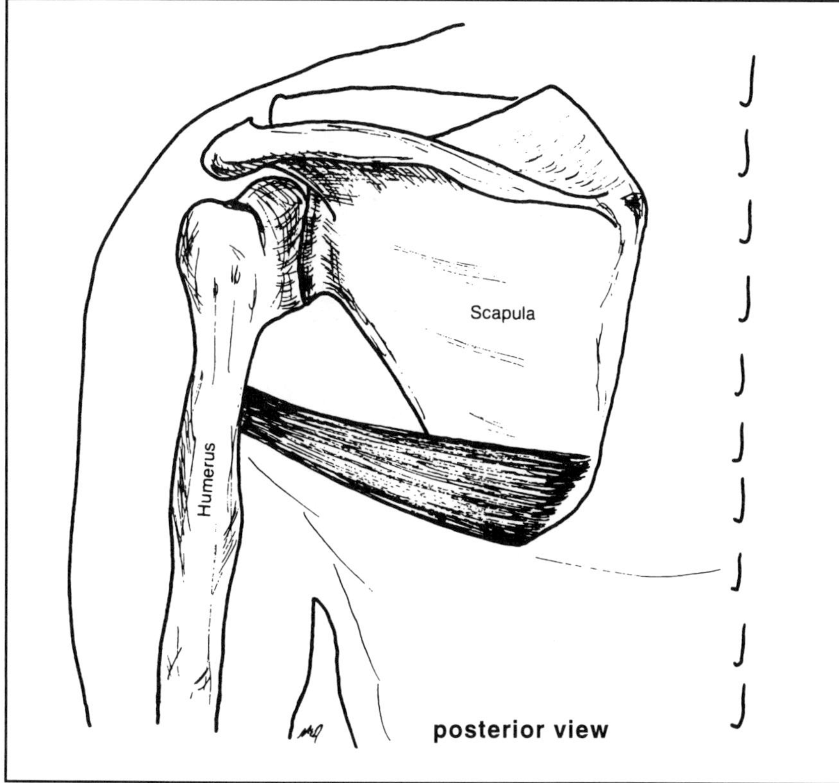

Teres Major

Fig. 3.22

Origin	Inferior angle of the scapula.
Insertion	Anterior aspect of the humerus, just medial to the tendon of the latissimus dorsi.
Innervation	Lower subscapular nerve.
Action	Extension, adduction, and internal rotation under special conditions (see below).

The relationship of the teres major to the three axes of the shoulder is the same as that of the latissimus dorsi; it has been thought, therefore, that it performs the same actions as the latissimus dorsi, and is frequently called the **latissimus dorsi's little helper**. This conception has been largely in error, however, because the teres major contracts only when resistance has been applied to the arm, and only when positions are reached and held in the ranges of movement in adduction, internal rotation, and extension. For example, when one performs a chin-up to a bent arm hang position, the latissimus dorsi will be strongly active during the lift of the body, but the teres major will be active only during the hang phase.

Infraspinatus and Teres Minor (infraspina'tus and te'res mi'nor)

These two muscles (Fig. 3.23) have identical actions and will be discussed together. They lie on the posterior surface of the scapula and are superficial except for a small portion which is covered by the posterior deltoid and the trapezius. They are two of the four rotator cuff muscles.

Infraspinatus and Teres Minor

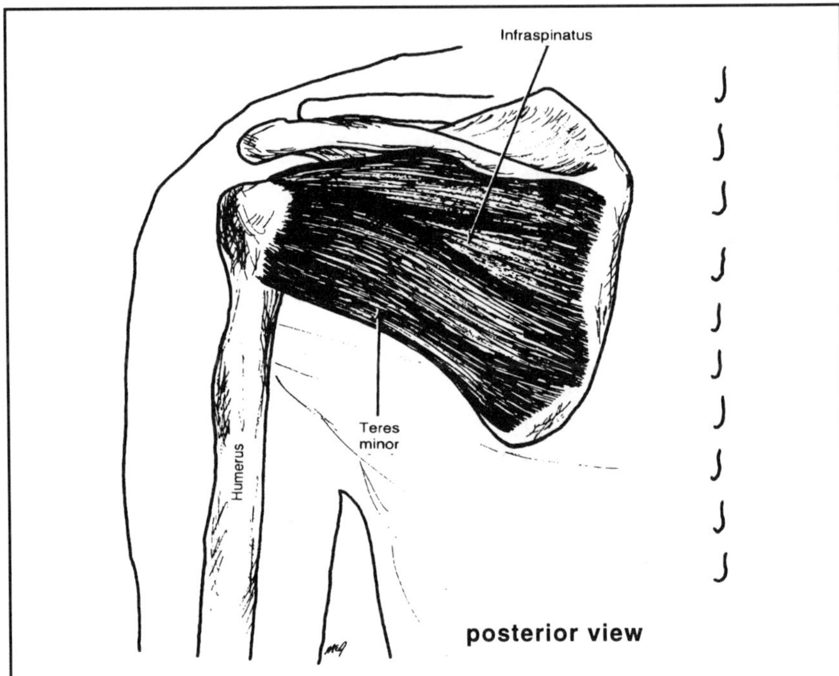

Fig. 3.23

Origin — Infraspinatus: Infraspinous fossa. Teres minor: Axillary border of scapula.
Insertion — Both muscles insert on the greater tuberosity and adjacent shaft of the humerus.
Innervation — Infraspinatus: Suprascapular nerve. Teres minor: Axillary nerve.
Action — External rotation, and horizontal abduction of the glenohumeral joint. They also participate in abduction and flexion by pulling downwardly on the greater tuberosity as the deltoid pulls upwardly on the middle of the shaft of the humerus.

The infraspinatus and teres minor pass posterior to the long axis of the shoulder joint regardless of the position of the humerus to become outward rotators and horizontal abductors. That they are not also extensors and adductors or abductors is explained by the fact that they pass directly over both the sagittal and frontal axes of the shoulder.

Palpation of these muscles may be accomplished easily on a subject who has inclined the trunk forward and hangs the arms downwardly. The palpating fingers are placed on the axillary border of the scapula below the posterior deltoid. The muscles will be felt to contract as the subject rotates the arms externally.

Subscapularis (subscapula'ris)

The subscapularis (Fig. 3.24), one of the rotator cuff muscles, is a triangular muscle located on the scapula and next to the rib cage. It can be palpated on oneself by placing the thumb in the axilla and underneath the scapula as a relaxed toe-touch position is assumed. The weight of the hanging arm pulls the scapula into abduction, making the anterior surface accessible to the thumb. The belly of the muscle can be felt to contract as the arms are internally rotated.

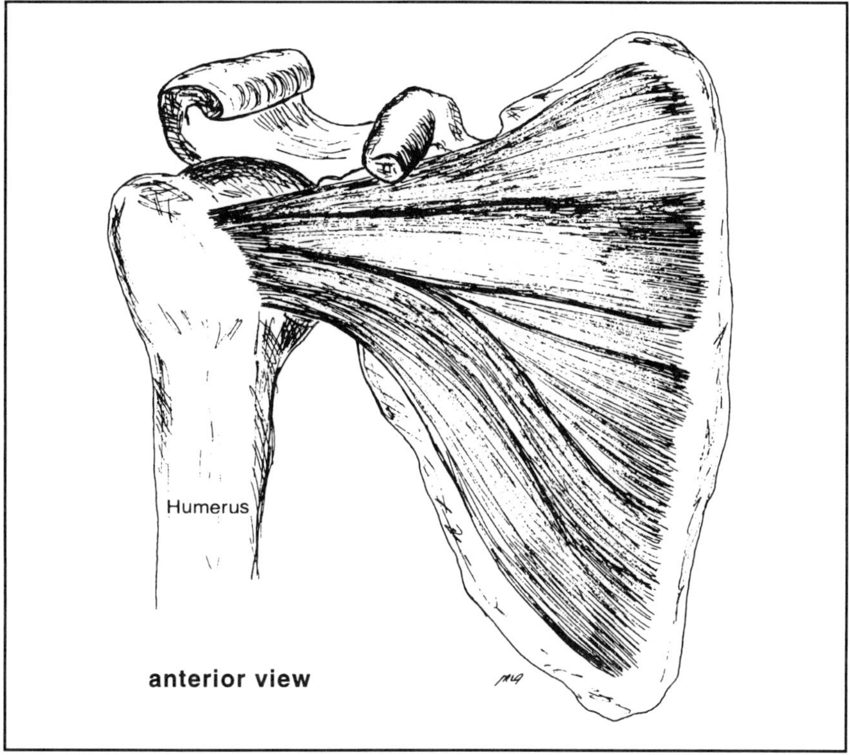

Subscapularis

Fig. 3.24

Origin —— Entire anterior surface of the scapula.
Insertion —— Lesser tuberosity of the humerus.
Innervation — Subscapular nerve.
Action —— Internal rotation of the glenohumeral joint. The muscle also acts with the infraspinatus and teres minor in participating with the deltoid during abduction and flexion.

The internal rotation function of the subscapularis can be recognized clearly by examining the relationship of the anterior surface of the scapula to the lesser tuberosity of the humerus. As the muscle courses between its two attachments, it crosses medial to the long axis and then wraps around the anterior aspect of the upper humerus to give it a very favorable line of pull for rotation.

Rotator Cuff

The rotator cuff is comprised of the supraspinatus, infraspinatus, teres minor, and subscapularis. These muscles are grouped together both because they all have rotational functions on the humerus, and because their tendons are interwoven into the capsule to form a musculotendinous cuff around the joint. They act together to hold the head of the humerus against the glenoid fossa and thus stabilize the joint against downward dislocation of the humerus. These muscles also perform with the deltoid during abduction and flexion of the shoulder joint. If the deltoid were to contract alone, its line of pull dictates that it would pull the humerus up against the acromion process. If the cuff muscles were to contract alone, they would depress the head of the humerus. Acting together, however, a force couple is produced and abduction and flexion of the joint fill occur (Fig. 3.25).

Mechanics of Abduction of the Glenohumeral Joint

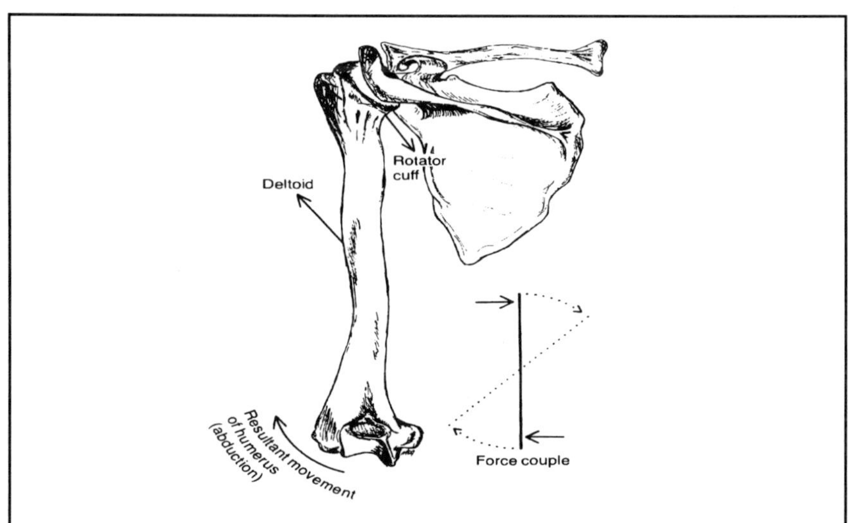

Fig. 3.25

Damage to the rotator cuff is frequently seen among persons who engage in repetitive movements in an overhand pattern. Using hammers, saws, and drills while holding the arm above the head are all examples of industrial tasks that can result in tears of the rotator cuff. In athletics, a host of activities may cause tears. Any overhand pattern that requires excessive abduction and external rotation, high velocity, great force, and repetition carries the risk of tearing a rotator cuff muscle. One need only think through a list of sports to recognize that the overhand pattern is used in badminton, tennis, volleyball, freestyle and butterfly swimming strokes, baseball, and softball to name a few.

In the past, rotator cuff tears were usually repaired surgically. Unfortunately, an individual's return to pre-surgery levels of activity was seldom noted. It is now recognized that successful rehabilitation lies in the early detection of vulnerability followed by establishment of muscular balance through exercise. If forceful and rapid external rotation and abduction of the humerus can be controlled and stabilized by muscular antagonists, injury may be prevented.

Biceps Brachii (bi'ceps bra'chii)

The biceps brachii (Fig. 3.26) lies on the anterior aspect of the upper arm. It is better known as a flexor of the elbow; however, it does cross the shoulder also and has, therefore, some ability to move the humerus. The biceps brachii is superficial, making it easily palpated and observed. It has two heads, the long and the short head.

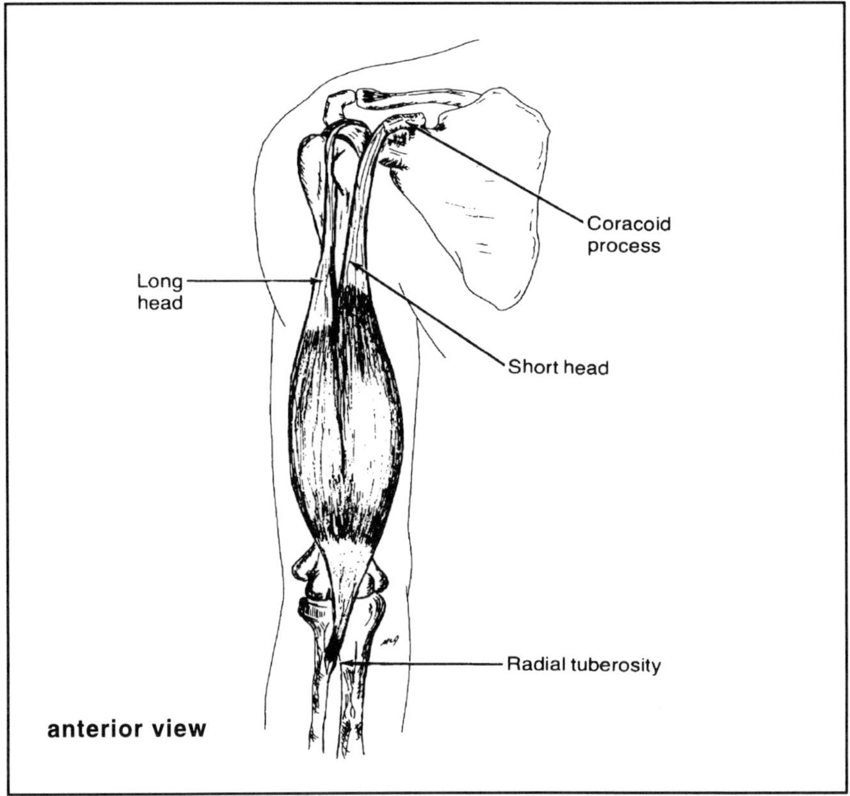

Fig. 3.26

Biceps Brachii

Origin — Long head: Upper rim of the glenoid fossa. Short head: Coracoid process of the scapula.
Insertion — Tuberosity of the radius.
Innervation — Musculocutaneous nerve.
Action — Long head: Abduction of the glenohumeral joint when the arm is outwardly rotated. Short head: Flexion, adduction, internal rotation, and horizontal adduction of the glenohumeral joint.

The line of pull of the biceps brachii at the shoulder joint is almost identical to that of the coracobrachialis and therefore the actions of the two muscles are similar, but are both of limited effectiveness. The actions of the biceps at the shoulder joint are enhanced, however, by maintaining the elbow in an extended position, thus putting the muscle slightly on the stretch.

Triceps Brachii -- Long Head (tri'ceps bra'chii)

The triceps brachii (Fig. 3.27) is located on the posterior aspect of the upper arm. As its name implies, it has three heads; one of these heads, the long head, crosses the shoulder joint and is, therefore, considered in the musculature of the shoulder joint. The triceps is superficial and is easily palpated and observed.

Triceps Brachii

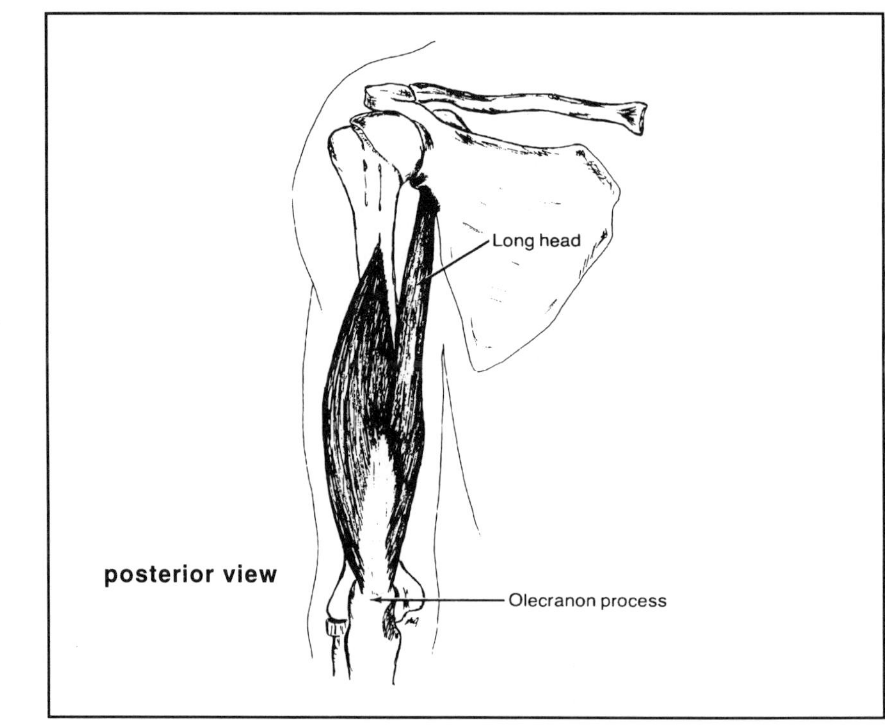

Fig. 3.27

Origin — Just inferior to the glenoid fossa.
Insertion — Olecranon process of the ulna.
Innervation — Radial nerve.
Action — Extension and adduction of the glenohumeral joint.

Comparison of the locations of the two attachments of the long head of the triceps indicates that it is ineffectual as a mover of the humerus around the long axis because it passes directly over the axis. The line of pull does pass slightly inferior to the sagittal axis for adduction, and slightly posterior to the frontal axis for extension. In both cases the line of pull produces a strong stabilizing component and a comparatively short angular component. It is to be expected, then, that the triceps is of limited effectiveness as a shoulder joint extensor or adductor. Its effectiveness can be increased, however, by placing the elbow in a flexed position to put the muscle on the stretch.

COMMENTS

The glenohumeral joint is surrounded by a relatively loose capsule. A number of factors contribute to the stability of the joint: the rotator cuff and deltoid muscles, the mechanical relationship between the glenoid fossa and the humeral head, and the glenohumeral ligaments. As one can see, the glenohumeral joint relies on static and dynamic elements so that joint integrity can be maintained throughout functional movements.

As the arm hangs by the side, the supraspinatus and superior glenohumeral and coracohumeral ligaments become taut. The plane of the glenoid fossa is tilted slightly upward. As the same time, a vertical force, produced by the weight of the hanging extremity, is tightening the superior joint capsule and pulling the head of the humerus into the upward-tilting glenoid fossa. The orientation of the glenoid, and the tightening of the supraspinatus and glenohumeral and coracohumeral ligaments provide static stability to the free hanging humerus. Studies conducted by Basmajian revealed that a contraction by the rotator cuff muscles is not necessary to prevent inferior subluxation of the joint while maintaining this dependent posture. As the arm begins to abduct, the muscles of the rotator cuff become active, and the tension on the superior joint capsule is lost. Support of the glenohumeral joint will then shift to the subscapularis and the middle and inferior glenohumeral ligaments. In extreme ranges of abduction, the axillary pouch of the inferior glenohumeral ligament will maintain the relationship between the humeral head and the glenoid.

As the extremity hangs freely at the side, the capsular structures of the glenohumeral joint lie in a forward and medial direction. Due to the orientation of these capsular fibers, a "twisting" type tension is produced during motion. During abduction in the frontal plane, tension of the capsular fibers increases; during flexion in the sagittal plane, the tension decreases. As the extremity progresses into abduction, the joint capsule pulls the head of the humerus into the glenoid fossa. With progressive abduction, the tension that is placed on the capsule will eventually pull the humerus into external rotation. This movement causes the greater tubercle of the humerus to clear the coracoacromial arch during abduction as well as uncoils the fibers of the joint capsule. If external rotation does not occur, abduction of the glenohumeral joint will be restricted due to impingement of the greater tubercle on the coracoacromial arch. The external rotation that occurs during abduction may be considered a passive act due to the arrangement of the capsular fibers. The active components that contribute to external rotation of the humerus are the infraspinatus and teres minor.

As stated previously, a powerful force couple relationship is established between the rotator cuff muscles and the deltoid during abduction. The force that is produced during abduction of the extremity, along with the active downward pull of the short rotator muscles (infraspinatus, teres minor, and subscapularis) establishes the muscle force couple needed to guide the humeral head within the glenoid fossa. When the extremity is in the dependent position (hanging freely), the muscular force of the deltoid is directed upward and outward, while the force of the short rotators is directed downward and inward with respect to the humerus. The force of the deltoid acts below the center of rotation, whereas the force transmitted by the short rotators acts above the center of rotation.

As abduction of the extremity progresses, the deltoid will become more active in pulling the humeral head into the glenoid cavity. In extreme ranges of abduction, the force of the deltoid will pull the humeral head downward. Abduction of the extremity is possible without the activity of the deltoid or supraspinatus muscles. Without activity of the deltoid, the combined action of the rotator cuff muscles produces about 50% of the force for abduction. If the function of the supraspinatus is absent, extreme ranges of abduction (above 90°) will be lost. It can be concluded, therefore, that both of these muscles are necessary to maintain normal glenohumeral function.

The long head of the biceps brachii muscle also assists with humeral head depression during abduction. The tendon of this muscle acts as a pulley around the superior aspect of the humerus. During external rotation, the bicipital groove faces laterally. In this position, the long head of the biceps brachii exerts a downward force on the humeral head and functions as a pulley to assist in abduction of the extremity.

The actions with which the muscles that move the humerus are credited can easily be deduced if their locations relative to the three axes of the shoulder joint are known. The procedure for learning muscle actions can be simplified even further by considering only the aspect of the shoulder on which the muscles are located. For example, the muscles which lie anterior to the frontal axis are generally those which lie on the anterior aspect of the shoulder. The same pattern holds true for the remaining muscles; thus, the four categories of anterior, posterior, superior, and inferior can be used -- each category being credited with performing the logical actions on the humerus.

A quiz for this material can be found in the back of this book on page 283.

Anterior Muscles	Flexion, horizontal adduction, internal rotation.
Anterior deltoid *Pectoralis major* *Subscapularis* *Biceps brachii*	*Coracobrachialis* *Latissimus dorsi* (internal rotation only) *Teres major* (internal rotation only)
Posterior Muscles	Extension, hyperextension, horizontal abduction, external rotation.
Posterior deltoid *Latissimus dorsi* *Teres major* *Teres minor/Infraspinatus*	*Triceps brachii* *Supraspinatus* (external rotation only) *Coracobrachialis* (extension only)
Superior Muscles	Abduction.
Middle deltoid *Biceps brachii*	*Supraspinatus* *Pectoralis major* - clavicular portion (abduction above 90 degrees)
Inferior Muscles	Adduction.
Latissimus dorsi *Teres major* *Pectoralis major* - sternal portion	*Coracobrachialis* *Biceps brachii* *Triceps brachii*

LABORATORY EXPERIENCES

1. Place the thumb and long finger along the scapular spine of a partner. While palpating, note the movements of the scapula as the arm is moved through the full range of flexion-extension, abduction-adduction, horizontal abduction-adduction, and internal-external rotation. Which of the actions of the humerus would be limited if each of the following scapular muscles were impaired?

   Pectoralis minor
   Part 2 of trapezius
   Levator scapula
   Serratus anterior

2. Categorize the muscles or muscle portions which move the humerus according to whether they are (1) superior to the sagittal axis, (2) inferior to the sagittal axis, (3) anterior to the front axis, (4) posterior to the frontal axis, (5) anterior to the long axis, or (6) posterior to the long axis. Notice that some muscles or muscle portions fall in one category only while others may be placed in two or even three categories. What actions will the muscles in the six categories perform?

3. Determine which of the muscles categorized in Experience #2 are superficial. Palpate these muscles on a partner as the humerus is moved against some resistance through full ranges of motion around the three axes. Does your palpation support your categorizations? For example, the anterior portion of the deltoid will have been categorized as being located anterior to the frontal axis and the long axis. As such, it should flex, horizontally adduct, and internally rotate the joint. Palpations should confirm these actions.

4. Place a partner in a chair facing the edge of a door so that the two door knobs can be grasped by the partner's right and left hands, respectively. Instruct the subject to extend the elbows and press down on the door knob held by the left hand and lift up on the door knob held by the right hand. Through palpation or observation, determine which portion of the left pectoralis major is active, and which portion of the right pectoralis major is active. Repeat your observations as the subject reverses the actions. Do your observations concur with the actions listed for the pectoralis major?

LABORATORY EXPERIENCES (CONTINUED)

5. Have a partner lie supine on a table and place electrodes on the belly of the biceps brachii. While monitoring the action potentials, have the partner flex the shoulder joint first with the elbow extended, then with the elbow fully flexed. Do your results agree with the actions noted for the biceps brachii as a mover of the humerus?

6. Repeat the above procedure on the long head of the triceps brachii of a partner who is lying prone on a table. Compare the action potentials of shoulder extension/elbow straight with those of shoulder extension/elbow flexed. What is your conclusion regarding optimum elbow position for the triceps as a mover of the humerus?

7. With a partner, determine whether the anterior portion of the deltoid acts as an adductor of the humerus. Be careful to eliminate the effects of gravity by having your partner take a supine lying position.

8. Analyze the movements of the humerus during the performance of a pushup. Based upon your analysis, determine which muscles will be involved, and by palpation or observation, confirm your determinations. What actions or exercises would you recommend to stretch these same muscles? Remember that to strengthen a muscle, its attachments must be pulled toward mid-muscle; to stretch a muscle, its attachments must be spread apart from each other.

9. Compare the actions of the humerus during the performance of a chin-up with supinated grip with those during the performance of a chin-up with pronated grip. According to the actions you have determined, list the muscles involved under each type of chin-up. Are the chin-ups alike or different with respect to muscle involvement?

THE ELBOW

The elbow is comprised of two joints formed by the articulation of the humerus with both the ulna and the radius. The trochlea of the humerus fits into the trochlear notch of the ulna to form a hinge joint, while the capitulum of the humerus articulates in gliding fashion with the head of the radius. Kinesiologically, the two joints can be thought of as one -- a hinge joint which permits rotation about a single axis represented by a line passing through the two epicondyles of the humerus. The only actions which can be performed by the elbow are flexion and extension (Fig. 4.1); as a consequence all muscles which cross the elbow will be either flexors or extensors of that joint. Muscles crossing the elbow posterior to the axis will be extensors, while muscles crossing the elbow anterior to the joint axis will be flexors.

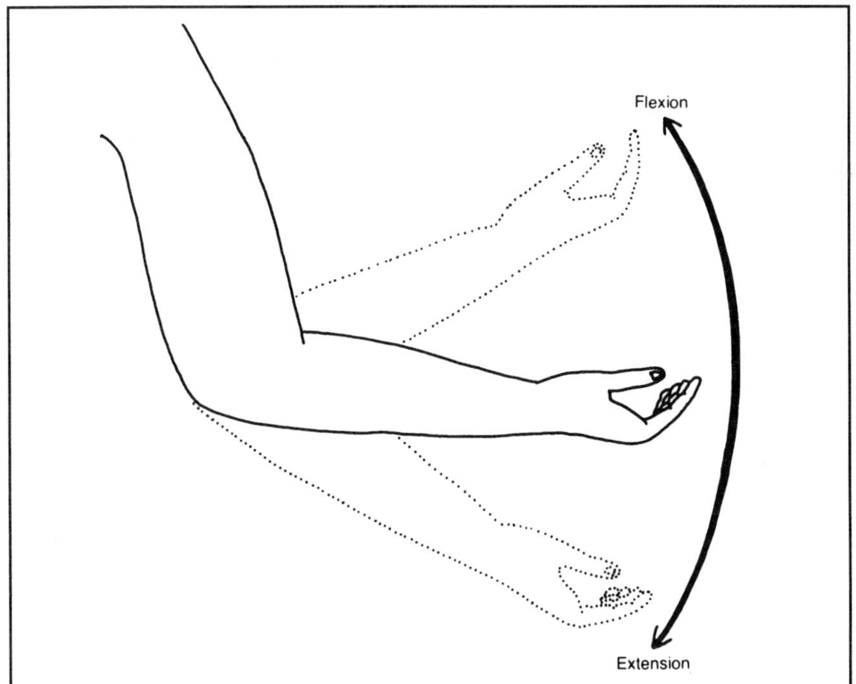

Fig. 4.1

Movements of the Elbow Joint

The major ligaments of the elbow joint are the ulnar and the radial collaterals (Fig. 4.2). The ulnar collateral ligament stabilizes the medial portion of the joint, and runs between the medial epicondyle of the humerus and the olecranon and coronoid processes of the ulna. The radial collateral ligament runs between a depression just below the lateral epicondyle and the annular ligament of the radioulnar joint.

Ligaments of Elbow

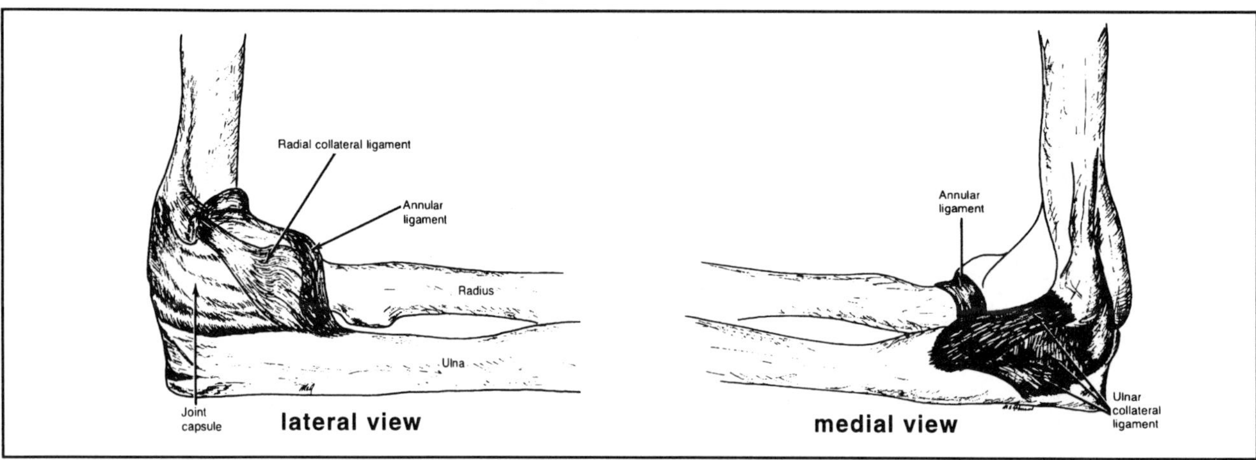

Fig. 4.2

The proximal radioulnar joint, a synovial joint, is formed by the head of the radius and the radial notch of the ulna. The joint is of the pivot variety and allows rotation about a long axis which is represented by a line passing through the head of the radius proximally and the head of the ulna distally (Fig. 4.3).

Axis of Radioulnar Joint

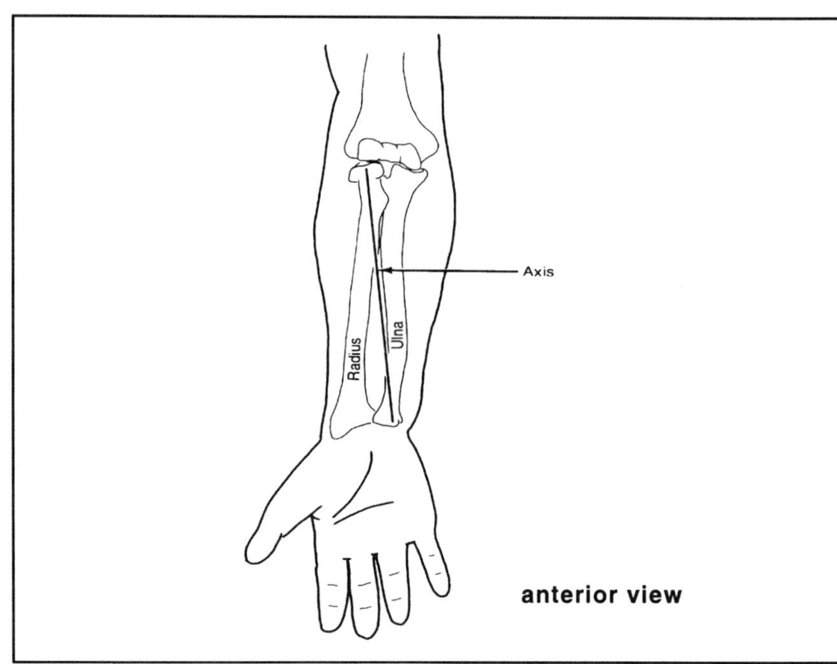

Fig. 4.3

The head of the radius is bound firmly to the ulna by the annular ligament which forms a ring within which the radius rotates (Fig. 4.2). When the radius is rotated outwardly, the radius and ulna are parallel and the palm of the hand faces forward (supination); when the radius is rotated inwardly, the radius crosses over the ulna and the palm of the hand faces backward (pronation).

The distal radioulnar joint, also of the synovial type, is the articulation between the head of the ulna and the radial notch. The joint is a pivot joint and permits the radius to rotate around the ulna in much the same fashion as is seen in the proximal joint of these two bones. A disc of fibrocartilage is interposed between the head of the ulna and the carpal bones to bind the radius and ulna firmly together.

Since both the proximal and distal radioulnar joints are pivot joints, they can permit only supination (external rotation of the radius) and pronation (internal rotation of the radius). Muscles which cross these two joints are, therefore, supinators or pronators. Supinators cross the joints posterior to the axis of rotation; pronators cross the joints anterior to the axis. When the forearm is midway between supination and pronation, it is said to be in neutral position.

The ligaments of the distal radioulnar joint are the palmar and dorsal radioulnar ligaments. These ligaments run between the radius and ulna on the palmar (anterior) and dorsal (posterior) sides of the joint, and are actually thickenings of the joint capsule.

BONE MARKINGS

Figure 4.4 notes the various bony landmarks pertinent to the kinesiology of the elbow. The illustration is intended only as review material and should be used with a skeleton for proper perspective.

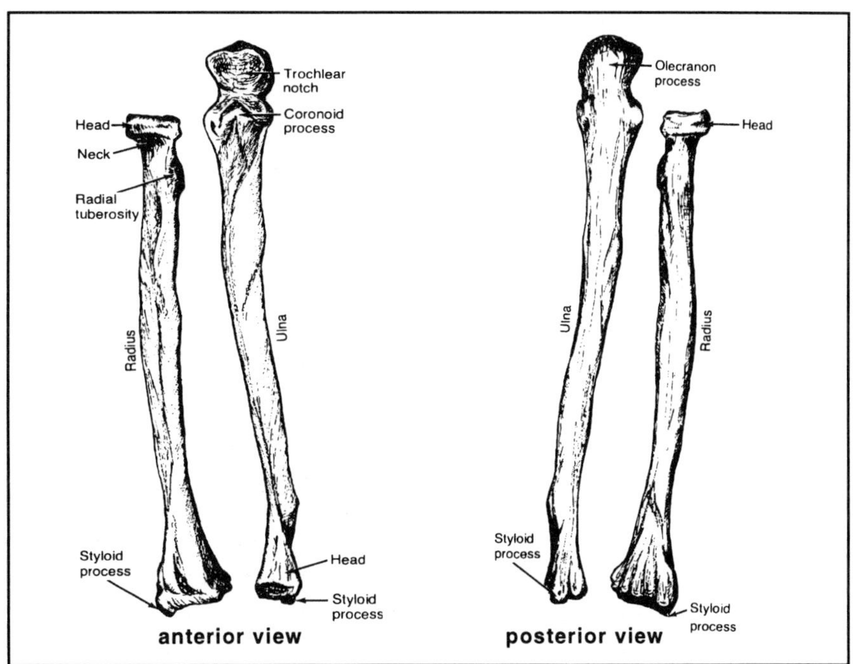

Bones of the Forearm

Fig. 4.4

MUSCULATURE

Biceps Brachii (bi'ceps bra'chii)

(See also muscles of shoulder joint, Chapter 3) The biceps brachii (Fig. 4.5) is a fusiform muscle located prominently on the front of the upper arm. It is superficial and can be easily palpated and observed.

Origin —— Long head: Upper rim of the glenoid fossa. Short head: Coracoid process of scapula.
Insertion —— Tuberosity of the radius.
Innervation — Musculocutaneous nerve.
Action —— Flexion of the elbow joint and supination of the radioulnar joints.

Biceps Brachii

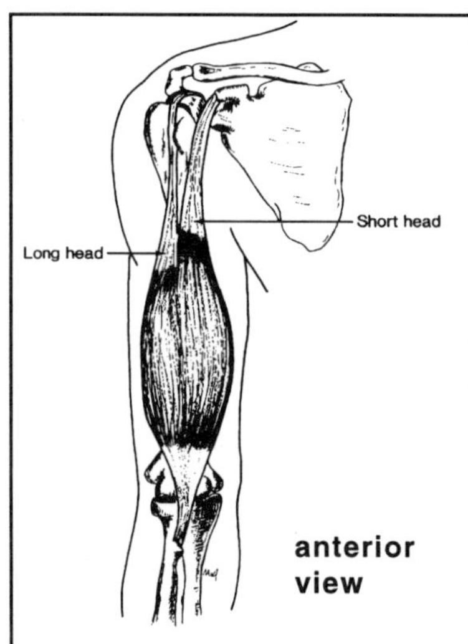

Fig. 4.5

The effectiveness of the biceps as a flexor of the elbow is shown in Figure 4.6. The muscle crosses the joint well in front of the axis regardless of the amount of flexion of the elbow. It will be seen, also, that as the forearm is moved through the range from full extension to full flexion, the force components of the pull of the biceps can vary in length. At full extension, the contracting biceps is accompanied by a strong stabilizing component and at full flexion there is a strong dislocating component. At approximately 90 degrees of elbow flexion, however, the only component provided by the biceps is the angular one. It follows, then, that when strength is desired during elbow flexion, the 90-degree angle of flexion is mechanically best. As the joint angulation changes from 90 degrees as it is either extended farther or flexed farther, the angular component decreases, giving way to the stabilizing or dislocating component, respectively.

It is important to note that the above discussion relates only to the **mechanics** of contraction and does not reflect any physiological property of the muscle. Because muscle tissue is contractile, extensible, and elastic, it has the ability to adjust itself in length -- an ability that materials with which the physicist and engineer work do not have. It is possible to require muscle tissue to so elongate that it cannot contract; it is also possible to shorten muscle tissue to the point at which no further contraction is possible. Hence, as a muscle contracts through its full range of shortening, it begins in a weakened condition, gradually becomes stronger, and then, as it approaches its shortest length, becomes weakened again. It can be seen, then, that if a muscle is required to elongate to accommodate hyperextension of a joint, the muscle contraction will be comparatively weak, both because of the mechanics of its attachments and because of its physiological properties. Similarly, the shortened muscle which

Insertion Angles of the Biceps Brachii at Various Degrees of Elbow Flexion

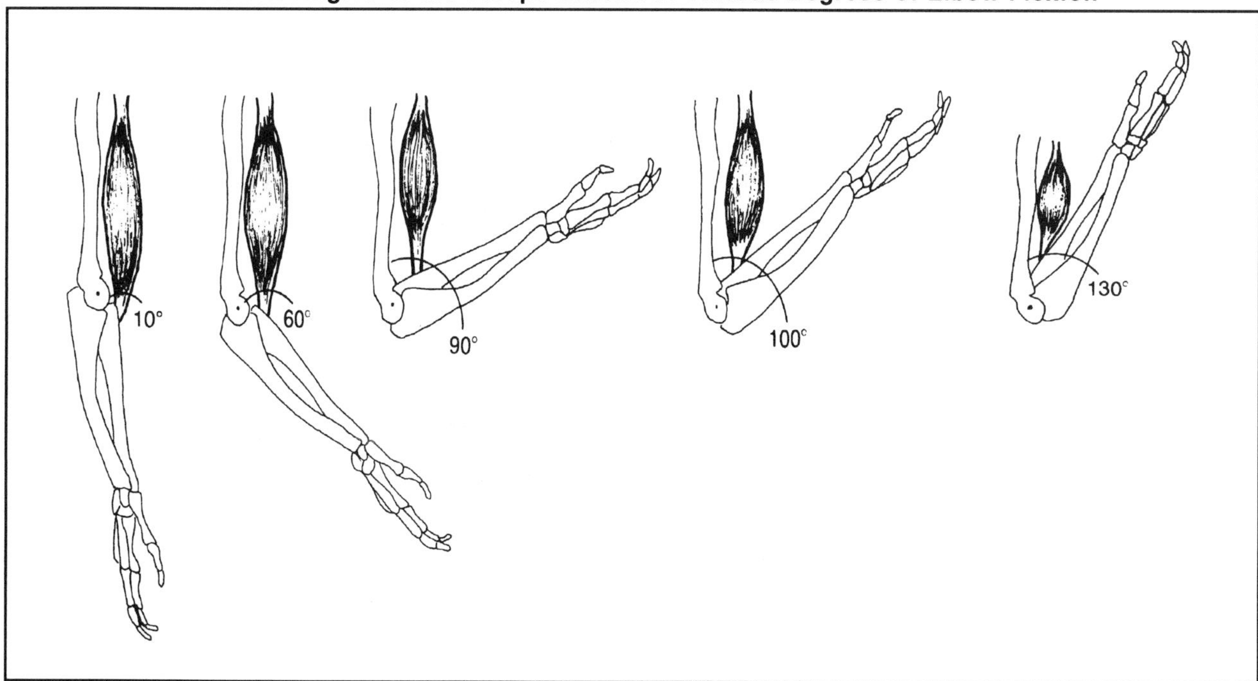

Fig. 4.6

accompanies a fully flexed joint is weak both mechanically and physiologically. Somewhere between the ends of the range continuum, peak strength is reached. Mechanically, that point occurs when the muscle inserts at 90 degrees; unfortunately, the physiological point of peak strength does not usually coincide, and is reached sooner, at approximately full extension of the joint. Figure 4.6 is presented to illustrate the difference between the two points of peak strength. The biceps brachii is used as the example; however, the example can be generalized to other muscles, and particularly those which can alter their angles of insertion.

In the above discussion, mention was made both of **joint angle** and **insertion angle.** These two angles, though somewhat complimentary, are not the same and must not be confused with each other. A joint angle is the angle formed by two articulating bones. An insertion angle is the angle between a bone and the muscle that attaches to the bone. The two angles are inversely related -- when the joint angle is large (full extension) the insertion angle is small. Conversely, a small joint angle (full flexion) is accompanied by a large insertion angle.

In summary, when a muscle or muscle group must exhibit maximum strength, position the joint so the angle of insertion is between 90° and the angle of insertion at which the joint is extended. For practical use, the rule can be simplified by first positioning the joint for the 90° insertion angle and then adjusting the position of the joint to put the muscle slightly on the stretch.

Brachioradialis (brachioradia'lis)

The brachioradialis (Fig. 4.7) is a fusiform muscle located on the radial border of the forearm. It is superficial and may be palpated readily by flexing the elbow and holding the forearm so that the thumb is up. When resistance is applied to the wrist, the brachioradialis is seen to contract just below the elbow.

Brachioradialis

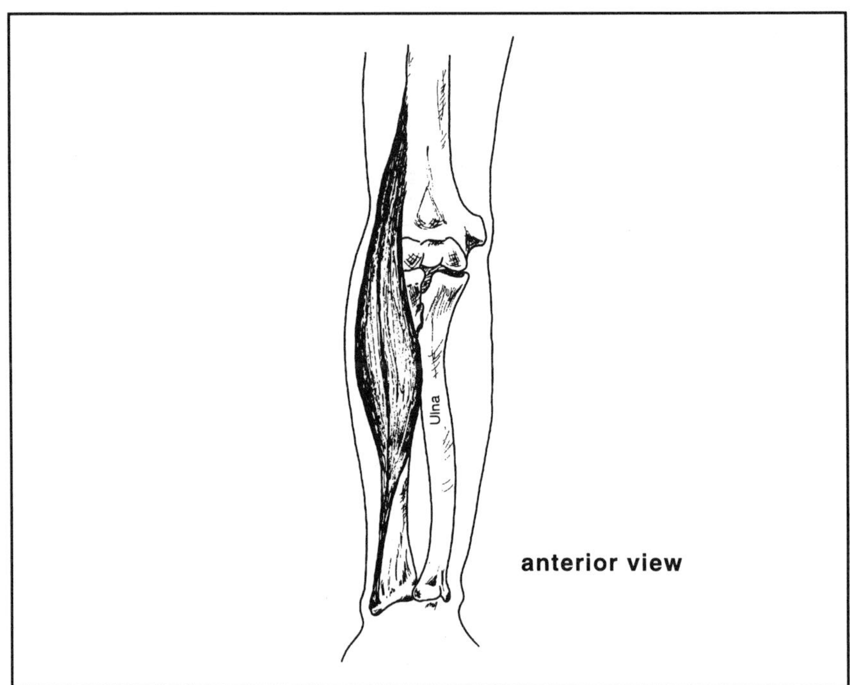

Fig. 4.7

Origin — Upper two-thirds of the supracondylar ridge of the lateral epicondyle of the humerus.
Insertion — Base of the styloid process of radius.
Innervation — Radial nerve.
Action — Flexion of the elbow; weak pronation to neutral position if forearm is supinated.

The distal attachment of the brachioradialis is considerably farther from the elbow than is the case with the other elbow flexors. The force arm and, therefore, the mechanical advantage afforded by this muscle is increased. Its proximal attachment is, however, much closer to the elbow than other flexors, and, because of this, the muscle lies very close to the joint axis. During contraction, then, the brachioradialis yields a small angular component at its distal attachment when compared to its large stabilizing component. This angular component can be lengthened slightly by placing the forearm in the neutral position so that the muscle will be made to pass farther anterior to the joint axis. The pull of the brachioradialis will, therefore, be strongest when the forearm is in neutral position.

Brachialis (brachia'lis)

The brachialis (Fig. 4.8), called the **workhorse of the elbow**, is a fusiform muscle located on the anterior aspect of the elbow. It may be palpated just lateral to the biceps when resistance is applied to the wrist.

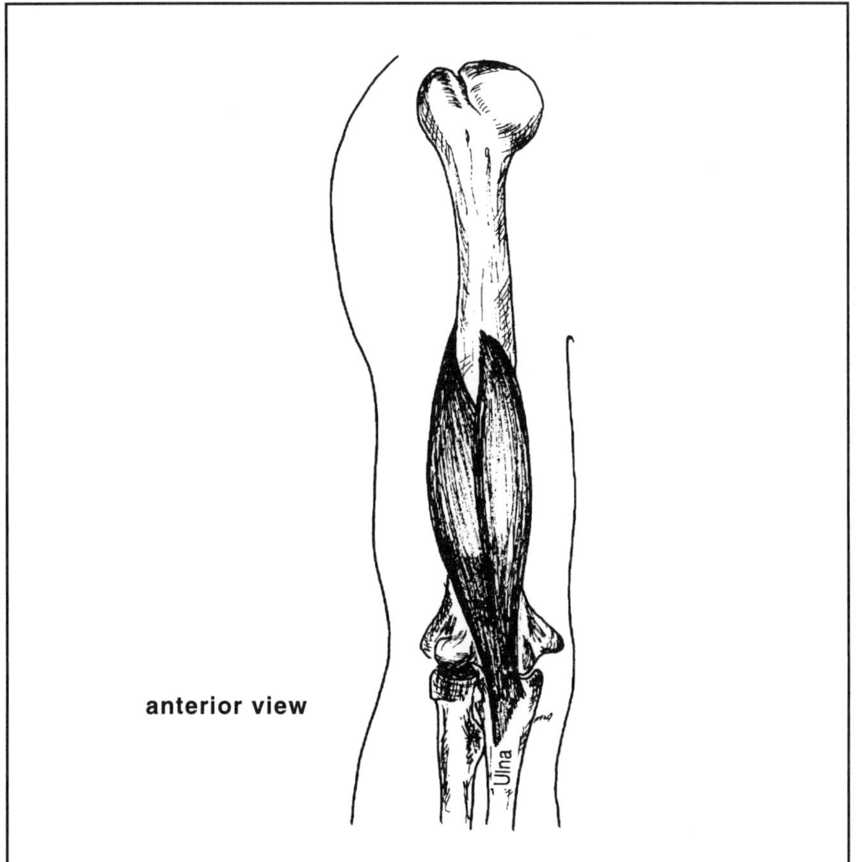

Brachialis

Fig. 4.8

Origin — Lower half of anterior surface of the humerus.
Insertion — Anterior surface of coronoid process of the ulna.
Innervation — Musculocutaneous nerve.
Action — Flexion of the elbow.

The brachialis crosses the elbow closer to the axis of flexion/extension than do the biceps or brachioradialis. Per unit of contraction, then, the brachialis is less favorably situated to provide force; however, since its distal attachment is on the ulna rather than the radius, forearm position is inconsequential to the effectiveness of its pull. Regardless of forearm position, degree of elbow flexion or amount of resistance, the brachialis is involved in the flexive action -- hence its name, workhorse of the elbow.

Pronator Teres (prona'tor te'res)

The pronator teres (Fig. 4.9) is located on the anterior and upper aspect of the forearm. Its distal portion is covered by the brachioradialis; however, the main muscle mass is superficial and may be palpated as the forearm is pronated against resistance with the elbow well-flexed. To help distinguish the pronator teres from surrounding musculature, place the thumb on the medial epicondyle and the long finger on the midpoint of the radius. A ridge of muscle will be seen running obliquely between the thumb and long finger when the forearm is pronated against resistance.

Origin — By two heads, one (humeral head) from the medial epicondyle of the humerus, and one (ulnar head) from the coronoid process of the ulna. The attachment to the medial epicondyle is by a common tendon which also supports the attachments of the flexor muscles of the forearm.
Insertion — Lateral surface of the radius near its midpoint.
Innervation — Median nerve.
Action — Pronation of the radioulnar joint; flexion of the elbow joint.

Pronator Teres

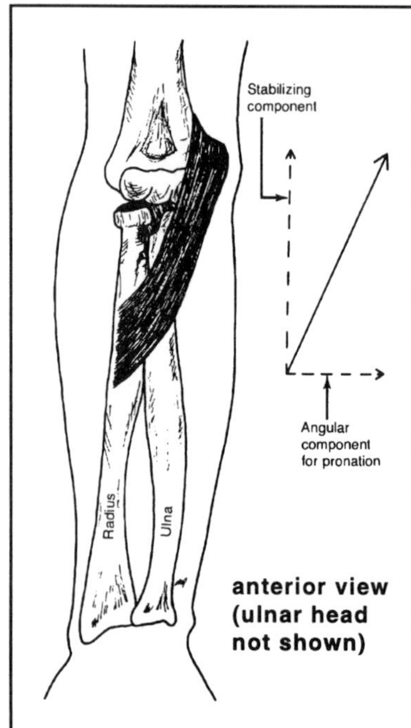

Fig. 4.9

The pronator teres is well anterior to the axis of the radioulnar joint. Its approximate angle of insertion on the radius is shown, together with its resolution to the two components, in Figure 4.9. The length of the angular component testifies to the high efficiency of the muscle as a pronator whereas the stabilizing vector indicates that contraction of this muscle will be accompanied by a force preventing any tendency of the radius to be dislocated as pronation is performed. Because of its strength and efficiency, the muscle does not participate when pronation is slow or unresisted.

The location of the pronator teres in relationship to the elbow axes can be seen easily through palpation. Regardless of forearm position, the muscle is quite close to the axis throughout the range of flexion, and is, therefore, inefficient as an elbow flexor when compared to the biceps, brachioradialis, and brachialis. As an elbow flexor, the pronator teres would be, at best, an assistant mover. Even then, its contraction may serve to neutralize the supinating tendency of the biceps rather than to contribute to the actual flexion of the joint.

Pronator Quadratus (prona'tor quadra'tus)

The pronator quadratus (Fig. 4.10) is a rhomboidal muscle located at the distal end of the forearm. It is a deep muscle and cannot be palpated.

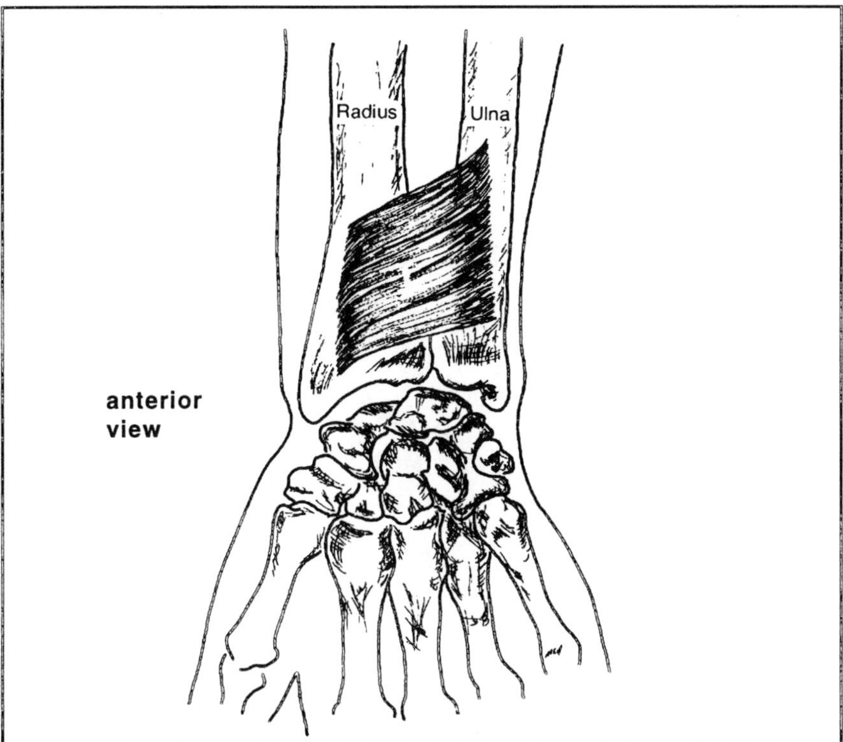

Pronator Quadratus

Fig. 4.10

Origin — Lower fourth of the palmar surface of the ulna.
Insertion — Lower fourth of the palmar surface of the radius.
Innervation — Median nerve.
Action — Pronation of the radioulnar joint.

The pronator quadratus is the primary mover for pronation. Its size and line of pull allow it to pronate the radioulnar joint without help when the action is performed slowly and without resistance. If speed is required, or if resistance is met, the quadratus will be aided by the pronator teres.

Triceps Brachii (tri'ceps bra'chii)

The triceps brachii (Fig. 4.11) is a three-headed muscle located superficially on the posterior aspect of the upper arm. Its lateral head may be palpated between the bulge of the deltoid and the lateral epicondyle; its long head may be palpated between the axilla and the olecranon process. The medial head is covered by the other heads and cannot be palpated.

Triceps brachii

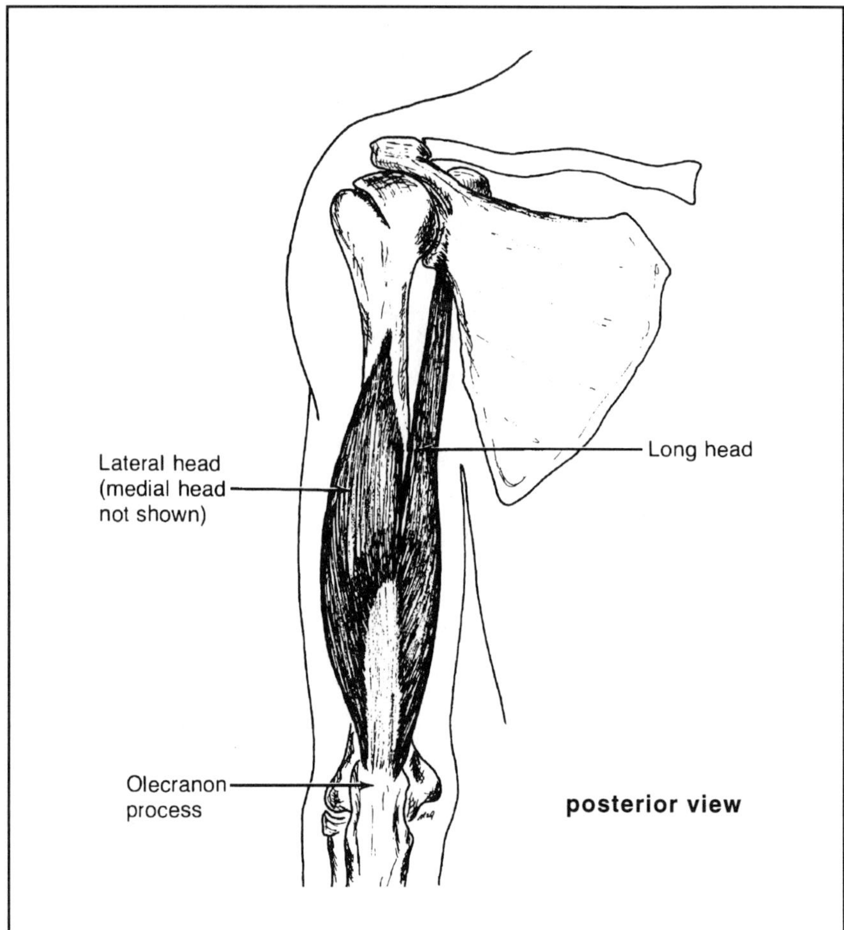

Fig. 4.11

Origin — Long head: Infraglenoid tuberosity of the scapula. Lateral head: Upper half of posterior surface of the humerus. Medial head: Lower two-thirds of the posterior surface of the humerus.
Insertion — Olecranon process of the ulna.
Innervation — Radial nerve.
Action — Extension of the elbow joint.

Figure 4.12 illustrates that the triceps, by virtue of its insertion on the olecranon process, applies force for first class leverage. The mechanical advantage is small (approximately .2) to favor speed over power; however, the size of the muscle as well as its angle of attachment on the olecranon give the triceps great power in spite of poor leverage.

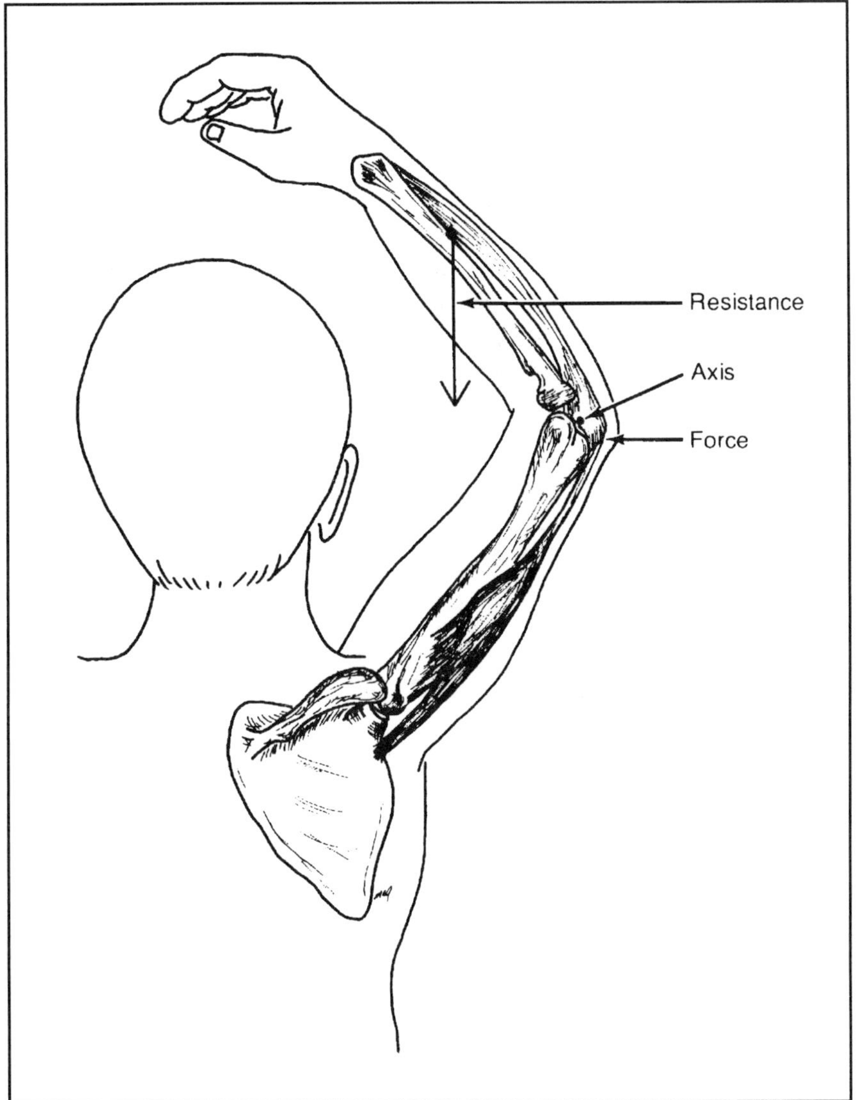

Fig. 4.12

First Class Leverage of the Triceps Brachii

Anconeus (ancone'us)

The anconeus (Fig. 4.13) is a small triangular muscle located on the upper and posterior aspect of the forearm. If the thumb and index finger are placed on the olecranon and lateral epicondyle, respectively, they will define the base of the equilateral triangle within which the anconeus may be palpated.

Anconeus of the Right Arm

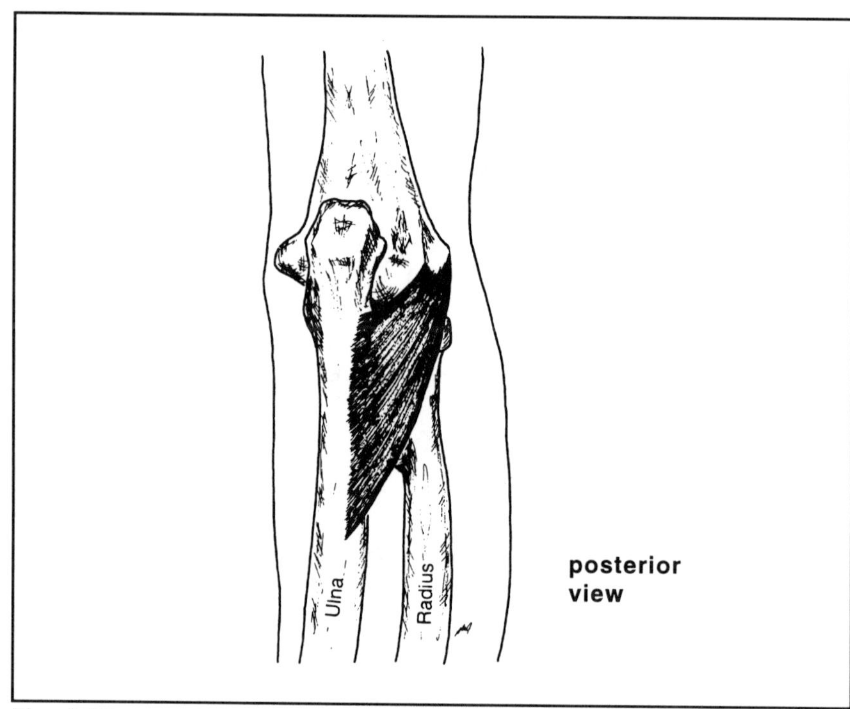

Fig. 4.13

Origin — Posterior surface of lateral epicondyle of the humerus.
Insertion — Lateral aspects of the olecranon and posterior face of upper ulna.
Innervation — Radial nerve.
Action — Extension of elbow joint.

As the anconeus courses between its two attachments, it comes very close to the elbow axis. This, in addition to its size, makes the muscle a weak extensor of the joint.

Supinator (supina'tor)

The supinator (Fig. 4.14), a longitudinal muscle of two layers, is located on the dorsum of the forearm. It is covered by the brachioradialis and the wrist extensors, and cannot be palpated.

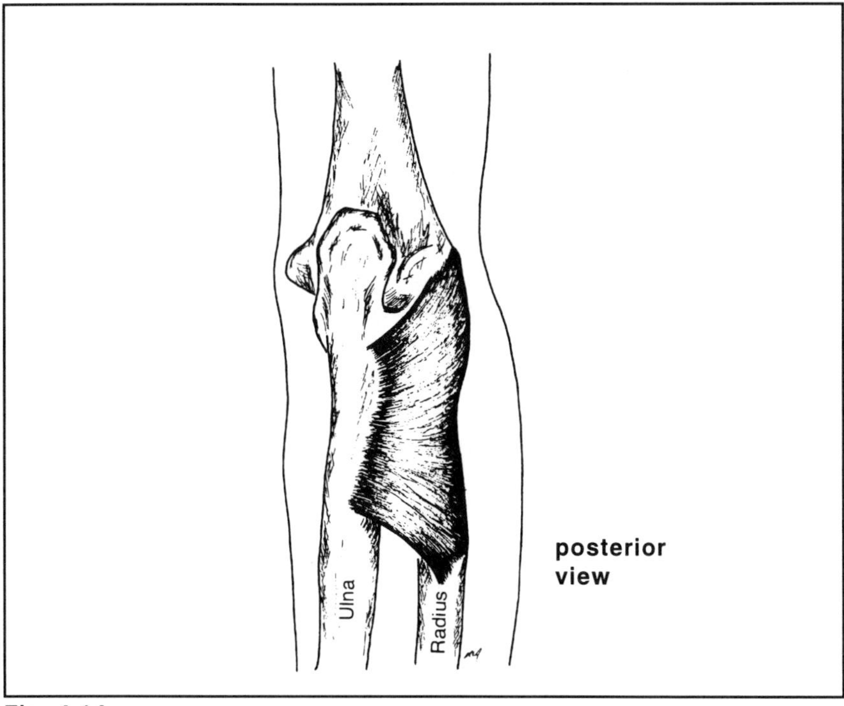

Supinator of the Right Arm

Fig. 4.14

Origin	Lateral epicondyle of the humerus; adjacent portion of the ulna; annular and radial collateral ligaments.
Insertion	Lateral surface of the upper third of the radius.
Innervation	Radial nerve.
Action	Supination of the radioulnar joint.

The supinator is in its best position to supinate the radioulnar joint when the elbow is extended, thus placing the muscle on the stretch. In this position, it requires assistance from the biceps brachii only when resistance is met. When the elbow is flexed, however, the supinator is shortened and must have the help of the biceps under all conditions except when supination is performed slowly and without resistance.

FOREARM MUSCLES

There are eight muscles of the forearm which originate on or just above the epicondyles of the humerus and insert distal to the wrist. The primary actions of these muscles are to move the hand around the wrist joint, or to flex or extend the fingers; however, they do cross the elbow joint, and it is necessary, therefore, to investigate their functions as movers of that joint.

It will be recalled that the axis of flexion-extension of the elbow passes through the two epicondyles of the humerus. Since the eight forearm muscles originate on or adjacent to these bony prominences, there is the possibility that the muscles cross the elbow in line with the axis and will not, therefore, be movers of that joint. Even if some of the muscles should cross the joint either anterior or posterior to the axis, they must, by virtue of their origins, be quite close to the axis, and cannot be powerful movers.

Careful examination of a skeleton will indicate that four of the eight forearm muscles -- the extensor carpi radialis longus, extensor carpi radialis brevis, palmaris longus, and flexor carpi radialis -- cross the elbow anterior to the axis and are, therefore, in a position to contribute somewhat to elbow flexion. Their contribution is only assistive, and is enhanced when wrist action is required simultaneously with elbow flexion. The origins, insertions, innervations, and additional actions of these muscles are discussed fully in Chapter 5.

COMMENTS

The elbow and radioulnar joints are admirably adapted to the innumerable requirements of daily living, work, and sport-related activities. The joints are structurally strong, yet allow for satisfactory range of movement. Surrounding musculature is both of the penniform and longitudinal types to meet the demands for strength as well as range of motion, and displays favorable mechanical advantage during both flexion-extension and pronation-supination.

Perhaps the versatility of the elbow region can best be appreciated when one considers the number of sports which involve action of the two joints. Movement patterns comprising activities from archery to waterskiing all require that specific degrees of motion of the elbow be performed with equally specific timing. Even motions which appear to be equivalent involve subtle differences in joint action. The overarm throw is an example. A shortstop and a quarterback both throw overarm but each uses the elbow differently; the javelin thrower exhibits yet a different pattern, as does the volleyball player delivering an overarm serve, the tennis player executing a smash, and the flyfisher making a cast.

Further respect for the elbow is earned when consideration is given to the size and weight of the objects we throw. Great muscular power is required to accelerate these objects to the point of release, and there is the inevitable stabilizing component which accompanies such forceful contractions. That the joints can withstand so constant a jamming of the articulating bones is, indeed, awesome.

A common ailment of the elbow is referred to as "epicondylitis" or "tendinitis" or, more commonly, as "tennis elbow". Symptoms can begin with a blow to the elbow or a twist of the forearm that produces a sudden sharp pain, but usually the complaint is one of an increasing ache in the elbow particularly after lifting objects or performing repetitive actions such as using a circular saw or hammer.

The causes of tennis elbow, whether located laterally or medially, are overuse and misuse of the forearm muscles that cross the elbow. By far the greatest incidence of tennis elbow pain is on the lateral side of the humerus and is caused by inflammation and microscopic tears of the extensor carpi radialis brevis and its tendon of origin. Medial tennis elbow results from forceful and repetitive contractions of the four wrist muscles that originate on the medial epicondyle.

To test for lateral tennis elbow, bend the elbow and hold the forearm pronated and parallel to the ground. Lift the hand against resistance. A sharp pain in the lateral elbow is indicative of tennis elbow. If pain in the vicinity of the medial epicondyle is felt when pressing the hand down against resistance, medial tennis elbow is indicated.

Treatment of tennis elbow includes relief of pain and inflammation through rest and anti-inflammatory medicines followed by exercises to strengthen the muscles and reestablish muscular balance around the joint. Surgery may be required for those few cases that do not respond to more conservative treatment.

A quiz for this material can be found in the back of this book on page 287.

LABORATORY EXPERIENCES

1. Place electrodes on the muscle bellies of the biceps brachii and brachioradialis of a partner. Monitor the action potentials as the partner performs arm curls with a two- or three-kilogram weight. Have the partner alternate between the supinated and pronated grips as the arm curls are performed. What conclusions can you make regarding the input of the two muscles relative to the types of arm curls?

2. While monitoring the action potentials of the biceps brachii, supinate the radioulnar joint slowly, and then rapidly. Are there differences in the activity of the muscle? Perform supination against resistance and note differences in the electromyographic record. Do your findings agree with the actions listed for the biceps brachii?

3. Using a cable tensiometer or other device which measures force, determine your maximum strength at 180, 120, 90 and 70 degrees of elbow flexion. At which joint angle are you strongest? Does this agree with the concepts of mechanical and physiological efficiency discussed in this chapter under actions of the biceps brachii?

THE WRIST AND HAND

5

The wrist and hand are comprised of over twenty bones and joints, and twenty-five muscles or muscle groups. Together, these joints and muscles become an important factor in the functional performance of everyday activities which we take for granted.

The anatomical terms that apply to the wrist and hand are somewhat different than those discussed in previous chapters. The thumb side of the hand is referred to as the radial surface while the ulnar surface is used to describe the small finger side of the hand. The anterior surface of the hand is commonly referred to as the palmar or volar surface. The posterior aspect is distinguished as the dorsal surface.

Landmarks on the palmar surface of the hand and wrist become extremely important in identifying underlying anatomical structures that may be impaired due to injury. These palmar landmarks also assist in the palpation of anatomical structures that are found in the hand and wrist. The palm is made up of the thenar eminence, found on the radial side of the hand, the hypothenar eminence on the ulnar side, and the midpalmar surface. The thenar eminence is associated with musculature that controls thumb movements whereas the hypothenar eminence is formed by muscles that assist in movement of the small finger. Creases that are found throughout the palmar surface stabilize the skin to the underlying palmar fascial plate, thus enabling frictional grasp.

At least two systems of labeling the carpal bones are commonly in use. In one system, the carpals are names the navicular, lunate, triquetrum, pisiform, multangulus major, multangulus minor, capitate, and hamate. In the second system, the multangulus major is called the trapezium, the multangulus minor is the trapezoid, and the navicular is the scaphoid. The first system is employed in this text.

The wrist joint (Fig. 5.1) is formed by the articulation of the radius and the articular disc with the navicular (scaphoid), lunate, and triquetrum bones. These latter three bones, along with the pisiform, form the proximal row of carpal bones and articulate, in turn, with the distal row -- the multangulus major (trapezium), multangulus minor (trapezoid), capitate, and hamate bones. It is clear that, in actuality, the wrist joint is comprised of several joints, some between the carpal bones, called **intercarpal joints,** one between the proximal and distal carpal rows called the **midcarpal joint**, and one between the radius and articular disc and the proximal row of carpals, called the **radiocarpal joint.** It is typical, however, to consider the joints as one and to refer to them collectively as the **wrist joint.**

Axes of the Wrist Joint

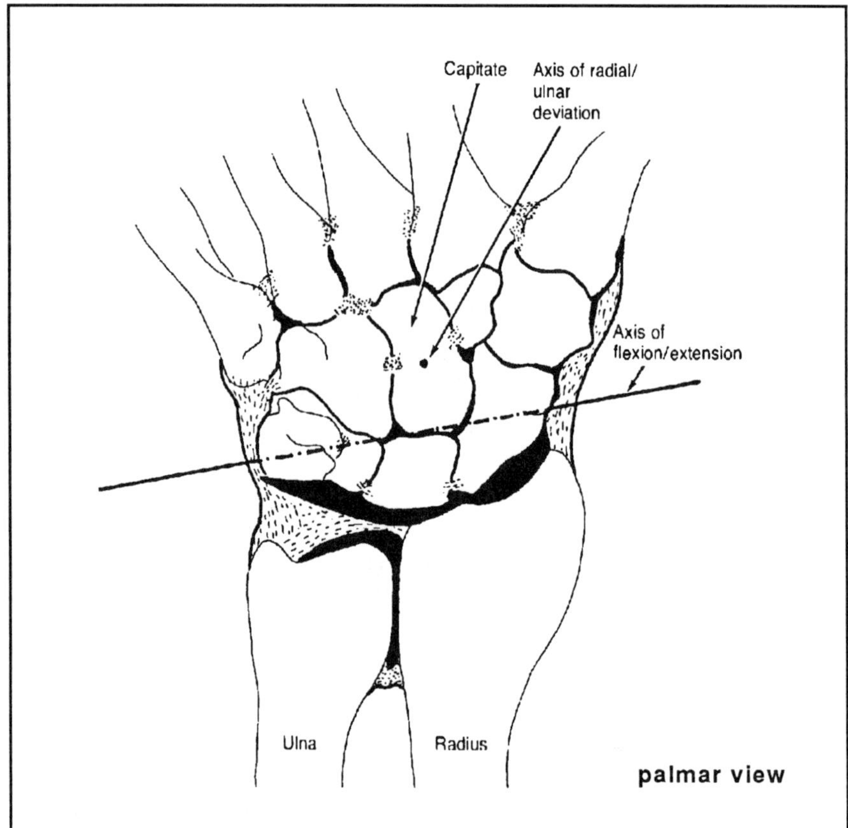

Fig. 5.1

The distal row of carpals articulates with the five metacarpals via the **carpometacarpal joints.** The metacarpals articulate, in turn, with the proximal phalanges by the **metacarpophalangeal joints,** and between themselves by the **intermetacarpal joints.** The joints between the phalanges are referred to as the **interphalangeal joints.**

BONE MARKINGS

Figure 5.2 is presented as a review of the bone markings of the wrist and hand which are relevant to the discussion of muscle origins and insertions. A skeleton should be used with the figure for best review.

Bones of the Wrist and Hand

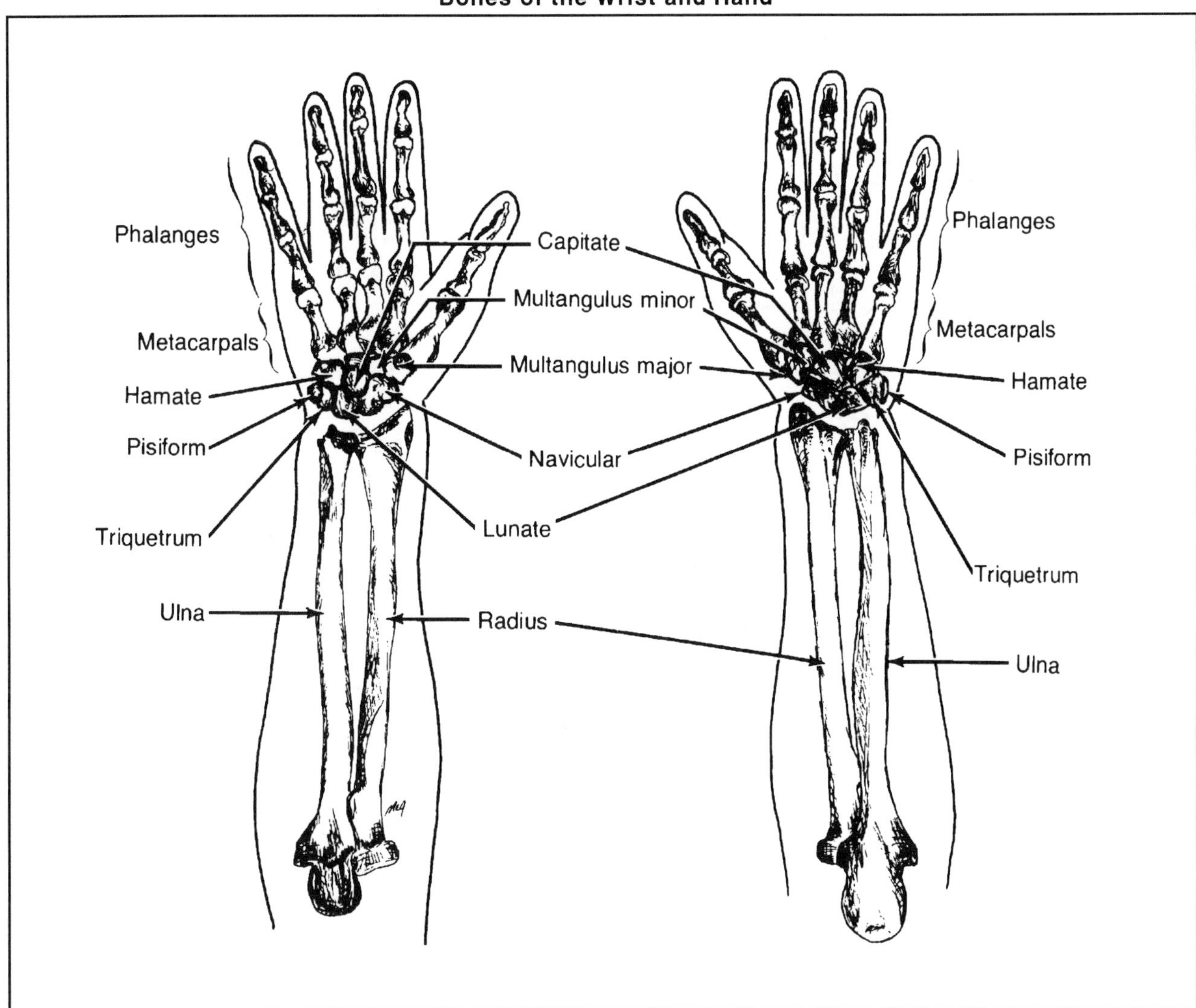

Fig. 5.2

JOINTS OF THE WRIST AND HAND

RADIOCARPAL JOINT

The radiocarpal joint is a condyloid joint and is found between the articular surface of the radius, the articular disc, and the navicular, lunate, and triquetrum. The articular disc extends from the distal radius to the ulna styloid. Only the lunate and triquetrum articulate with this disc, while the navicular and lunate articulate with the radius. Not only does the articular disc act as a shock absorber for the wrist joint, it also maintains a mechanical relationship between the carpal bones and the ulna. With the articular disc intact, the radius will bear 60% of the axial load and the ulna will bear 40% during functional activities. If the articular disc is injured, the radius will compensate by transmitting most of the force on itself (95%) while the ulna is only able to transmit a small percentage of the force (5%).

The radiocarpal joint provides for rotation about two axes. One, the frontal axis, passes through the wrist just distal to the styloid processes of the radius and ulna (Fig. 5.1), and is the axis for flexion and extension. The second axis is a sagittal one and passes through the capitate bone at a right angle to the palm (Fig. 5.1). Movements of the hand which require rotation around the sagittal axis are radial deviation and ulnar deviation. Sequential combination of movements around the two axes results in circumduction.

The major ligaments of the radiocarpal joint are the volar and dorsal radiocarpal ligaments, the palmar ulnocarpal ligament (not shown), and the radial and ulnar collateral ligaments. The palmar radiocarpal ligament (Fig. 5.3) courses medially between the palmar surfaces of the radius and articular disc, all the bones on the proximal carpal row, and the capitate; it also blends with the palmar intercarpal ligaments. The palmar ulnocarpal ligament is a small ligament that blends in with the ulnar collateral and palmar radiocarpal ligaments. It extends from the distal ulna and attaches to the lunate and triquetrum. The dorsal radiocarpal ligament (Fig. 5.4) is attached proximally to the dorsal surface of the radius and disc, and distally to only the proximal row of carpal bones. The dorsal radiocarpal ligament is thinner and more membranous than its palmar counterpart. Due to the orientation of these ligaments, they ensure that the carpals follow the radius throughout forearm rotation. During pronation, the dorsal radiocarpal ligament is functional with the radius; during supination, the palmar radiocarpal ligament carries the wrist with the radius.

The collateral ligaments of the wrist (Fig. 5.3) are, as their names imply, on the radial and ulnar sides of the joint. The radial collateral ligament is attached proximally to the styloid process of the radius and distally to the navicular and multangulus major. The ulnar collateral ligament attaches to the styloid process of the ulna and the articular disc, and runs distally to the nonarticular surface of the triquetrum and pisiform.

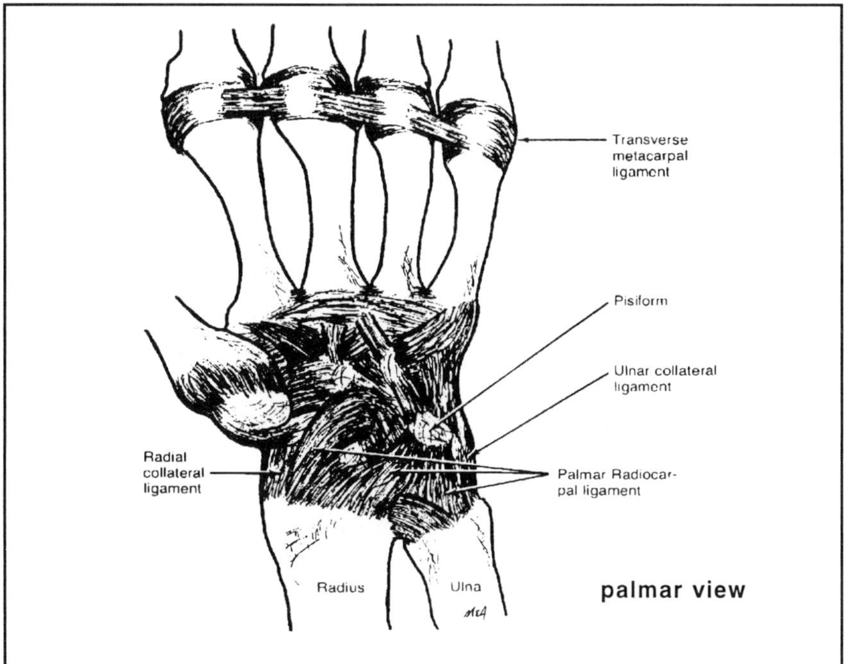

Fig. 5.3

Ligaments of the Wrist

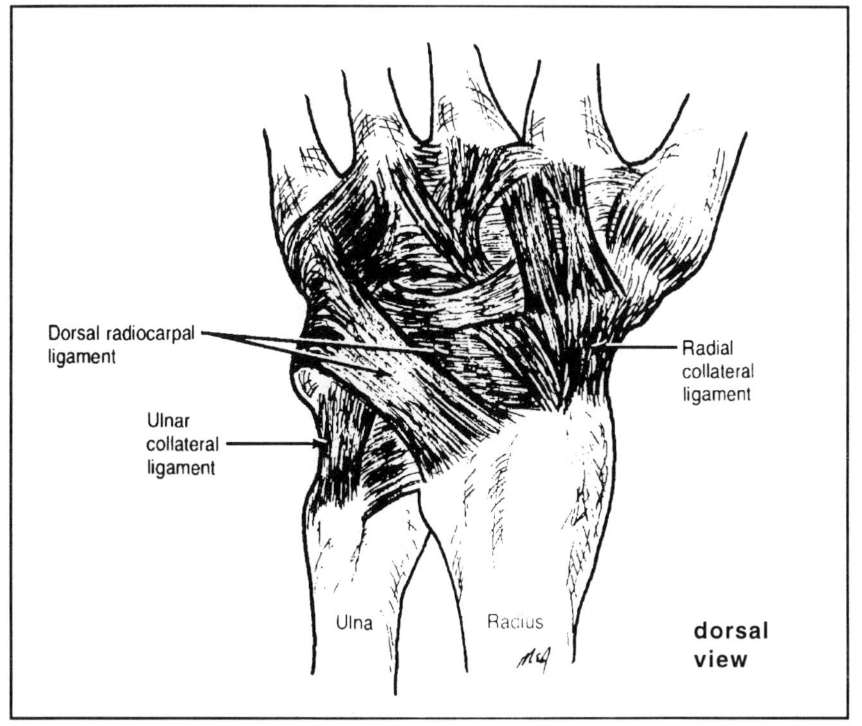

Fig. 5.4

Ligaments of the Wrist

The joint capsule is encased by the five ligaments of the wrist joint and thus covers the articular surfaces of the radius and articular disc, and the carpal bones. In order to provide for ease of motion the capsule is quite loose and presents numerous folds, especially when the wrist is flexed.

INTERCARPAL AND MIDCARPAL JOINTS

The intercarpal joints are those articulations between the individual bones and between the two rows of bones as well. All of the joints are synovial; however, they are nonaxial and permit only a gliding motion between adjacent bones in each row. The palmar and dorsal intercarpal ligaments connect the carpal bones within each row as well as between rows. Small interosseous intercarpal ligaments may also be found binding adjacent bones within each row. The pisotriquetral joint is considered separate from the intercarpal joints. Because of the location of the pisiform on the palmar triquetrum, it does not take part in direct intercarpal movements.

The articulating cavity between the two carpal rows is known as the **midcarpal** joint. Two compound **sellar** (saddle-shaped) joints are actually formed within this joint cavity. The first joint is made up of the navicular, lunate, and triquetrum articulating with the capitate and hamate. The second articulation occurs between the navicular, multangulus major, and multangulus minor. Dorsal and palmar intercarpal ligaments are found binding these joints; however, interosseous ligaments are not found connecting the bones between the distal and proximal rows. Due to the ligamentous architecture of the midcarpal joint, more motion is permitted at this joint than at the intercarpal joints.

The collateral ligaments are located along the two sides of the hand and are continuous with the radial and ulnar collateral ligaments of the wrist joint. The interosseus ligaments join the articular surfaces of adjacent carpals.

In addition to the ligamentous tissues discussed above, there are structures of the carpals known as the **flexor retinaculum** and **extensor retinaculum** (Fig. 5.5). The flexor retinaculum is comprised of two bands previously known as the **palmar carpal ligament** and the **transverse carpal ligament**. The proximal portion of the flexor retinaculum may be located at the distal skin crease of the wrist. The structure is a dense, wide band that inserts on the radial side of the wrist to the crest of the multangulus major, the tubercle of the navicular, and sometimes the styloid process of the radius. Its ulnar attachment includes the hook of the hamate and the pisiform. The proximal portion forms the border on the palmar side of the **carpal tunnel** which is an opening at the wrist through which the flexor digitorum profundus, flexor digitorum superficialis, and the flexor pollicis longus run as well as the median nerve. It acts as a pulley across the palmar wrist confining and redirecting the median nerve and the long flexor tendons of the digits.

The extensor retinaculum extends across the dorsal surface of the wrist forming a roof for the extensor tendons but attaching between the tendons to form six individual extensor compartments. The fibers of the retinaculum insert on the pisiform and the triquetrum on the ulnar side. On the radial side, the extensor retinaculum blends in with the flexor retinaculum. As with the flexor retinaculum, the extensor retinaculum acts as a pulley mechanism for the extensor tendons.

Flexor Retinaculum

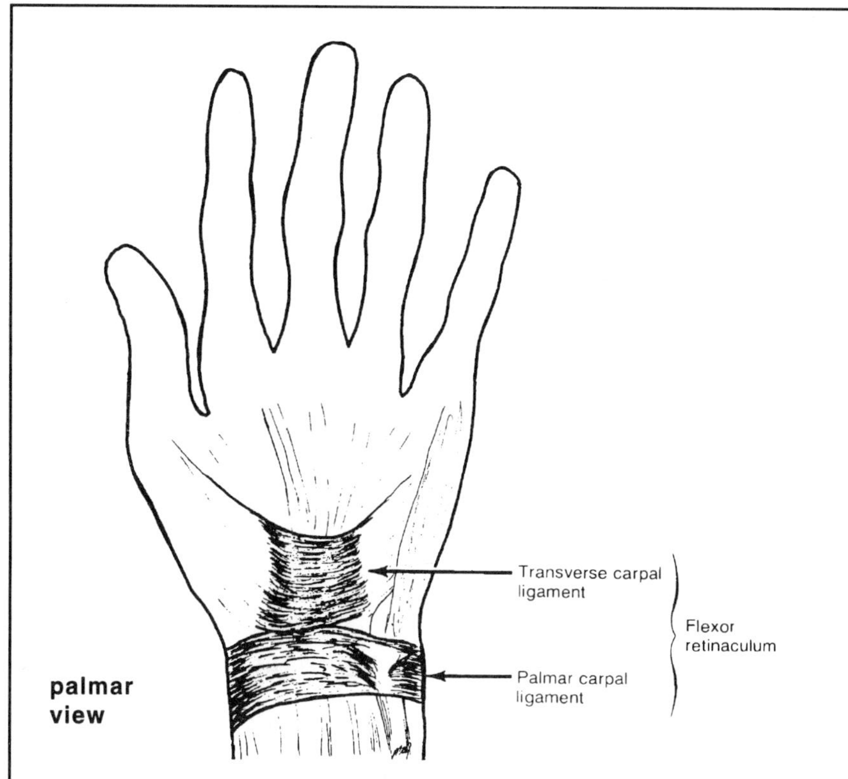

Fig. 5.5

Each extensor tendon is surrounded by a synovial sheath as it passes through its compartment formed by the retinaculum. The first dorsal compartment is found on the radial side of the wrist and forms the tunnel for the abductor pollicis longus and extensor pollicis brevis. The next compartment contains the extensor carpi radialis longus and brevis. The extensor pollicis longus may be found in the third dorsal compartment. The fourth dorsal compartment contains the extensor indicis and extensor digitorum. The extensor digiti minimi is housed in the fifth compartment while the sixth compartment forms a tunnel for the extensor carpi ulnaris.

Wrist Movements

During wrist extension, approximately 50° of motion occurs at the radiocarpal joint and 35° occurs at the midcarpal joint. A slight pattern of radial deviation and forearm pronation is noted during wrist extension. Increased midcarpal motion is noted during wrist flexion (50°) and less movement is noted at the radiocarpal joint (35°). Slight ulnar deviation and forearm supination is present during wrist flexion.

During radial deviation, movement is noted to occur primarily at the midcarpal joint. The proximal carpal row is noted to move toward the ulna while the distal row moves toward the radius. Movement of the wrist during ulnar deviation occurs primarily at the radiocarpal joint.

CARPOMETACARPAL JOINTS

The carpometacarpal (referred to as CMC) joints are formed by the articulations of the distal row of carpal bones with the base of the five metacarpals. The first CMC joint, that articulation between the multangulus major and the metacarpal of the thumb, is a saddle-shaped (sellar) joint and allows rotation around two axes; however, these axes are somewhat offset from the cardinal planes of motion and, therefore, are not perpendicular to the bones or to each other. This arrangement allows for motion at right angles to the palm, parallel to the palm, and across the palm. One of these axes runs through the base of the first metacarpal and slants toward the base of the ring finger (Fig. 5.6). When the metacarpal moves around this axis, the actions of abduction and adduction are performed. These actions can easily be repeated by the individual, but care must be taken to restrict action at the knuckle joint of the thumb, and to concentrate attention on the CMC joint. If difficulty is encountered, the actions can be enhanced by placing just the ulnar half of the palm down on a table. Pointing the thumb alternately at the floor and ceiling will produce abduction and adduction at the CMC joint.

Axes of the Saddle Joint of the Thumb

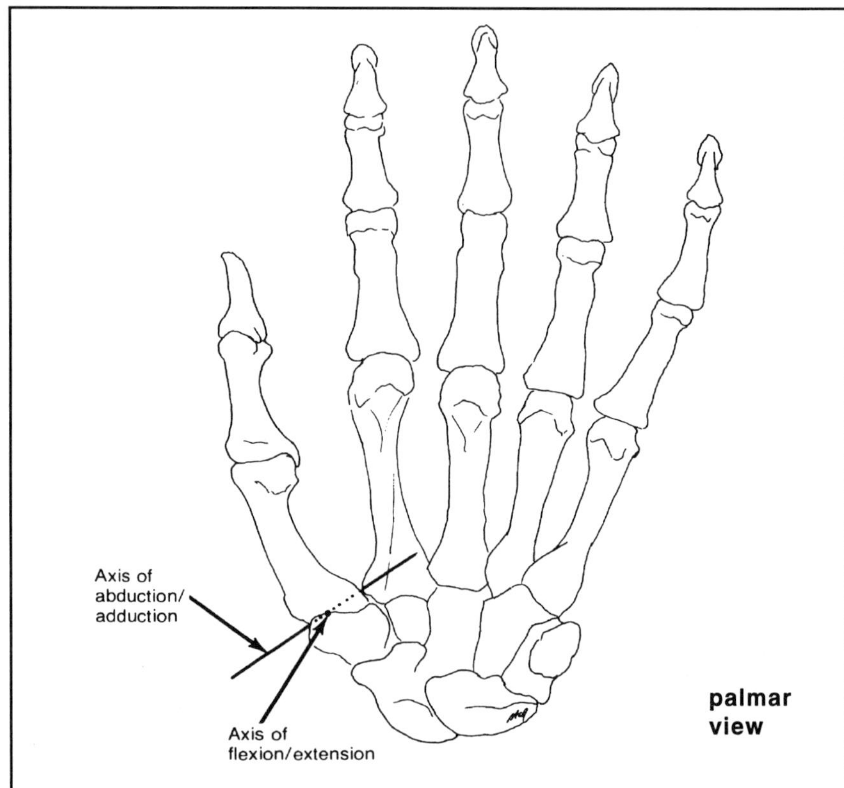

Fig. 5.6

The second axis of the first CMC joint goes through the multangulus major but is at an approximate right angle to the palm (Fig. 5.6). Flexion and extension are performed around this axis. These movements occur in a plane that is parallel to the palm.

In addition to flexion/extension and abduction/adduction, the CMC joint of the thumb can allow for actions known as **opposition** and **reposition (retroposition)** (Fig. 5.7). These actions are most easily thought of as partial circumductions. If the left hand is held with the palm toward the face, and the thumb circumducted counter-clockwise, the movement described as opposition will be seen to occur as the thumb approaches the palm. Reposition will be performed if the direction of circumduction is reversed. Opposition and reposition are not, therefore, pure actions of the CMC joint of the thumb, but are rather combination actions comprised of flexion and abduction (opposition), and extension and adduction (reposition). The axis of these two actions is, similarly, a combination axis which is aligned between those of flexion/extension and abduction/adduction.

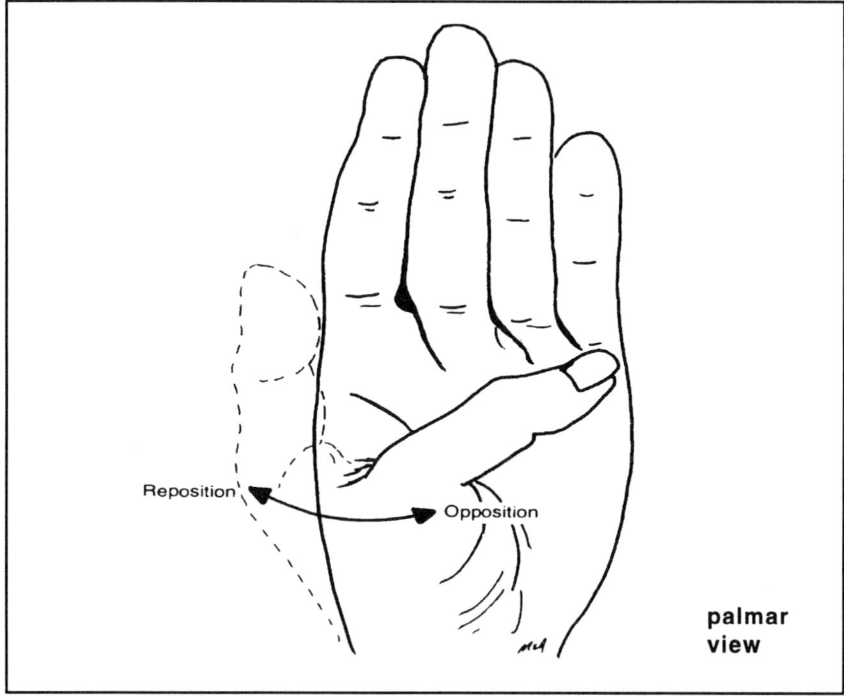

Opposition and Reposition of the Saddle Joint of the Thumb

Fig. 5.7

The joint capsule of the first CMC joint is thick but loose; however, the joint is reinforced by two strong ligaments known as the lateral and ulnar ligaments. The lateral ligament can be found attached to the radial base of the first metacarpal and multangulus major. The ulnar ligament extends from the ulnar base of the first metacarpal to the distal portion of the multangulus major. The dorsal and palmar aspects of the first CMC joint are reinforced by corresponding dorsal and palmar ligaments. The thenar muscles as well as the extrinsic flexors and extensors that cross this CMC joint also provide support to this very mobile joint. Even though the first CMC joint is able to adopt a variety of positions with respect to the palmar surface of the hand, the joint capsule is strong enough to prevent dislocations from occurring.

Carpometacarpal joints two through five articulate the metacarpal bones of the four fingers with adjacent carpal bones. These joints are synovial and are classified as modified saddle joints. Movement at these joints is slight, and of a gliding nature, because of the presence of ligaments connecting the bones on their dorsal and palmar surfaces (Fig. 5.3 and Fig. 5.4) as well as between their adjacent surfaces. The ligaments are the dorsal ligaments, palmar ligaments, and interosseus ligaments, respectively. The joint capsule, a continuation of the intercarpal capsule, aids in restricting joint movements.

Motion at the second through fifth CMC joints is least in joints two and three, and greatest in joint five. The limited mobility present at the second and third CMC joints allows the index and middle fingers to stabilize themselves and work in unison with the thumb during fine prehensile movements. The mobility present in the fourth and fifth CMC joints permits the hand to cup itself around objects for grasping. Movement contribution of the latter joint may be observed as an attempt is made to touch the base of the thumb to the base of the small finger. The fifth metacarpal will be seen to exhibit limited opposition and reposition (Fig. 5.8).

Opposition and Reposition of the Fifth Carpometacarpal Joint

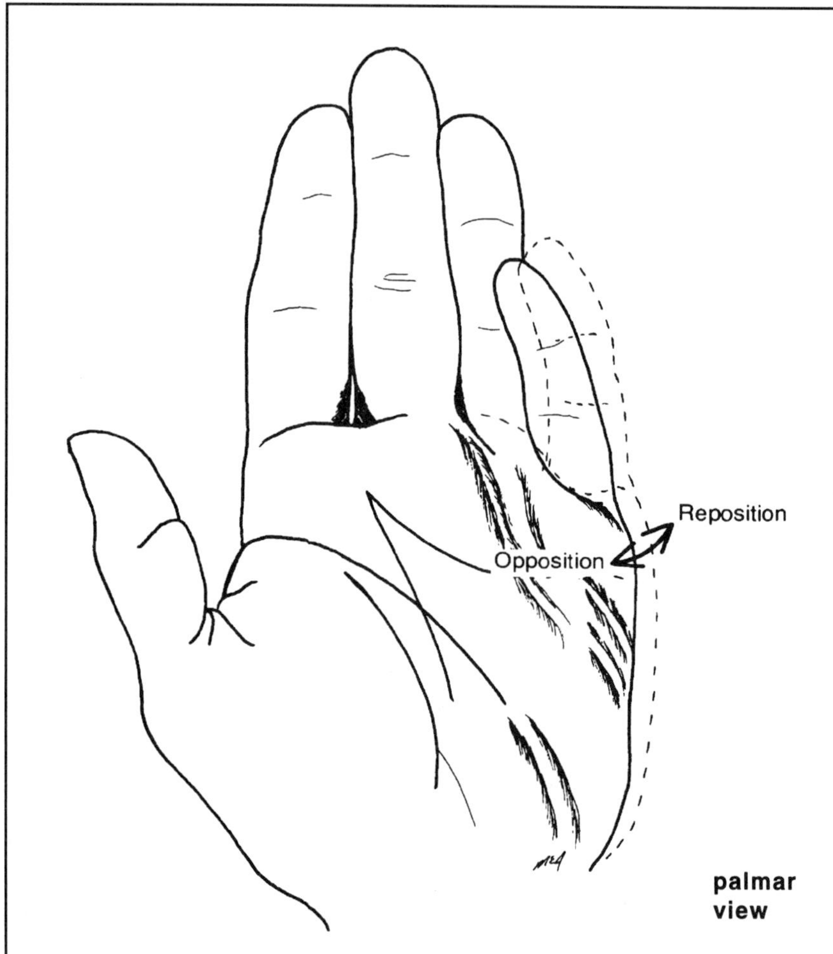

Fig. 5.8

INTERMETACARPAL JOINTS

The intermetacarpal joints (known as IM joints) are formed by the bases of the second, third, fourth, and fifth metacarpals. The bones are united by dorsal, palmar, and interosseus ligaments, and are encased in a joint capsule continuous with that of the intercarpal and carpometacarpal joints. Movements permitted by these joints are slight and are of a gliding nature. Most movement occurs between the fourth and fifth metacarpals during opposition and reposition at the fifth CMC joint.

METACARPOPHALANGEAL JOINTS

The metacarpophalangeal (abbreviated *MCP*) joints are formed by the heads of the five metacarpal bones, and the proximal phalanx of the thumb and four fingers. The joints are condyloid and allow for flexion/extension around an axis passing from side to side through the joints, and for abduction/adduction around an axis passing from palmar to dorsal surfaces (Fig. 5.9). A small amount of rotation may also be observed at the proximal phalanx during MCP abduction/adduction and flexion/extension because of the irregular spherical surface of the metacarpal head moving with the concave surface of the base of the proximal phalanx. This phenomenon of rotation may be observed during pulp-to-pulp pinch movements between the thumb and digits. As flexion of the MCP joints increases during these pinch movements, more rotatory movements are available thus allowing greater lateral movement of the proximal phalanx of each finger.

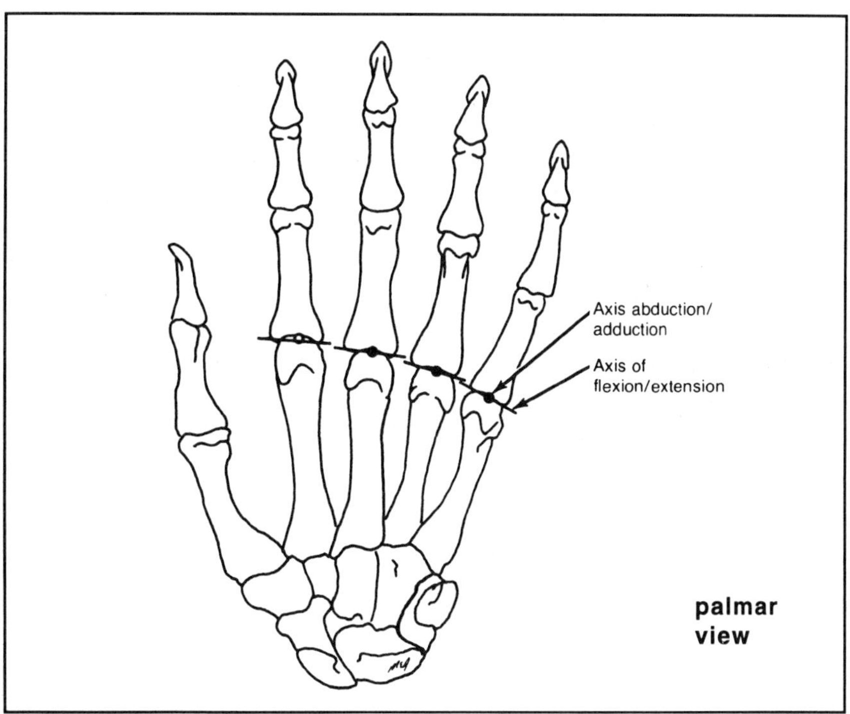

Fig. 5.9

Axes of the Metacarpophalangeal Joints

Observation of one's hand will indicate that these movements are much freer in the MCP joints of the hand than they are in the thumb. In fact, it may be necessary to stabilize the first metacarpal to fully observe motion at that MCP joint. Abduction and adduction are particularly difficult to perform, leading one to conclude that the first MCP joint is more of a modified hinge joint than a true condyloid joint.

The ligaments of each MCP joint are one **volar plate** (palmar ligament) and two **collateral ligaments** (radial and ulnar collateral ligaments). There is also the deep **transverse metacarpal ligament** (Fig. 5.3) which runs between the heads of the four metacarpals of the hand. This ligament is primarily responsible for limiting sideward spread of the metacarpals; however, since it blends with the palmar ligaments, it has some slight contribution to the integrity of the MCP joints. The palmar, radial, and ulnar capsules of each joint are formed by the deep surfaces of the ligaments. Dorsally, the capsule of each MCP joint is covered by an extension of the long extensor tendon known as the **extensor mechanism**. The extensor mechanism is discussed more fully below.

The volar plate has a thin membranous origin at the head of the palmar metacarpal and a thick fibrocartilaginous insertion at the palmar base of the proximal phalanx. This arrangement increases the cavity of the MCP joint during flexion, and also restricts the amount of hyperextension that can occur during extension of the metacarpophalangeal joint.

The collateral ligaments originate on the dorsal side of the metacarpal and extend obliquely to insert on the palmar base of the proximal phalanx. One ligament is found on each side of the MCP joint (radial and ulnar sides). During flexion of the MCP joint, the collateral ligaments become taut and prevent side-to-side movements from occurring at the joint. In extension, the collateral ligaments become slack, permitting abduction/adduction and some rotational movements at the MCP joint.

It has been noted that the movements at the MCP are flexion/extension and abduction/adduction. The movements of abduction and adduction (Fig. 5.10) require further explanation in that it is conventional to use the long finger of the hand as the reference position for these actions. When the fingers or thumb are spread away from the long finger, abduction is occurring. When the fingers are closed on the long finger, adduction is occurring. Side to side movements of the long finger are referred to as **radial deviation** (radial flexion) and **ulnar deviation** (ulnar flexion), as shown in Fig. 5.10.

Movements of the Fingers in the Frontal Plane

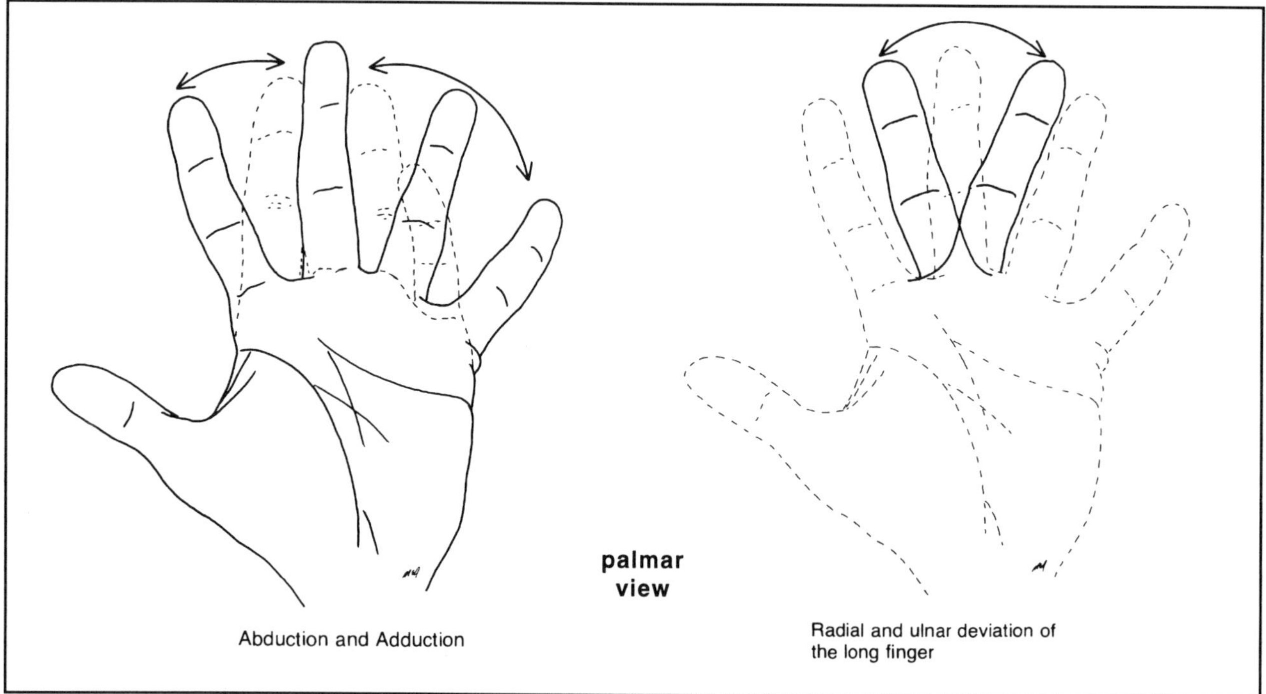

Fig. 5.10

INTERPHALANGEAL JOINTS

The interphalangeal joints are those joints between the phalanges of the fingers and thumb. There are two interphalangeal joints in each finger; the joint between the proximal and middle phalanges is the proximal interphalangeal (abbreviated *PIP*) joint, and the joint between the middle and distal phalanges is the distal interphalangeal (*DIP*) joint. Since there is only one such joint in the thumb, it is referred to simply as the interphalangeal (*IP*) joint of the thumb.

All of the interphalangeal joints are of the hinge type, and permit flexion and extension around axes which pass from side to side through the joints. The ligaments of the joints are the **volar plate**, and the **radial and ulnar collateral** ligaments. These ligaments are arranged in similar fashion to those of the MCP joints while the extensor hood protects the dorsal aspect of the interphalangeal joints. As in the MCP joint, the volar plates of the interphalangeal joints restrict hyperextension. However, unlike the MCP joint, the collateral ligaments of the interphalangeal joints restrict side-to-side movements during flexion and extension. Along with the volar plates, the collateral ligaments also assist in limiting extension at the interphalangeal joints.

Compared to the MCP joint, little hyperextension is present at the PIP joint. The volar plate is stronger here and is further reinforced by attachment of the flexor sheath. At the DIP joint, the volar plate is weaker thus permitting greater hyperextension during pinching movements between the thumb and digits.

During flexion, limited rotation of the interphalangeal joints may be observed. As the MCP, PIP, and DIP joints are flexed, the three digits on the ulnar side of the hand may be seen converging toward the thumb. The range of flexion at the interphalangeal joints is noted to increase finger by finger to the ulnar side. In other words, the range of flexion at the interphalangeal joints of the index finger will be less than the range of flexion at the interphalangeal joints of the small finger.

THE EXTENSOR MECHANISM

The extensor mechanism, also referred to as the extensor hood, extensor expansion, extensor apparatus, or dorsal finger apparatus, is a complex structure that deserves further discussion. The extensor tendon is a superficial, flat structure that has an excursion which is considerably less than that of the flexor tendons. These tendons are not surrounded by a synovial sheath and, when injured, have a high incidence of becoming adherent to underlying bones and joints. When the excursion of the tendon is compromised in this way, it is more difficult to compensate for the loss of its length than would be the case for a flexor tendon.

The extrinsic extensor system (Fig. 5.11a and b) runs along the dorsum of the digit and has four sites of insertion. The most proximal insertion is at the level of the MCP joint on the sagittal bands. The base of the proximal phalanx serves as the second insertion site. The next site is located at the base of the middle phalanx and is commonly referred to as the central slip. The distal site of insertion is at the base of the distal phalanx and is called the terminal insertion. When the extensor digitorum contracts, force is distributed across all three phalanges of each finger.

Extensor Mechanism

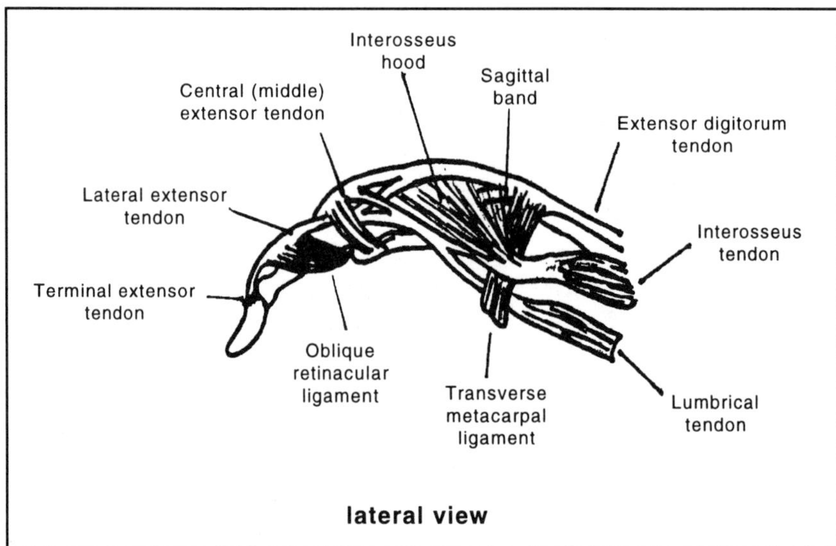

Fig. 5.11a

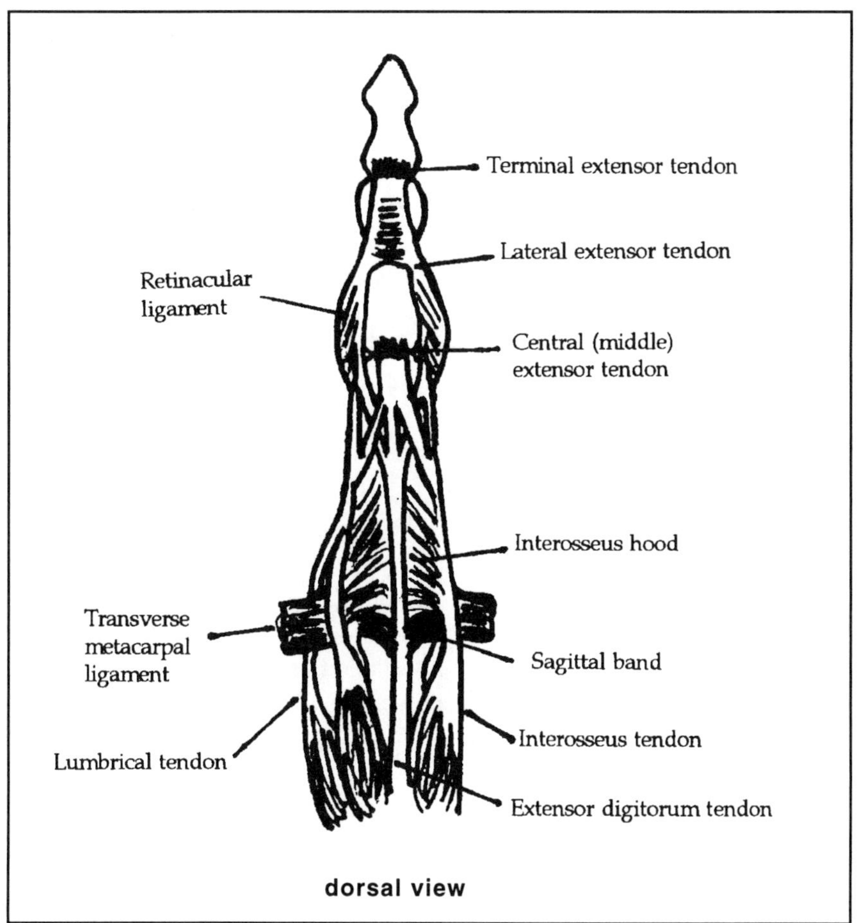

Fig. 5.11b

Extensor Mechanism

The interossei and lumbricales are also responsible for extension at the IP joints. The tendinous insertions of these muscles begin to converge onto the extensor mechanism, at the level of the middle phalanx, where they form a junction and insert with the central slip and the terminal insertion. These intrinsic muscles lie to the palmar side of the flexion/extension axis at the MCP joints and are, therefore, flexors of the joints. As they progress distally along the digits, the tendons begin to assume a dorsal orientation to the flexion/extension axis of the PIP and DIP joints and now, act as extensors of these joints. Extension of both interphalangeal joints occurs simultaneously and is caused by an active pull on the extensor mechanism by the interossei or lumbricales. Extension of the IP joints can only occur if there is tension at the extensor digitorum; otherwise, the interossei and lumbricales would not have a firm base on which to execute their pull.

The thumb has one interphalangeal joint which is extended by extrinsic extensor muscles (extensor pollicis longus and extensor pollicis brevis) in a fashion similar to that of the extensor mechanism. As in the digits, intrinsic muscles also assist with extension of the IP joint of the thumb. This extension is produced by the dorsal expansion of the abductor pollicis brevis and adductor pollicis.

MUSCLES OF THE WRIST AND HAND

The twenty-five muscles or muscle groups which are movers of the joints of the wrist and hand have been categorized as extrinsic and intrinsic muscles. The extrinsic muscles are those which have their muscle bellies between the elbow and the wrist, and their tendinous insertions in the hand. These fifteen muscles may be further grouped into extrinsic flexor and extensor muscles of the wrist and hand. The extrinsic extensor muscles make up the six dorsal compartments discussed earlier in this chapter. The extrinsic muscles are:

Extrinsic Flexor Muscles	***Extrinsic Extensor Muscles***
Flexor Carpi Ulnaris (FCU) Flexor Carpi Radialis (FCR) Palmaris Longus (PL) Flexor Pollicis Longus (FPL) Flexor Digitorum Superficialis (FDS) Flexor Digitorum Profundus (FDP)	Extensor Pollicis Brevis (EPB) Abductor Pollicis Longus (APL) Extensor Carpi Radialis Longus (ECRL) Extensor Carpi Radialis Brevis (ECRB) Extensor Pollicis Longus (EPL) Extensor Digitorum (ED) Extensor Indicis (EI) Extensor Digiti Minimi (EDM) Extensor Carpi Ulnaris (ECU)

The intrinsic muscles are the ten muscles or muscle groups which originate and insert within the hand. Four of the intrinsics are thumb or thenar muscles and form the palmar muscle mass on the radial side of the hand called the **thenar eminence**. Three intrinsics are movers of the small finger and form the **hypothenar eminence** which is the fleshy part of the palm on the ulnar side of the hand. The remaining intrinsics are muscle groups located between the metacarpals. The intrinsics are:

Lumbricales **Interossei** (palmar and dorsal) **Adductor Pollicis** (AP)	***Thenar Muscles***	***Hypothenar Muscles***
	Abductor Pollicis Brevis (APB) Opponens Pollicis (OP) Flexor Pollicis Brevis (FPB)	Abductor Digiti Minimi (ADM) Flexor Digiti Minimi (FDM) Opponens Digiti Minimi (ODM)

EXTRINSIC FLEXOR MUSCLES

Flexor Carpi Ulnaris (flex'or car'pi ulna'ris)

The flexor carpi ulnaris (Fig. 5.12) is a superficial muscle located on the palmar aspect of the ulna. Its tendon is palpable just proximal to the pisiform bone when a firm fist is made or when one is asked to flex the wrist.

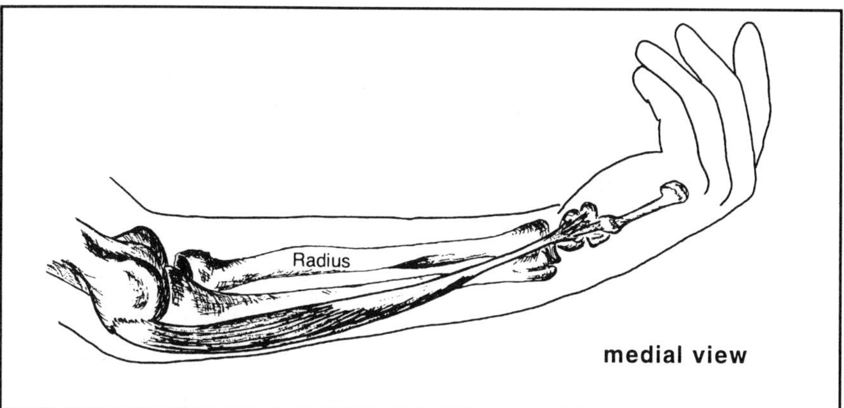

Flexor Carpi Ulnaris

Fig. 5.12

Origin	By two heads, humeral and ulnar, from the medial epicondyle of the humerus by the common flexor tendon, and the upper two-thirds of the dorsal border of the ulna including the olecranon process.
Insertion	Pisiform and hamate bones, and the palmar surface of the base of the fifth metacarpal.
Innervation	Ulnar nerve.
Action	Flexion and ulnar deviation of the wrist joint.

The flexor carpi ulnaris crosses the wrist joint anterior to the flexion/extension axis and to the ulnar side of the deviation axis, and, therefore, contributes significantly to both flexion and ulnar deviation. In the latter action, it shares responsibility with the extensor carpi ulnaris and, in so doing, neutralizes that muscle's tendency to extend the wrist as it contracts. This muscle is needed during activities which require sustained power grip (i.e., hammer or axe stroke).

Flexor Carpi Radialis (flex'or car'pi radia'lis)

The flexor carpi radialis (Fig. 5.13) is a slender muscle on the palmar aspect of the forearm. Its tendon is palpable on the radial side of the tendon of the palmaris longus, and is particularly prominent when one performs resisted radial deviation and flexion.

Flexor Carpi Radialis

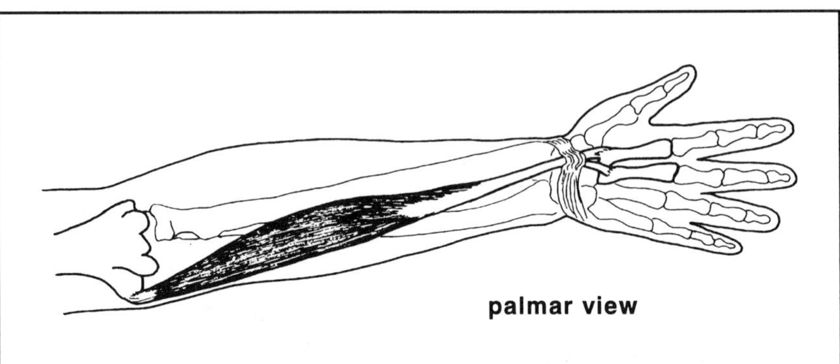

Fig. 5.13

Origin — Medial epicondyle of the humerus by the common tendon.
Insertion — Palmar surface of the base of the second metacarpal with a slip to the base of the third metacarpal.
Innervation — Median nerve.
Action — Flexion and radial deviation of the wrist joint.

The flexor carpi radialis crosses the wrist joint anterior to the flexion/ extension axis and to the radial side of the radial and ulnar deviation axis. Even though the muscle is well located to perform its two actions, it is only 60% as strong as the flexor carpi ulnaris.

Palmaris Longus (palma'ris lon'gus)

The palmaris longus (Fig. 5.14) is a small fusiform muscle located superficially on the palmar aspect of the forearm. The muscle is absent in 10 to 15 percent of people, but, if it is present, is easily palpated and observed between the flexor carpi radialis and flexor carpi ulnaris at the wrist when the thumb is opposed to the small finger with the wrist flexed.

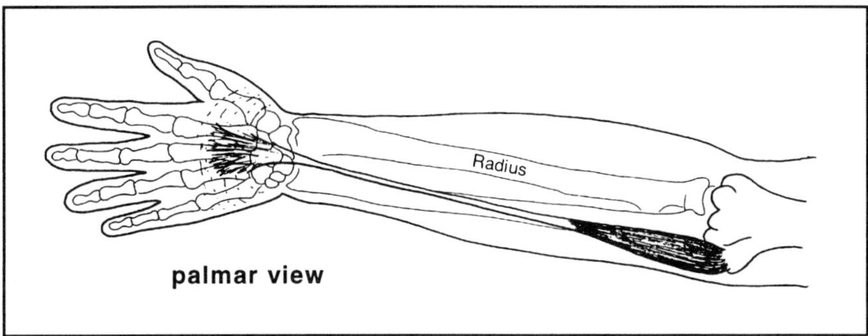

Palmaris Longus

Fig. 5.14

Origin ——	Medial epicondyle of the humerus, by the common flexor tendon.
Insertion ——	Flexor retinaculum.
Innervation –	Median nerve.
Action ——	Flexion of the wrist joint.

The palmaris longus is in a favorable position to flex the wrist since it crosses the wrist joint farther from the flexion/extension axis than any other flexor. The muscle is so small, however, that, even with its long force arm, it can contribute only weak flexion to the joint. Because of its insertion into the flexor retinaculum, the palmaris longus assists in the cupping movements of the palm during grasp.

Flexor Pollicis Longus (flex'or pol'licis lon'gus)

The flexor pollicis longus (Fig. 5.15), a penniform muscle, lies deep on the radial side of the forearm. Its tendon can be palpated on the palmar surface of the thumb between the MCP and IP joints as the IP joint is flexed.

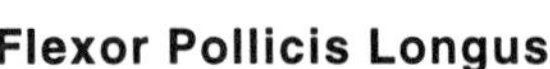

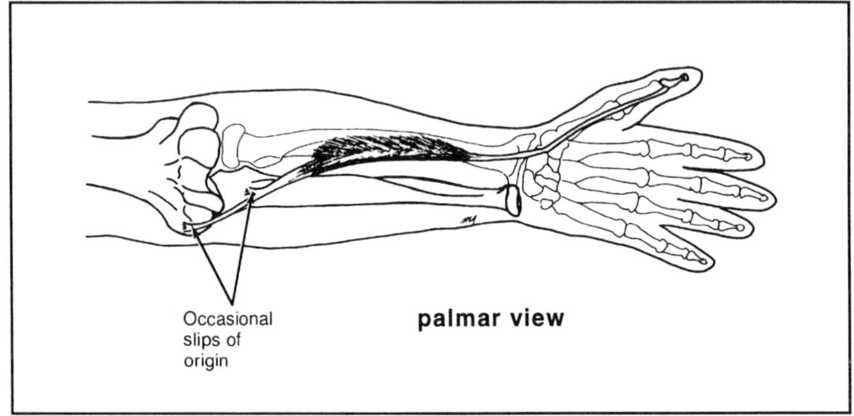

Fig. 5.15

Origin	Palmar surface of the middle half of the radius.
Insertion	Palmar surface of the base of the distal phalanx ofthe thumb.
Innervation	Anterior interosseous branch of the median nerve.
Action	Flexes the interphalangeal joint, and by continued contraction, flexes the metacarpophalangeal joint of the thumb; flexes the carpometacarpal joint when resistance is applied.

The tendon of the flexor pollicis longus crosses the IP and MCP joints of the thumb to the palmar side of the flexion/extension axes of those joints to act as a flexor. In addition, the tendon passes to the ulnar side of the CMC axis of flexion/extension to act as a flexor of that joint. The muscle is not credited with wrist joint movement because it lies quite close to both wrist axes and because its contraction powers are largely spent by the time it flexes the three joints of the thumb.

Flexor Digitorum Superficialis (flex'or digito'rum superficia'lis)

The flexor digitorum superficialis (Fig. 5.16) is the largest of the flexor muscles of the forearm group. Its tendons can be palpated and observed on the palmar surface of the wrist between the tendons of the flexor carpi radialis and the flexor carpi ulnaris. The tendons may be seen to move within their sheaths as the fingers are flexed to make a fist.

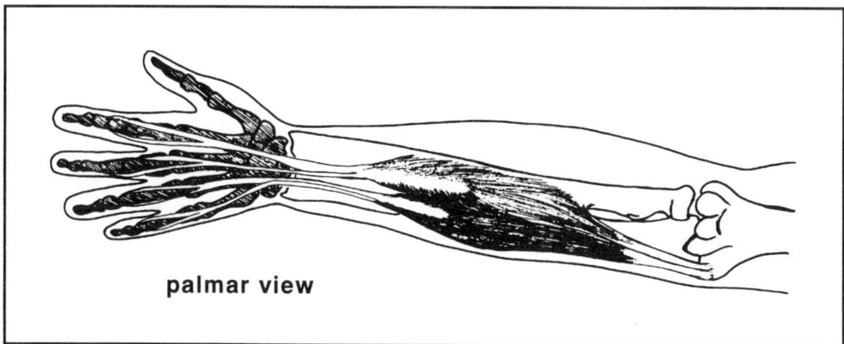

Flexor Digitorum Superficialis

Fig. 5.16

Origin ——	By three heads -- humeral, ulnar, and radial -- from the medial epicondyle of the humerus by the common flexor tendon; the medial aspect of the coronoid process; and the oblique line of the radius.
Insertion ——	By four tendons to the sides of the base of the middle phalanges of the four fingers.
Innervation—	Median nerve.
Action ——	Flexion of the metacarpophalangeal and proximal interphalangeal joints of the four fingers; assists in flexion of the wrist.

The flexor digitorum superficialis crosses the wrist, metacarpophalangeal , and proximal interphalangeal joints anterior to the flexion/extension axes of these joints. When all of these joints are flexed, the superficialis has contracted to its shortest length; conversely, when these joints are extended, the muscle is stretched to its fullest.

This muscle may be tested by asking one to flex the PIP joint of one of the four fingers (i.e., the index finger). The other three fingers must be stabilized by the examiner so that profundus function is occluded as the four digits share a common muscle belly. When performing flexion of the PIP joint of the index finger, stabilizing these remaining digits will produce isolated action of the flexor digitorum superficialis at that joint.

Flexor Digitorum Profundus (flex'or digito'rum profun'dus)

The flexor digitorum profundus (Fig. 5.17) lies deep on the palmar surface of the forearm. Its tendons are deep also as they cross the wrist and hand and cannot be palpated.

Flexor Digitorum Profundus

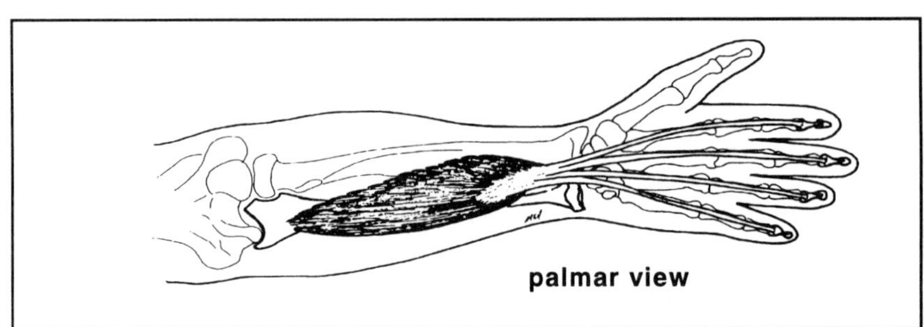

Fig. 5.17

Origin — Upper three-fourths of the ulna.
Insertion — By four tendons, to the base of the distal phalanx of each of the four fingers.
Innervation — Index, middle, and 1/2 ring finders by the anterior interosseous branch of the median nerve; 1/2 ring finger and small finger by the ulnar nerve.
Action — Flexion of the distal interphalangeal joints of the four fingers and, by continued contraction, flexes the proximal interphalangeal joints, then the metacarpophalangeal joints, and finally the wrist joint.

The flexor digitorum profundus provides a line of pull which is to the palmar side of the flexion/extension axis of each of the joints it crosses. Its only action at these joints is, therefore, flexion which progresses sequentially from the most distal of the joints (the DIP joint) to the most proximal (wrist joint). The strength of its contraction lessens progressively from joint to joint since the muscle must become gradually shorter; it, therefore, can contribute only weakly to wrist flexion. Its contribution at the wrist can be enhanced, however, by holding the MCP and IP joints of the fingers in extension to prevent excessive shortening of the fibers. This should be remembered when testing for range of motion of the wrist. Instruct the patient to extend the fingers when measuring for flexion. The action of the flexor digitorum profundus may be observed when one is asked to flex the DIP joint with the PIP joint stabilized in extension.

Unlike the flexor digitorum superficialis, the flexor digitorum profundus has only a single muscle belly, and tends to cause movement in all fingers simultaneously. This can be seen easily as one attempts to flex all joints of the long finger. Invariably, the ring finger moves also, as would the index and small fingers were it not for the neutralizing action of the extensor indicis and extensor digiti minimi. The profundus to the index finger has a relatively small connection with the profundus to the middle finger, however, and for the most part, is independent. The flexor digitorum profundus of the middle, ring, and small fingers have little independence from one another, and therefore tend to move simultaneously.

EXTRINSIC EXTENSOR MUSCLES

Extensor Pollicis Brevis (exten'sor pol'licis bre'vis)

The extensor pollicis brevis (Fig. 5.18) lies beneath and to the radial side of the extensor pollicis longus. Its tendon emerges to be superficial as it crosses the wrist joint and may be palpated and observed on the radial side of the extensor pollicis longus during forced extension of the thumb. These two tendons form the "anatomical snuff box" of the hand.

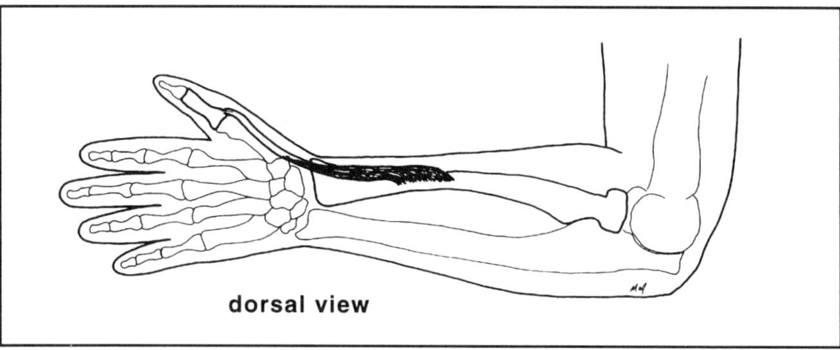

Extensor Pollicis Brevis

Fig. 5.18

Origin —— Dorsal surface of the radius at its midpoint.
Insertion —— Dorsal surface of the base of the proximal phalanx of the thumb.
Innervation — Deep radial nerve.
Action —— Extension of the metacarpophalangeal joint of the thumb; extension of the carpometacarpal joint; radial deviation of the wrist.

The actions of the extensor pollicis brevis differ from those of the extensor pollicis longus in three respects: (1) the tendon of the extensor pollicis longus crosses the wrist joint posterior to the axis of flexion/extension to become a wrist extensor; the tendon of extensor pollicis brevis crosses directly over that axis and is ineffective as an abductor or adductor of that joint; (2) the tendon of the extensor pollicis longus passes dorsal to the axis of abduction/adduction of the carpometacarpal joint to act as an adductor; the tendon of extensor pollicis brevis crosses directly over the axis and is ineffective as an abductor or adductor of that joint; (3) the tendon of the extensor pollicis brevis does not cross the IP joint of the thumb as does the tendon of extensor pollicis longus. The brevis has, therefore, no action at that joint.

Abductor Pollicis Longus (abduc'tor pol'licis lon'gus)

The abductor pollicis longus (Fig. 5.19) is a deep muscle lying on the dorsal aspect of the forearm just distal to the supinator. Its tendon is superficial as it crosses the wrist joint and may be palpated to the palmar side of the tendon of the extensor pollicis brevis when the thumb is forcefully abducted.

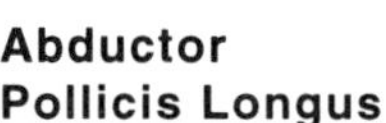

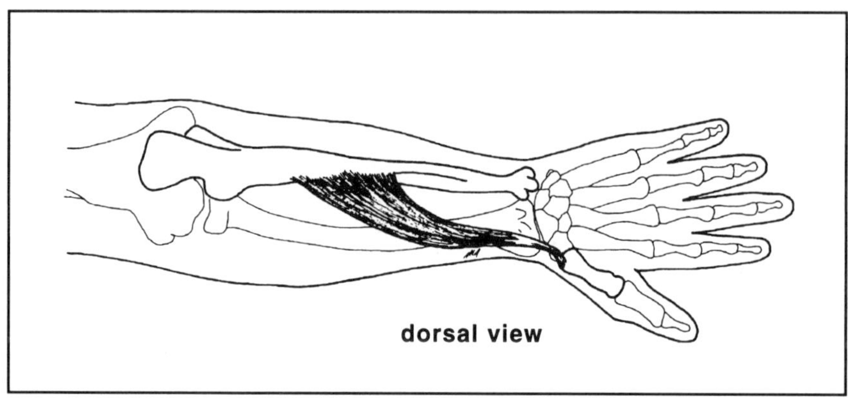

Fig. 5.19

Origin	Middle third of the dorsal surface of the radius and ulna.
Insertion	Radial side of the base of the first metacarpal.
Innervation	Deep radial nerve.
Action	Abduction and extension of the carpometacarpal joint of the thumb and, by continued contraction, radial deviation and flexion of the wrist joint.

The abductor pollicis longus crosses only the wrist joint and CMC joint of the thumb. Its tendon is centered directly above the flexion/extension axis of the wrist when in anatomical position, but as the wrist is flexed the tendon "bowstrings" below the axis which allows it to contribute to increased flexion. The muscle is well to the radial side of the deviation axis of that joint. The tendon is to the radial side of the abduction/adduction axis of the CMC joint to become an abductor and, because of its insertion on the radial side of the metacarpal is able to pull the thumb into extension. In summary, contraction of the abductor pollicis longus will cause abduction and extension of the CMC joint followed by radial deviation and flexion of the wrist joint.

Extensor Carpi Radialis Longus (exten'sor car'pi radia'lis lon'gus)

The extensor carpi radialis longus (Fig. 5.20) is a partially superficial muscle located on the dorsal surface of the forearm. Its muscular portion may be palpated just above the elbow as the wrist is forcefully extended. Its tendon is prominent also during this action and can be palpated over the dorsiradial aspect of the wrist.

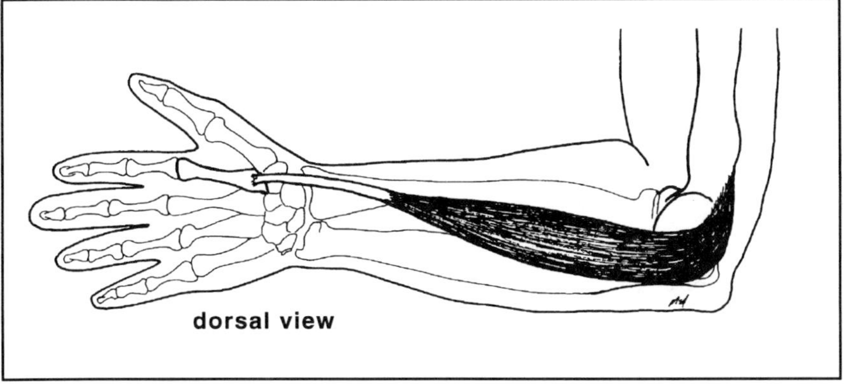

Extensor Carpi Radialis Longus

Fig. 5.20

Origin	Distal third of the supracondylar ridge; lateral epicondyle of the humerus by the common extensor tendon.
Insertion	Dorsal surface of the base of the second metacarpal.
Innervation	Radial nerve.
Action	Extension and radial deviation of the wrist joint.

The actions of the extensor carpi radialis longus are logical ones, and follow from the location of the muscle to the wrist axes as it crosses that joint. It is posterior to the flexion/extension axis and to the radial side of the deviation axis. It is most effective as a wrist extensor when the elbow is extended.

Extensor Carpi Radialis Brevis (exten'sor car'pi radia'lis bre'vis)

The muscular portion of the extensor carpi radialis brevis (Fig. 5.21) is covered in its proximal part by the extensor carpi radialis longus. It is superficial on the dorsal surface of the middle forearm and may be palpated there if care is taken not to confuse it with the extensor digitorum. Its tendon is also difficult to identify because it is crossed by the tendons of the abductor pollicis longus and the extensor pollicis longus, but it can usually be felt proximal to its insertion if the thumb is placed in the palm of the hand and alternately flexed and relaxed at its interphalangeal joint. In addition, it may be palpated on the dorsiradial aspect of the wrist during fisted wrist extension.

Extensor Carpi Radialis Brevis

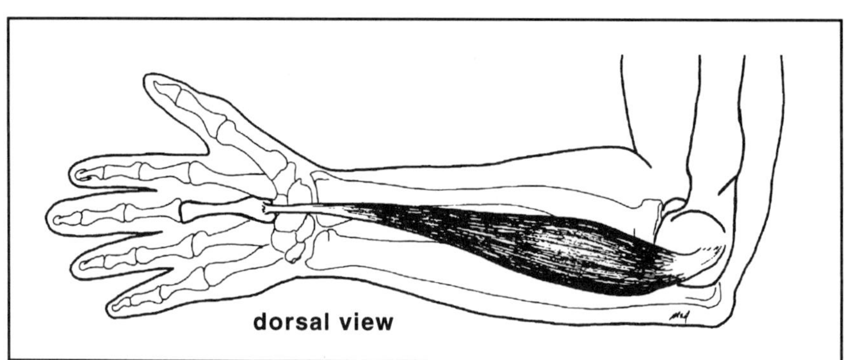

Fig. 5.21

Origin ——	Lateral epicondyle of the humerus by the common extensor tendon; and radial collateral ligament.
Insertion ——	Dorsal surface of the base of the third metacarpal.
Innervation —	Radial nerve.
Action ——	Extension and weak radial deviation of the wrist joint.

The extensor carpi radialis brevis crosses well posterior to the flexion/extension axis of the wrist; however, it courses very close to the deviation axis and thus has scant contribution to radial deviation. The method of palpating the tendon of this muscle attests to its central location in the wrist, because as the thumb is brought toward the palm and then flexed, the palmaris longus contracts to tense the flexor retinaculum. The extensor carpi radialis brevis contracts to prevent the palmaris longus from also flexing the wrist. There is some evidence that "tennis elbow" is caused by inflammation and microscopic tears of this muscle in the vicinity of its origin. The extensor carpi radialis longus lies over the origin of the brevis and, until recently, has effectively hidden it as one of the causes of tennis elbow pain. Tennis elbow is discussed more fully in Chapter 4.

Extensor Pollicis Longus (exten'sor pol'licis lon'gus)

The extensor pollicis longus (Fig. 5.22) is located on the dorsal surface of the forearm. Its muscular portion is difficult to palpate; however, its tendon is clearly prominent when the thumb is fully extended. This tendon may also be evaluated by placing the palmar surface of the hand on a table; from this position the thumb is lifted off the table.

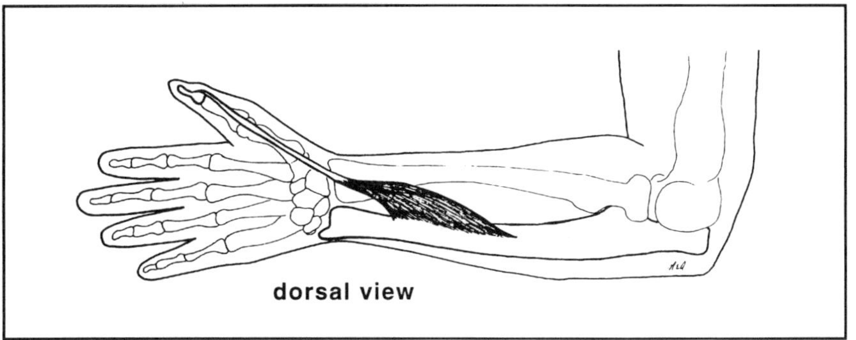

Extensor Pollicis Longus

Fig. 5.22

Origin — Middle third of the ulna on its dorsal surface.
Insertion — Dorsal surface of base of distal phalanx of the thumb.
Innervation — Deep radial nerve.
Action — Extension of the metacarpophalangeal and interphalangeal joints of the thumb; reposition (adduction and extension) of the carpometacarpal joint; contributes to wrist extension and radial deviation.

The actions of the extensor pollicis longus are several and at first sight may seem difficult to learn. All the actions are straight forward, however, when the respective muscles are viewed with reference to the axes of the joints they cross. At the wrist joint, the tendon of the extensor pollicis longus courses posterior to the flexion/extension axis and to the radial side of the deviation axis to perform the actions of extension and radial deviation. At the CMC joint, the tendon passes to the radial side of the flexion/extension axis to perform extension, and dorsal to the abduction/adduction axis to act as an adductor. The reposition function results from the fact that reposition is a combination movement comprised of adduction and extension. At the metacarpophalangeal and interphalangeal joints, the tendon passes dorsal to the flexion/extension axes to extend the joints.

Extensor Digitorum (exten'sor digito'rum)

The extensor digitorum (extensor digitorum communis) (Fig. 5.23) is a fusiform muscle located on the dorsal surface of the forearm. It can be palpated in its entirety except where it is covered proximally by the extensor carpi radialis longus. Its four tendons are easily observed and palpated as they cross the second, third, fourth, and fifth metacarpophalangeal joints; they are particularly prominent when the metacarpophalangeal joints are fully extended to arch the hand.

Extensor Digitorum

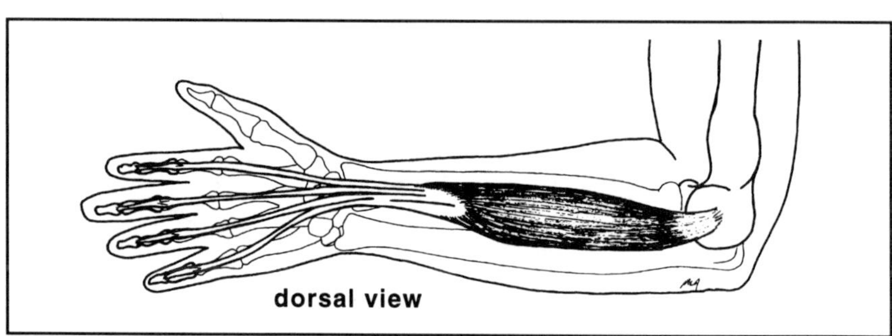

Fig. 5.23

Origin	Lateral epicondyle of the humerus by the common extensor tendon.
Insertion	By four tendons to the bases of the second and third phalanges of the four fingers.
Innervation	Deep radial nerve.
Action	Extension of the metacarpophalangeal joint, and the proximal and distal interphalangeal joints of the four fingers; and if contraction is continued, extension of the wrist joint.

The extensor digitorum crosses more joints than any other muscle of the forearm group. If all of these joints -- wrist, metacarpophalangeal, proximal interphalangeal, and distal interphalangeal -- are simultaneously extended, the muscle is contracted to its shortest length and is only weakly responsive at the wrist joint. Strength will be quickly restored, however, if the extensor digitorum is lengthened by flexing the PIP and DIP joints of the fingers.

Simultaneous flexion of the wrist, MCP, PIP and DIP joints forces the extensor digitorum to stretch to its fullest; in fact, the extensor digitorum is unable to lengthen sufficiently to allow full flexion at all joints, as can be observed if a firm fist is made followed by an attempt to fully flex the wrist. Full flexion of the wrist can only be performed if the fingers are allowed to uncurl. This principle is used in self-defense to disarm opponents, since by forcing the wrist into flexion, the grip on the weapon is loosened. It is important to remember this principle, also, when testing for range of motion of the wrist. Unless the patient is instructed to uncurl the fingers while flexing the wrist, the measurement will be less than true.

Extensor Indicis (exten'sor in'dicis)

The extensor indicis (extensor indicis proprius) (Fig. 5.24) is a long slender muscle lying deep on the dorsal aspect of the forearm. Its tendon is superficial and can be observed running on the ulnar side of but parallel to the tendon of the extensor digitorum as it approaches the base of the index finger.

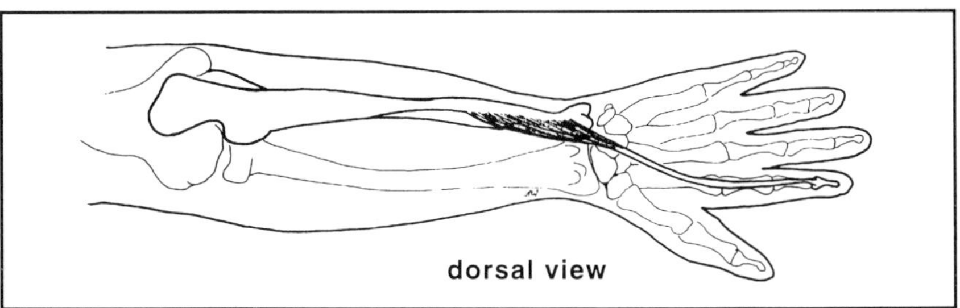

Extensor Indicis

Fig. 5.24

Origin —	Dorsal surface of the lower half of the ulna.
Insertion —	Ulnar side of the tendon of the extensor digitorum opposite the second metacarpophalangeal joint.
Innervation —	Deep radial nerve.
Action —	Extension of the second metacarpophalangeal joint with contribution to adduction of that joint. Through the extensor hood, the muscle contributes also to extension of the proximal and distal interphalangeal joints of the index finger. Continued contraction of the muscle assists in wrist extension.

Contraction of the extensor indicis results initially in extension of the MCP joint of the index finger, followed by extension of the PIP and DIP joints and finally extension of the wrist joint. If the MCP joint is held in flexion, however, the muscle's ability to extend the IP joints and then the wrist will be enhanced; if the MCP and IP joints are all held in flexion, the muscle will become an effective wrist extensor. The extensor indicis may be seen acting alone when one is asked to extend the index finger with the other digits flexed into the palm.

That the extensor indicis contributes to adduction of the index finger can be observed by forcefully extending the index finger at the MCP and IP joints. As noted above under palpation procedures, the tendon of the extensor indicis runs parallel to but on the ulnar side of the tendon of the extensor digitorum. The muscle is, thus, just to the ulnar side of the abduction/adduction axis, making it a weak adductor.

Extensor Digiti Minimi (exten'sor dig'iti min'imi)

The extensor digiti minimi (Fig. 5.25) is a long slender muscle located to the ulnar side of the extensor digitorum. The muscle emerges to become superficial slightly proximal to the wrist; its tendon can be palpated and observed on the dorsum of the hand, and especially at the fifth MCP joint when the small finger is extended against resistance. The extensor digiti minimi may be seen acting alone when one is asked to extend the small finger with the remaining digits flexed into the palm.

Extensor Digiti Minimi

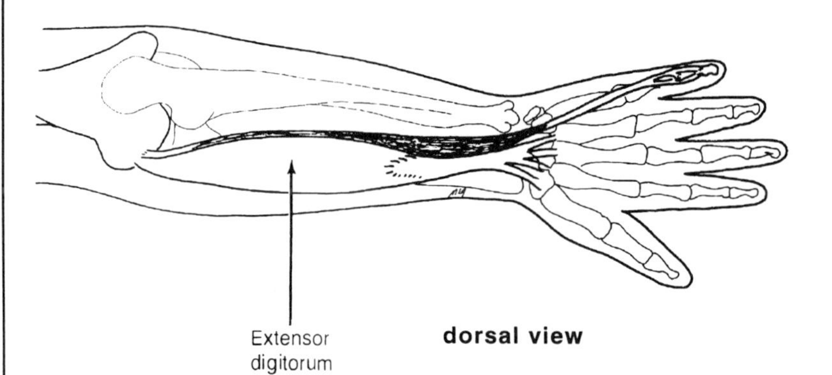

Fig. 5.25

Origin — Proximal tendon of the extensor digitorum.

Insertion — Tendon of the extensor digitorum at a point just distal to the fifth metacarpophalangeal joint.

Innervation — Deep radial nerve.

Action — Extension of the fifth metacarpophalangeal joint and, with continued contraction, contributes to wrist extension. The muscle also extends the two interphalangeal joints of the small finger by acting upon the hood of the extensor mechanism.

Extensor Carpi Ulnaris (exten'sor car'pi ulna'ris)

The extensor carpi ulnaris (Fig. 5.26) is located superficially on the ulnar side of the dorsum of the forearm. Its muscular portion may be palpated next to the anconeus as the wrist is forcefully extended. Its tendon will be prominent just distal to the ulnar styloid process if a fist is made as the wrist is extended and ulnarly deviated.

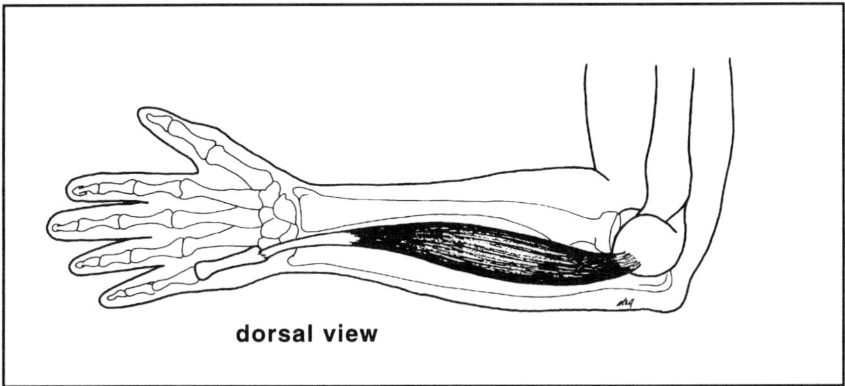

Extensor Carpi Ulnaris

Fig. 5.26

Origin	Lateral epicondyle of the humerus by the common extensor tendon; and the middle third of the dorsal border of the ulna.
Insertion	Ulnar side of the base of the fifth metacarpal.
Innervation	Deep radial nerve.
Action	Extension and ulnar deviation of the wrist joint.

Crossing to the posterior and ulnar sides of the two axes of the wrist joint, the extensor carpi ulnaris is well located to perform its actions. Its ability in ulnar deviation is particularly efficient because the wedge-like flare at the base of the fifth metacarpal increases the angle of the muscle's attachment. This muscle provides stability to the head of the ulna during wrist movements. It is a more effective wrist extensor when the forearm is supinated and a stronger ulnar deviator of the wrist when the forearm is pronated.

INTRINSIC MUSCLES

Flexor Pollicis Brevis (flex'or pol'licis bre'vis)

The flexor pollicis brevis (Fig. 5.27) is comprised of both a deep portion and a superficial portion. The superficial fibers may be palpated along the ulnar border of the thenar eminence during resisted flexion of the metacarpophalangeal joint of the thumb.

Origin	Deep head: Ulnar surface of first metacarpal. Superficial head: Multangulus major (trapezium) and adjacent portion of flexor retinaculum.
Insertion	Deep head: Ulnar side of the palmar surface of the base of the proximal phalanx of the thumb. Superficial head: Radial side of the palmar surface of the proximal phalanx of the thumb.
Innervation	Deep head: Deep ulnar nerve. Superficial head: Median nerve.
Action	Both heads: Flexion of the metacarpophalangeal joint of the thumb. Deep head: Adduction of the metacarpophalangeal joint of the thumb. Superficial head: Flexion of the carpometacarpal joint.

Flexor Pollicis Brevis

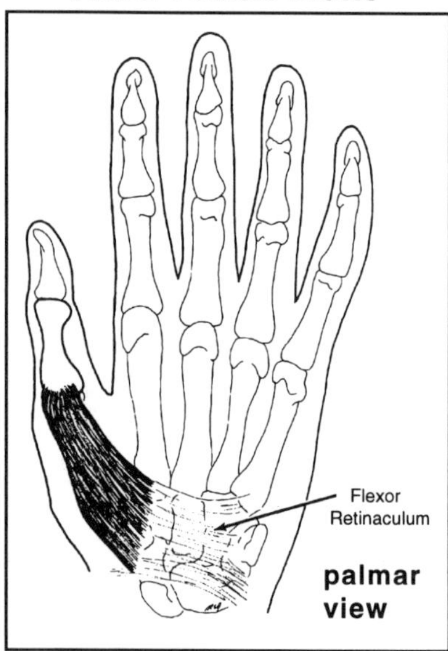

Fig. 5.27

The two heads of the flexor pollicis brevis, with their insertions on the palmar surface of the proximal phalanx, cross the flexion/extension axis of the MCP joint well to the palmar side to become effective flexors of that joint. The deep head of the muscle, as it courses between its two attachments, crosses only the MCP joint, and is located to the ulnar side of the abduction/adduction axis of the MCP joint to be additionally active as an adductor of that joint. The superficial head crosses both the MCP and CMC joints of the thumb. At the latter joint, the muscle lies to the palmar side of the flexion/extension axis, and slightly medial to the opposition/reposition axis, to function as both a flexor and a weak opposer. Being inserted on the radial side of the proximal phalanx, the muscle would appear to be capable of abducting the metacarpal joint; however, study of a skeleton will confirm that the muscle runs directly across that axis and cannot contribute significantly to any side-to-side movement at that joint. A small portion of the flexor pollicis brevis and adductor pollicis attaches on the extensor expansion of the thumb and therefore they contribute to extension of the interphalangeal joint.

Abductor Pollicis Brevis (abduc'tor pol'licis bre'vis)

The abductor pollicis brevis (Fig. 5.28) is the most superficial muscle of the thenar eminence. It may be palpated in the center of the eminence during resisted abduction of the carpometacarpal joint of the thumb.

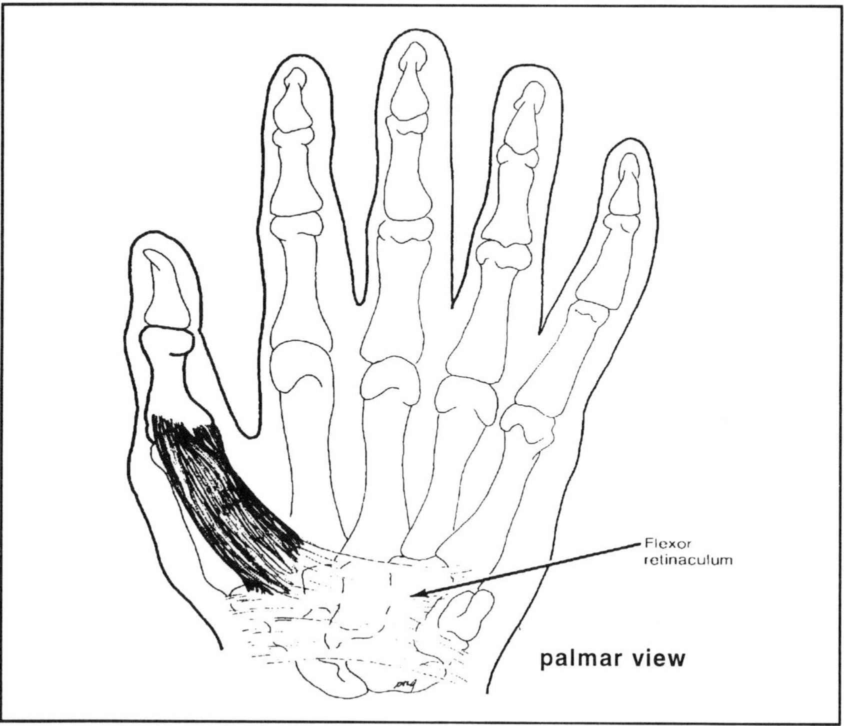

Abductor Pollicis Brevis

Fig. 5.28

Origin	Multangulus major (trapezium) and navicular (scaphoid) bones, and adjacent portion of flexor retinaculum.
Insertion	Radial side of the base of the first phalanx of the thumb.
Innervation	Median nerve.
Action	Abduction of the carpometacarpal joint of the thumb; flexion and abduction of the metacarpophalangeal joint of the thumb.

The abductor pollicis brevis and the superficial head of the flexor pollicis brevis have similar lines of pull; however, the origin of the abductor pollicis brevis is somewhat more to the radial side of the hand than the flexor pollicis brevis. By this slight lateral displacement, the abductor pollicis brevis is made to be ineffectual as a mover around all but the abduction/adduction axis of the CMC joint; and, being well to the palmar side of this axis, it is a strong abductor. At the MCP joint, the muscle crosses both to palmar side of the flexion/extension axis and to the radial side of the abduction/adduction axis. Since the muscle must share its strength between both axes, it is only an assistive mover in either of the actions of flexion or abduction.

Opponens Pollicis (oppo'nens pol'licis)

The opponens pollicis (Fig. 5.29) is located beneath the abductor pollicis brevis. It is superficial along the radial border of the thenar eminence next to the first metacarpal and can be palpated when the thumb is pressed firmly against the tip of the long finger.

Opponens Pollicis

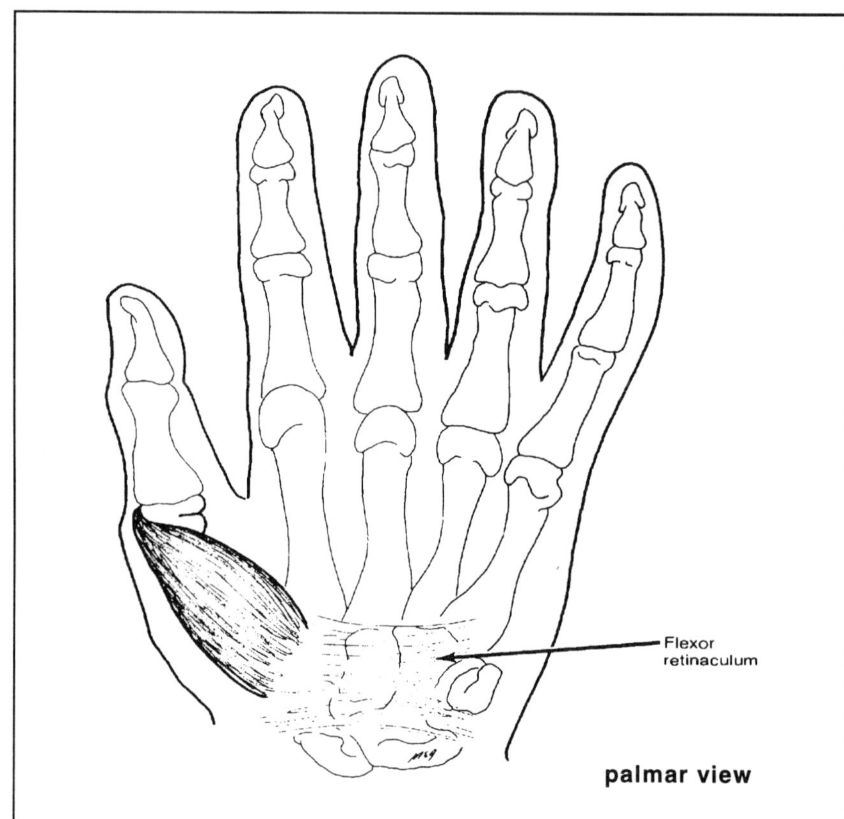

Fig. 5.29

Origin —— Multangulus major (trapezium) and adjacent portion of flexor retinaculum.
Insertion —— Radial surface of entire length of the first metacarpal.
Innervation— Medial nerve.
Action —— Opposition of the carpometacarpal joint of the thumb; contributes to abduction and flexion of that joint.

The opponens pollicis is triangular in shape and located so that its uppermost fibers are in a favorable position to cause flexion of the CMC joint, while its lowermost fibers are situated to cause abduction. When the muscle contracts, it performs both actions, and opposition results.

Adductor Pollicis (adduc'tor pol'licis)

The adductor pollicis (Fig. 5.30) lies deep in the palm of the hand but emerges to be superficial just before its insertion. It can be palpated between the first and second metacarpals as the thumb is pressed firmly against the tip of the index finger. This muscle may also be evaluated by asking one to hold a piece of paper between the thumb and radial aspect of proximal phalanx of the index finger.

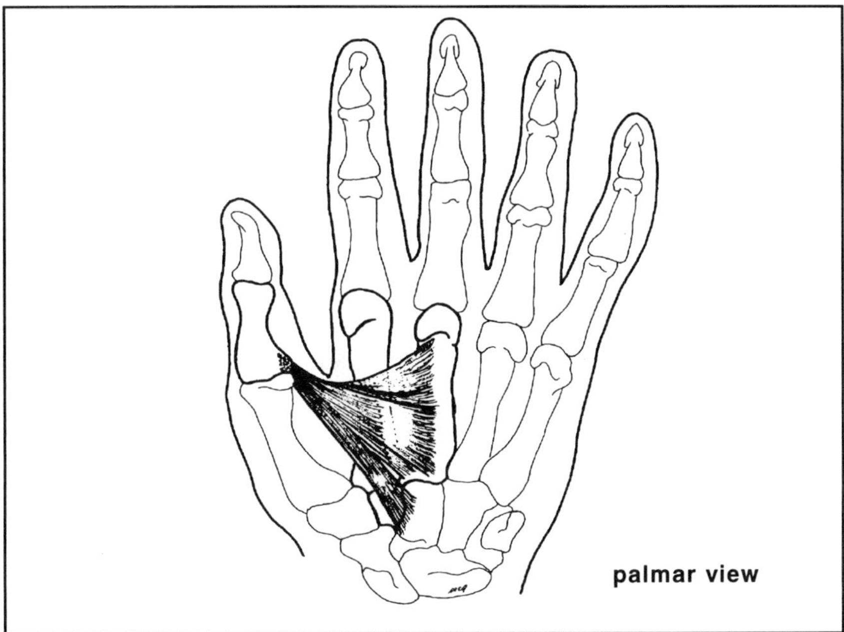

Adductor Pollicis

Fig. 5.30

Origin	By the oblique and transverse heads, from the capitate and bases of the second and third metacarpals, and the distal two-thirds of the third metacarpal.
Insertion	Both heads converge to insert on the ulnar side of the proximal phalanx of the thumb.
Innervation	Deep palmar branch of the ulnar nerve.
Action	Adduction and flexion of the carpometacarpal joint of the thumb.

The adductor pollicis is favorably located to flex the first CMC joint regardless of the position of the thumb. Its ability to adduct the CMC joint is greatest when the joint is fully abducted and diminishes gradually as the muscle pulls the metacarpal closer and closer to the palm. When the thumb is positioned even with the palm, the adductor pollicis is no longer effective since its two attachments are then aligned with the abduction axis. A small portion of the adductor pollicis and flexor pollicis brevis attaches on the extensor expansion of the thumb and therefore they contribute to extension of the interphalangeal joint.

Abductor Digiti Minimi (abduc'tor dig'iti min'imi)

The abductor digiti minimi (Fig. 5.31) is superficial on the ulnar border of the hypothenar eminence. It may be palpated next to the fifth metacarpal during resisted abduction of the small finger.

Abductor Digiti Minimi

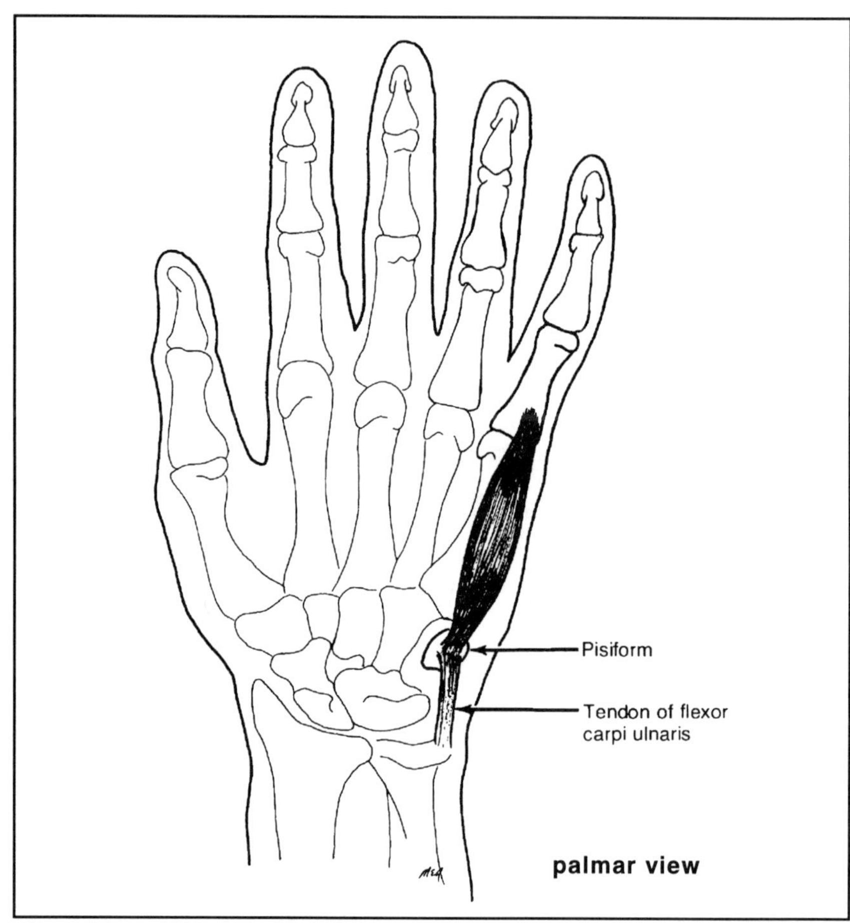

Fig. 5.31

Origin — Pisiform bone and tendon of the flexor carpi ulnaris.
Insertion — By two tendinous slips, to the ulnar side of the base of the proximal phalanx of the small finger, and the ulnar surface of the aponeurosis of the extensor digiti minimi.
Innervation — Ulnar nerve.
Action — Abduction and flexion of the metacarpophalangeal joint of the small finger.

The line of pull of the abductor digiti minimi is much more favorable for abduction than it is for flexion since the muscle is farther from the abduction/adduction axis than it is from the flexion/extension axis of the joint. The muscle's primary function is, therefore, to abduct; it is only assistive as a flexor.

Flexor Digiti Minimi Brevis (flex'or dig'iti min'imi bre'vis)

The flexor digiti minimi brevis (Fig. 5.32) runs parallel to and on the radial side of the abductor digiti minimi. It is superficial, but palpation is difficult because it is easily confused with the abductor digiti minimi.

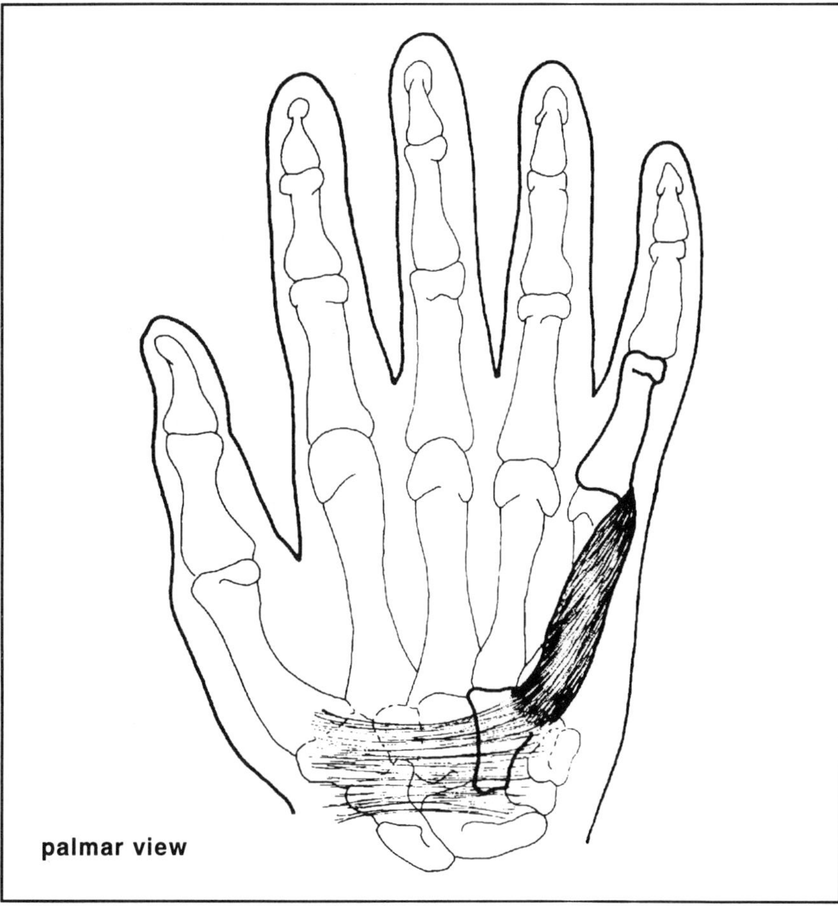

Fig. 5.32

Origin	Hook of the hamate and adjacent portion of the flexor retinaculum.
Insertion	Ulnar surface of the base of the proximal phalanx of the small finger.
Innervation	Ulnar nerve.
Action	Flexion of the metacarpophalangeal joint of the small finger.

The flexor digiti minimi brevis crosses to the palmar side of the axis of flexion/extension of the fifth MCP joint to be a flexor of that joint; however, its oblique direction across the hypothenar eminence aligns it with the abduction/adduction axis to permit no side-to-side action.

Opponens Digiti Minimi (oppo'nens dig'iti min'imi)

The opponens digiti minimi (Fig. 5.33) lies beneath the abductor digiti minimi and the flexor digiti minimi brevis in the hypothenar eminence. It is not palpable.

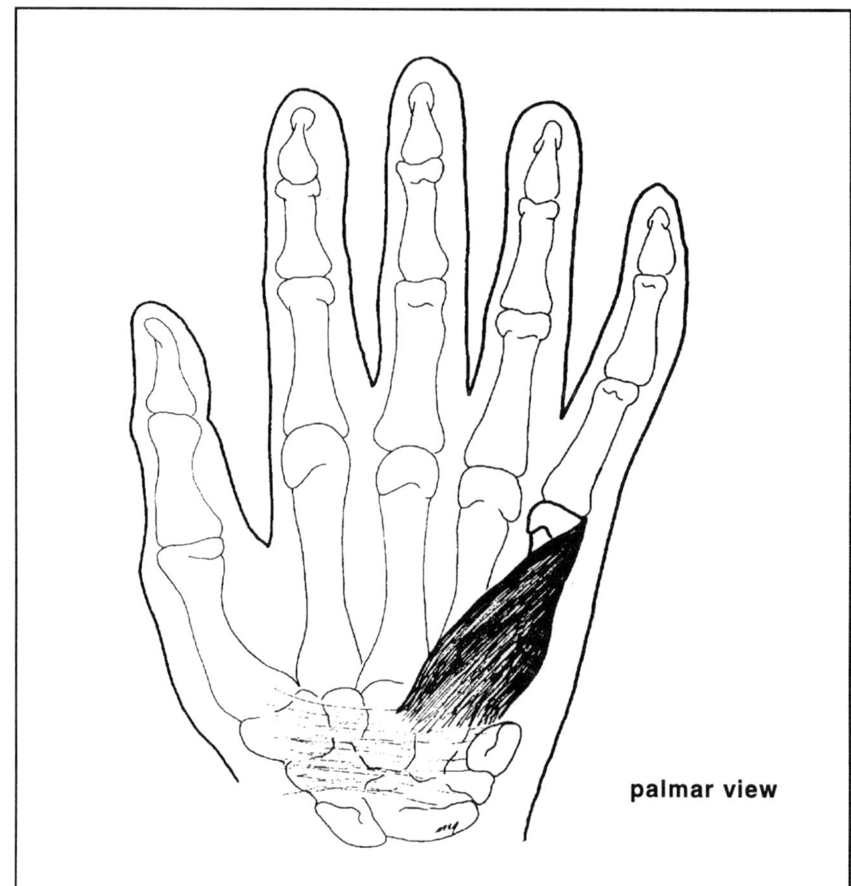

Fig. 5.33

Origin	Hook of the hamate and adjacent portion of the flexor retinaculum.
Insertion	Ulnar border of the entire length of the fifth metacarpal.
Innervation	Ulnar nerve.
Action	Opposition of the carpometacarpal joint of the small finger.

The proximal fibers of the opponens digiti minimi are well situated to flex the fifth CMC joint while the distal fibers are more favorably placed to adduct that joint. Contraction of the muscle thus causes the metacarpal to move in both directions simultaneously, and opposition results.

Dorsal Interossei (dor'sal interos'sei)

The dorsal interossei (Fig. 5.34) are four muscles located superficially on the dorsum of the hand. As their name implies, they lie between the metacarpals and, except for the first dorsal interosseous, are difficult to palpate. Dorsal interosseus 1 lies between the thumb and the 2nd metacarpal and can be observed as a firm fist is made. This muscle also lends stability to the first CMC joint during lateral pinch and power grip.

Origin ——	Each of the four muscles arises by two heads from adjacent sides of the metacarpals.
Insertion ——	Base of the proximal phalanx and aponeurosis of the tendons of the extensor digitorum on the radial aspect of the index finger, the radial and ulnar sides of the long finger, and the ulnar side of the ring finger.
Innervation —	Deep palmar branch of the ulnar nerve.
Action ——	Abduction of the second and fourth metacarpophalangeal joints; radial and ulnar deviation of the third metacarpophalangeal joint; flexion of the second, third and fourth metacarpophalangeal joints; extension (through the extensor hood) of the interphalangeal joints of the index, long, and ring fingers.

The dorsal interossei are particularly well-located to perform their abduction/adduction and deviation actions, since they display a relatively long force arm by virtue of the flair at the bases of the proximal phalanges. The muscles perform their strongest flexion actions at the MCP joints with extension of the PIP and DIP joints during the pinch grasp when the thumb and fingers are used to pick up a small object such as a pin or a coin. The muscles are also very active during a power grip. Ability to abduct the index finger is an easily administered test of the ulnar nerve.

Dorsal Interossei

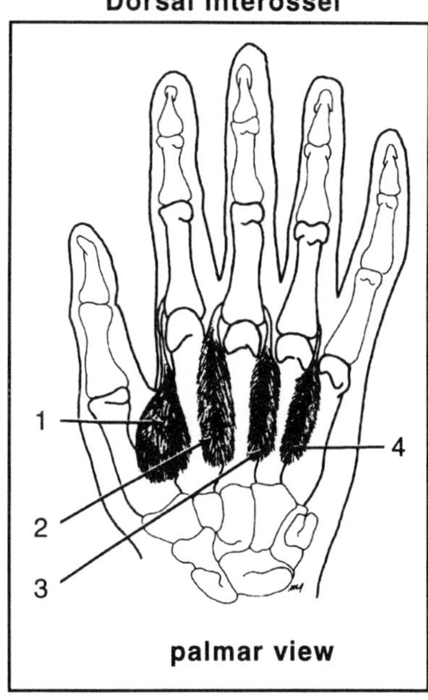

Fig. 5.34

Palmar Interossei (pal'mar interos'sei)

The palmar interossei (Fig. 5.35) are three in number and are located beneath the dorsal interossei. They are not palpable.

Palmar Interossei

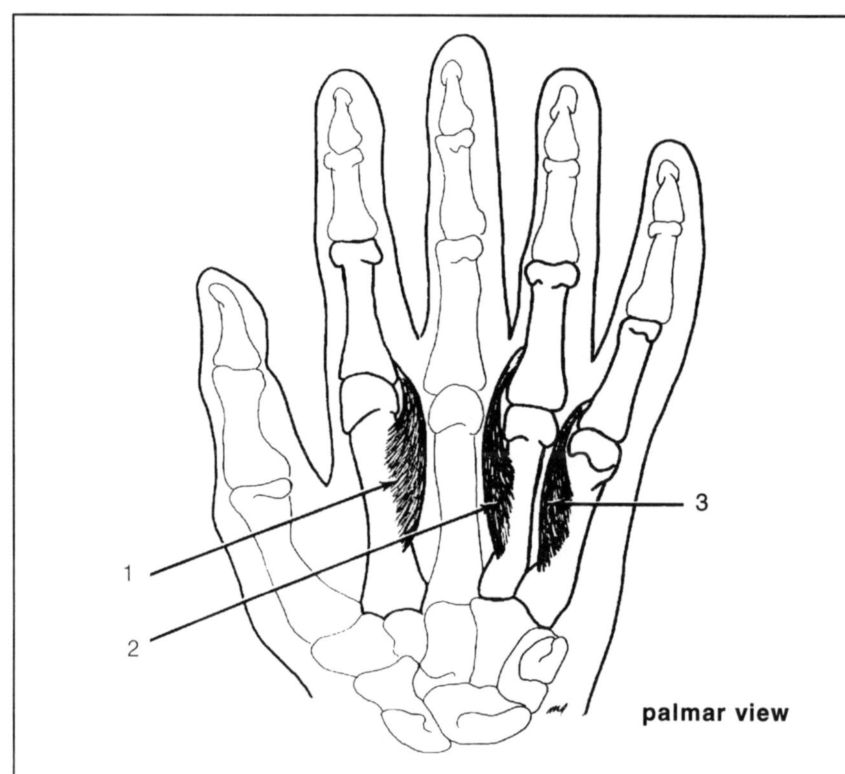

Fig. 5.35

Origin — First palmar interosseus: Ulnar surface of the second metacarpal. Second palmar interosseus: Radial surface of the fourth metacarpal. Third palmar interosseus: Radial surface of the fifth metacarpal.

Insertion — Base of the proximal phalanx and the aponeurosis of the tendons of the extensor digitorum on the ulnar side of the index finger; the radial side of the ring finger; and the radial side of the small finger.

Innervation — Deep palmar branch of the ulnar nerve.

Action — Adduction and flexion of the metacarpophalangeal joints of the index, ring, and small fingers; extension (through the extensor hood) of the interphalangeal joints of those fingers.

The flexion and extension functions of the palmar interossei and the dorsal interossei are similar; however, the palmar interossei are somewhat farther from the flexion/extension axis of those joints than are the dorsal interossei. The palmar muscles have, therefore, greater efficiency as flexors. The adduction action of the palmar set follows from their medial locations with respect to those axes.

Lumbricales (lumbrica'les)

The lumbricales (Fig. 5.36) comprise four muscles located around the tendons of the flexor digitorum profundus. They are deep in the palm and cannot be palpated.

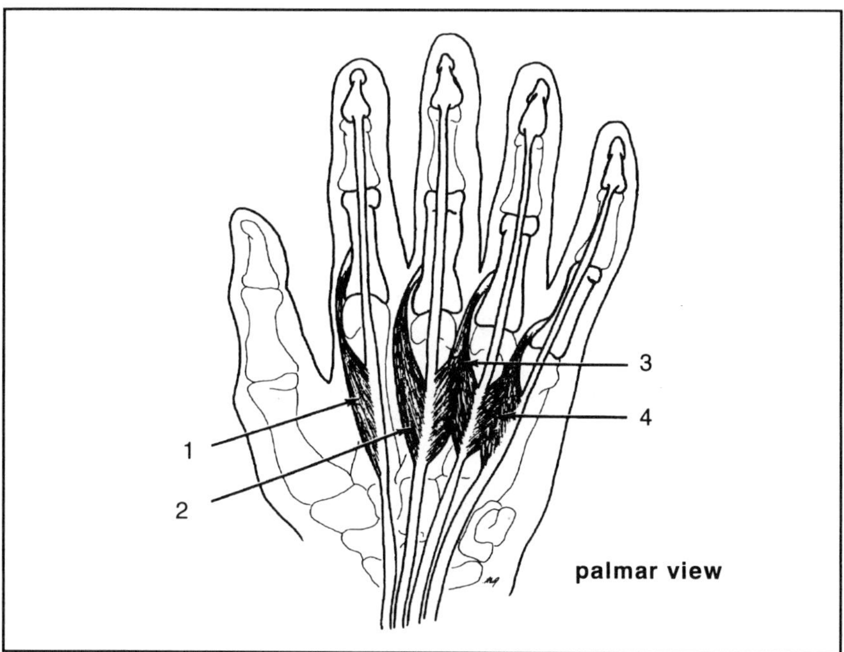

Lumbricales

Fig. 5.36

Origin	From the four tendons of the flexor digitorum profundus.
Insertion	Aponeuroses of the tendons of the extensor digitorum. After passing to the radial sides of the metacarpals, the points of insertion are opposite the metacarpophalangeal joints.
Innervation	Lumbricales one and two: Median nerve. Lumbricales three and four: Deep palmar branch of ulnar nerve.
Action	Flexion of the second through fifth metacarpophalangeal joints; extension through the extensor hood of the interphalangeal joints of the four fingers.

The lumbricales are primarily involved in extending the IP joints of the fingers since their contractions pull the extensor hood proximally to tighten the entire mechanism. A secondary result of their contractions is to produce slack in the profundus tendons so that extension of the IP joints will be allowed.

The lumbricales pass to the palmar side of the flexion/ extension axis of the MCP joints as they course between their two attachments, and can be expected to make some contribution in the flexing of those joints. Their effectiveness is limited, however, since they do not have a firm origin on the profundus tendons, and is displayed more as neutralizing action against the extensor digitorum rather than as observable flexion of the joints.

ARCHITECTURE OF THE HAND

Throughout the performance of daily activities, one can see that the hand is able to assume a variety of positions and shapes. During grasping activities, for example, the hand will conform itself to the shape of the object in question while a flattening of the palmar surface occurs when the object is released. It is the flexion of the digits that increases the cupping and grasping ability of the hand, and it is their extension that flattens the hand.

The skeletal composition of the hand may be divided into fixed and mobile units (Fig. 5.37). The fixed unit of the hand includes the distal row of carpal bones and the metacarpals of the index and long fingers. These structures are firmly attached to each other by the intercarpal ligaments and the configuration of the four distal carpal bones.

Fixed and Mobile Units of the Hand

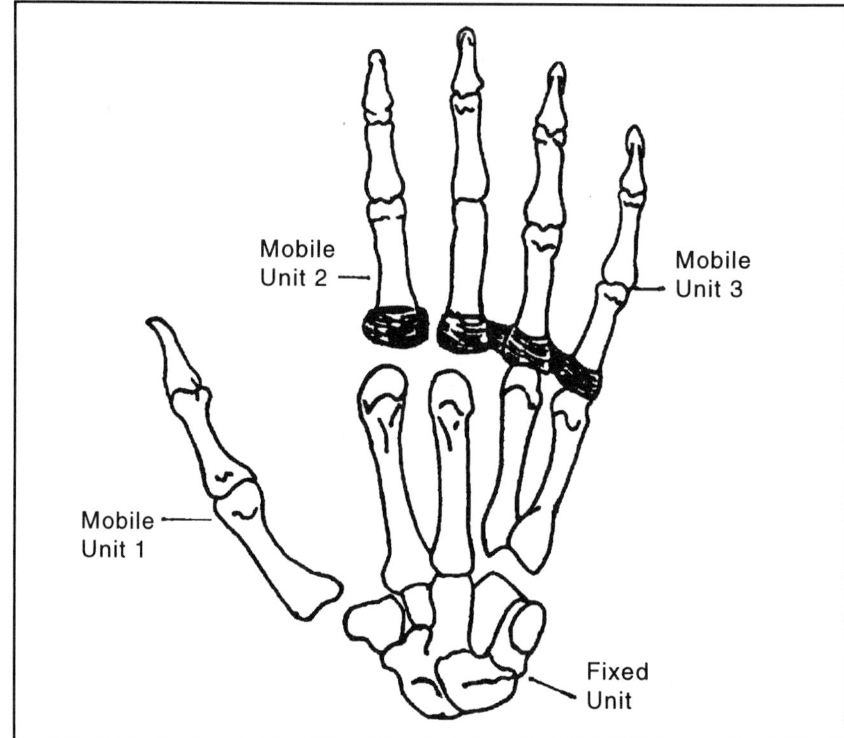

Fig. 5.37

The mobile units of the hand consist of three components: (1) the thumb, (2) the phalanges of the index finger, and (3) the phalanges of the long, ring, and small fingers and the fourth and fifth metacarpals. These structures move around the fixed unit of the hand. The thumb possesses the greatest latitude of the mobile units as it moves around the multangulus major. Second in ability to move is the index finger as it moves around the second metacarpal independently of the other fingers. Least movement is seen in the third component as it functions around its base on the head of the third metacarpal and the hamate.

The third mobile component -- the ulnar side of the hand along with the long finger -- functions as a moveable structure around which object manipulation by the thumb and index finger is permitted. This can easily be seen as one holds and writes with a pen or pencil. In addition, the third mobile unit, because of the several joints comprised by it, is vital to performance of the power grip; i.e. holding and using a hammer or power saw.

The hand and wrist are composed of three functional arches (Fig. 5.38). Two transverse arches (carpal and metacarpal) and one longitudinal arch are traditionally depicted; however, the oblique arches of opposition between the thumb and the four fingers may also be considered as separate functional arches.

Arches of the Hand

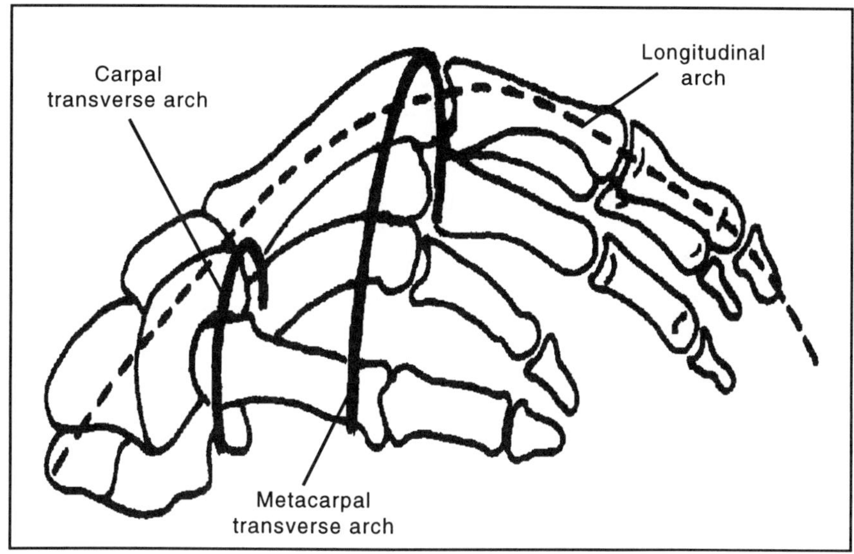

Fig. 5.38

The transverse carpal arch may be subdivided into its proximal and distal carpal portions. The proximal portion, made up of the proximal row of carpals, communicates with the radius and the distal row of carpals. This portion of the arch is more mobile than the distal portion because the bones of the proximal row enjoy their own distinct articulations with surrounding bones. Movement of the distal portion is rather rigid, occurring primarily between the metacarpals of the index and long fingers. The capitate is the center point of the distal portion.

The heads of metacarpals one through five form the transverse metacarpal arch. Because of the mobility of the first and fifth metacarpals, this arch has the ability to deepen or flatten the palmar concavity of the hand. As the thumb and small finger move toward each other in opposition, the curvature of the palm increases. During reposition of the thumb, the palm becomes flat. The center of this arch is the head of the third metacarpal.

The longitudinal arch is composed of a fixed unit, a metacarpal and its adjacent carpal, and a mobile unit, the phalanges. Each digit possesses its own longitudinal arch that is centered around its MCP joint. The stability of the MCP joint is essential, therefore, to the maintenance of functional integrity of both the longitudinal and transverse metacarpal arches. Excessive hyperextension or instability at the MCP may collapse the arch system. As a result, thumb and small finger opposition and sequential digital flexion and extension may become difficult or even lost.

For a more in-depth discussion of the architecture of the hand, the reader is referred to the excellent works of Raoul Tubiana. Complete citations appear in the bibliography.

PALPATIONS

The following chart presents the sites and actions to perform for palpating the extrinsic and intrinsic muscles of the wrist and hand.

Extrinsic Flexor Muscles

MUSCLE	ACTION TO PERFORM	PALPATION SITE
Flexor Carpi Ulnaris	Pinch fingertips together or flex the wrist	Proximal to the pisiform
Flexor Carpi Radialis	Resisted radial deviation and flexion	Radial side, tendon of palmaris longus
Palmaris Longus	Pinch tip of thumb to tip of small finger and flex the wrist	Center of wrist, palmar surface
Flexor Pollicis Longus	Flex and extend the IP joint of the thumb	Palmar surface between IP and MCP joints
Flexor Digitorum Superficialis	Stabilize three fingers and flex the PIP joint of the free finger	Note flexion at the PIP joint of finger being tested
Flexor Digitorum Profundus	Stabilize PIP joint in extension	Flex the DIP joint

Extrinsic Extensor Muscles

MUSCLE	ACTION TO PERFORM	PALPATION SITE
Extensor Pollicis Brevis	Extend the thumb forcefully	Radial part of anatomical snuff box
Abductor Pollicis Longus	Abduct the CMC joint of thumb	Palmar side of anatomical snuff box
Extensor Carpi Radialis Longus	Extend the wrist	Dorsiradial aspect of wrist
Extensor Carpi Radialis Brevis	Make a fist and extend the wrist	Dorsiradial aspect of wrist
Extensor Pollicis Longus	Place palmar surface of hand on table; lift thumb off table	Ulnar part of anatomical snuff box
Extensor Digitorum	Extend wrist and MCP joints	Tendons seen on dorsal surface of hand
Extensor Indicis	Extend the index finger with remaining digits flexed into palm	Ulnar side of tendon of ext. digitorum at 2nd MCP joint
Extensor Digiti Minimi	Extend the small finger with remaining digits flexed into palm	Ulnar side of tendon of ext. digitorum at 5th MCP joint
Extensor Carpi Ulnaris	Make a fist, extend and ulnarly deviate the wrist	Distal to styloid process of ulna

Intrinsic Muscles

MUSCLE	ACTION TO PERFORM	PALPATION SITE
Flexor Pollicis Brevis	Flex the 1st MCP joint against resistance	Ulnar border of thenar eminence
Abductor Pollicis Brevis	Abduct the CMC joint of the thumb against resistance	Center of the thenar eminence
Opponens Pollicis	Press tip of thumb to tip of long finger	Radial side of thenar eminence
Adductor Pollicis	Press thumb against tip of index finger; or, hold piece of paper between thumb & radial aspect of the proximal phalanx of index finger	Palmar surface between 1st and 2nd metacarpals
Abductor Digiti Minimi	Abduct the small finger against resistance	Ulnar border of hypothenar eminence
Flexor Digiti Minimi Brevis	Flex the 5th MCP joint against resistance	Radial side of abductor digiti minimi
Opponens Digiti Minimi	Cannot palpate	
Dorsal Interossei	Make a fist	Dorsal surface between 1st and 2nd metacarpals
Palmar Interossei	Cannot palpate	
Lumbricales	Cannot palpate	

TESTING FOR NERVE FUNCTION

As has been demonstrated in previous pages, the 25 muscles or muscle groups are innervated by only three nerves; i.e., median, ulnar, and radial. Knowledge of muscle actions together with muscle innervation can be of immeasurable help when diagnosing possible nerve injury. The procedure used by diagnosticians is relatively simple, albeit slightly reversed from the thought processes emphasized heretofore. For example, material specific to a given muscle, say the flexor carpi radialis, has been presented in this text first as its attachments (medial epicondyle of the humerus by the common tendon -- palmar surface of the base of the second metacarpal with a slip to the base of the third metacarpal), its actions (flexion and radial deviation of the wrist joint), and finally, its innervation (median nerve). The diagnostician, however, begins by establishing the actions that are weak or missing around a joint (the wrist in our example). Having noted a weakness in the patient as flexion and radial deviation are performed, the diagnostician considers the nerve supply of the muscles that flex the wrist and radially deviate it (median and radial nerves). Since the patient shows no weakness or limited range of motion in wrist extension; thus, the radial nerve is ruled out. The nerve involved must be the median nerve, but which muscle is affected? Is it the flexor carpi radialis, flexor digitorum superficialis, flexor digitorum profundus, or the palmaris longus? Since neither the flexors of the fingers nor the palmaris longus radially deviate the wrist, the muscle of concern must be the flexor carpi radialis. Confirmation of this conclusion can be made by palpating the tendon just proximal to its insertion and noting that there is a tendency toward ulnar deviation as the wrist is flexed. The textbook method, then, presents muscles by origin, insertion, innervation, and action. The diagnostician analyzes actions, determines innervation, and confirms by palpating at or between origin and insertion.

By grouping the muscles innervated by the median, ulnar, or radial nerve, one can expect irregular postures of the hand, or weaknesses, or even physical differences that are the result of nerve impairment. If the median nerve is involved, atrophy of the thenar eminence is expected because the median nerve supplies two and one-half of the four muscles which form the eminence. Likewise, the thumb will be pulled into a position of outward rotation since the thenar muscles are incapable of balancing the pull of their antagonists. The "benediction" posture of the hand in which the index and long fingers are extended while the other two digits are curled is frequently seen. The flexor digitorum superficialis and radial portion of the flexor digitorum profundus are unable to balance the pull of the extensors of the index and long fingers. The ring and small fingers are not affected because the ulnar nerve supplies the ulnar portion of the flexor digitorum profundus. Atrophy of the muscle mass associated with the common tendon of the medial epicondyle is expected. Most of the extrinsic muscles that are innervated by the median nerve (as well as the pronator teres) originate there.

Muscle testing to determine impairment of the median nerve can occasionally lead to spurious conclusions because of the body's unparalleled ability to substitute actions of healthy muscles for involved muscles. The following tips are offered to aid in making the correct diagnosis.

Testing for Impairment of the Median Nerve

1. The flexor digitorum profundus is normally innervated by both the median and ulnar nerves. Anomalies may occur in which the flexor digitorum profundus is almost all or entirely innervated by the ulnar nerve. Finger flexion could, therefore, be performed even though the median nerve is not intact.

2. When the forearm is supinated, the brachioradialis can pronate it (weakly) to neutral position at which point gravity can complete the action. In this event, the pronator teres should be evaluated by palpation. The pronator quadratus cannot be palpated, however, and may be mistaken for causing the pronation.

3. When the thumb and wrist are strongly hyperextended, flexion of the interphalangeal joint can be caused by passive pull of the abductor pollicis longus on the tendon of the flexor pollicis longus. This muscle test should be done with the thumb held next to the radial border of the hand.

4. Flexion of the metacarpophalangeal joints can be caused by the interossei and lumbricales 3 and 4. Lumbrical 2 may also be involved as a rather common anomaly is innervation of lumbrical 2 by the ulnar nerve. Nevertheless, this action can be performed even though the median nerve is not functioning.

5. When opposition is performed by a healthy hand, a well-shaped "O" is formed when the thumb pulp meets the pulp of the small finger. If the opponens pollicis is inoperative, the first metacarpal is not pulled away from the plane of the palm and the result will be a flexion of the thumb across the palm to touch the radial side of the small finger. This action is caused by the adductor pollicis and the ulnar head of the flexor pollicis longus, both of which are innervated by the ulnar nerve.

6. The abductor pollicis longus can easily substitute for the abductor pollicis brevis during abduction of the CMC joint of the thumb. To test for median nerve, stabilize the first metacarpal and abduct the MCP joint.

Evidence of ulnar nerve impairment may include atrophy of the hypothenar eminence, "hollows" between the metacarpals, "claw" hand particularly on the ulnar side of the hand, and a posture of abduction-extension of the small finger. Atrophy of the eminence and "hollows" between the metacarpals are the result of atrophy of the three hypothenar muscles, the interossei, and lumbricales 3 and 4. The "claw" hand posture results from the inability of the interossei muscles and the lumbricales 3 and 4 to balance the pull of the extensor digitorum over the MCP joints and the flexor digitorum superficialis and flexor digitorum profundus over the IP joints. The posture of the small finger is caused by the unopposed pull of the extensor digiti minimi against the absence of an adductor to that finger.

When testing for ulnar nerve lesion, one should proceed with the following cautions.

Testing for Ulnar Nerve Impairment

1. Evaluate adduction of the thumb by keeping the thumb in contact with the palm. The abductor pollicis brevis can substitute to cause adduction but it will be accompanied by some abduction which causes the thumb to move away from the palm. Efforts to substitute the flexor pollicis longus will be easily recognized as the first MCP joint will hyperextend under the pull of the flexor pollicis longus which will simultaneously cause flexion of the IP joint (Froment's sign).

2. In the absence of the interossei and lumbricales 3 and 4, the tendons of the extensor digitorum, extensor indicis, and extensor digiti minimi can substitute to cause weak abduction of the fingers. This is particularly true for the index and small fingers. Concentrate the test, therefore, on the long finger by placing the hand palm down on the table and performing radial and ulnar deviation without lifting the finger from the table.

3. Finger adduction can be caused by substitute muscles such as the flexor digitorum superficialis, flexor digitorum profundus, and even the extensor tendon of the index finger. A conclusive test can be given, however, by adducting the small finger. There are no muscles to substitute for this action.

4. Impairment of the ulnar nerve limits flexion of the MCP joints; however, compensatory actions of the lumbricales 1 and 2 and the flexor digitorum superficialis should be recognized and not evaluated falsely. Flexion of the third and fourth MCP joints which is accompanied by flexion of the PIP joints is indicative of flexor digitorum superficialis activity.

5. The IP joints of the ring and small fingers can be extended only by the extensor digitorum and the interossei and lumbricales of those fingers. Lesions of the ulnar nerve render the interossei and lumbricales ineffectual. One need only hyperextend the wrist and MCP joints to block (by shortening) the extensor digitorum from further action and then attempt to extend the IP joints. Inability to do so indicates involvement of interossei and lumbricales.

Radial nerve function is difficult to evaluate because of the many muscle substitutions that can be made. "Drop hand" is a posture often seen. There are no wrist extensors to balance the wrist flexors. Atrophy of the muscle mass in the vicinity of the lateral epicondyle may be noted as well as a wasting of tissue on the dorsal aspect of both the upper arm and forearm. Hints for muscle testing are offered below.

Testing for Impairment of the Radial Nerve

1. Gravity should be eliminated when testing for elbow extension.
2. The supinating action of the biceps brachii can easily be mistaken for the supinator.
3. Hold your hand in a relaxed posture and allow it to flex passively. While ensuring that the wrist continues to relax, slowly make a fist. Notice the marked extension of the wrist to anatomical position. This is caused by a passive pull of the tendons of the extensor digitorum rather than any muscular activity. If the fingers are held extended, the wrist itself cannot be extended if the radial nerve is impaired.
4. Extension of the PIP and DIP joints of the fingers may be caused by passive pull of the tendons of the extensor digitorum if the wrist is in a flexed position.

MOVEMENT PATTERNS OF THE HAND

Grips - Power and Precision

The movements of the hand can be divided into two categories: **power grip** and **precision** or **prehension grip**. **Power grip** is a forceful act in which all of the digits assume a position of sustained flexion that varies in degree with the shape, size, and weight of the object being held. The digits will hold the object against the palm while the partially opposed thumb applies counter pressure. The radial and ulnar borders of the palm act as buttresses as the digits maintain a flexed position around the object. While the hand remains stable, power is produced by movements at the wrist, forearm, and elbow. Examples of power grips include **cylindrical grip, hook grip**, **spherical grip**, and **fisted grip**.

Cylindrical grip is one in which the entire hand is wrapped around an object while the thumb is used to provide stability and power (holding a soft drink can). A grip in which the interphalangeal joints, and sometimes the metacarpophalangeal joints, are flexed around an object is called a **hook grip**. The thumb is not involved in this grip. This grip is commonly used when one carries a briefcase.

The **spherical grip** involves opposition of the thumb and partial flexion of the digits around a sphere. The grip assumed when grasping a ball is illustrative of the spherical grip. In the **fisted grip**, all digits are flexed tightly around a narrow object (i.e., gripping a golf club).

Precision or **prehension grip** is an activity which requires dynamic movements. It is here that object manipulation occurs between the opposing thumb and remaining digits -- mainly the index and long fingers. The palm of the hand is usually not involved in precision activities. Positional adjustments are influenced by sensory input from the digits. Three types of prehension grips are commonly described. The first, known as **three-point chuck** or **three-fingered pinch**, involves opposition and pulp-to-pulp pinch between the thumb, index, and long fingers. This pattern is used for picking up and holding objects (i.e., pencil). **Lateral**, **key**, or **pulp-to-side pinch**, does not require opposition from the thumb. During this act of prehension, the thumb presses against the radial surface of the proximal phalanx of the index finger. Holding a key, coin, or card is an example of this prehension pattern. The third prehension grip is **tip pinch** or **tip-to-tip prehension**. This prehension pattern involves opposing and positioning the tip of the thumb to the tip of the index finger. Tip pinch is primarily used for holding and/or picking up small objects such as a pin. This pinch involves a variety of muscles and movements, and is used only in acitivites requiring fine motor coordination.

COMMENTS

Of the muscles of the wrist and hand, the larger ones originate above the wrist. When implements are gripped over long periods of time, the forearm muscles of the preferred arm hypertrophy and are often responsible for a considerable difference in the girth of the two arms. Hand size may differ, also, because of hypertrophy of the intrinsic muscles. The degree of hypertrophy is related to the weight of the implement used and, therefore, to the size of the grip on the implement. Hammers used for various tasks vary in both weight and grip size. A comparison of the grips of different hammer sizes will suffice to illustrate the mechanics involved in executing the power grip with the hand.

The heaviest of the three hammers has the largest grip. When the hand grasps the grip, both the flexors and the extensor contract forcefully. This may seem unusual since the flexors are the gripping muscles; however, it must be remembered that when the flexors contract they tend to cause wrist flexion as well as flexion of the joints of the hand. Neutralization must be provided by the extensors in order to maintain a straight wrist. The more forceful the grip, the more neutralization is required of the extensors.

A tack hammer is a light hammer and has a small grip -- small enough to allow the entire distal phalanx of the thumb to overlap that phalanx of the long finger. The metacarpophalangeal joints, as well as the interphalangeal joints, are required to flex to acute angles in order to grip the hammer, and there is an accompanying loss of strength of the flexor muscles. Since the hammer is so light, however, the loss is not critical. Far more important than the strength loss is the fact that the extensor digitorum is near its maximum length when the joints of the hand are flexed to such an extent. When wrist flexion is required to execute a stroke, the small amount of extensibility remaining to the muscle is limiting to the range of motion. To offset this disadvantage, the worker may grip the hammer with only the first two or three fingers. By allowing the remaining finger or fingers to be free, the extensor digitorum is given some slack, and wrist flexion will be enhanced.

Even though the above application of grip mechanics has been specific to the use of a hammer, the concepts can be generalized to other situations in which objects must be held or swung. When power is the most important requirement, the size of the object to be gripped should allow for an approximate 90-degree angle at the metacarpophalangeal joints. If the object is small in circumference, wrist flexion will be limited unless one or two fingers can be relieved of their gripping responsibilities and are allowed to curl passively. Large objects such as footballs and softballs cannot be gripped securely, but they can be thrown with a great deal of wrist "snap." As a side comment, it is noted that the baseball pitcher is faced with a serious problem of grip mechanics. A baseball is small enough to permit the hand to close around it to the extent that wrist flexion will be limited. To compensate, the pitcher grips the ball with the fingers and thumb in such a way that the metacarpophalangeal joints are extended. The responsibility of gripping the ball is, thus, relegated to the digits in order to afford the extensor digitorum some slack which can be used subsequently to permit the wrist "snap" at the time of ball release.

A quiz for this material can be found in the back of this book on page 289.

LABORATORY EXPERIENCES

1. Determine, through the use of a goniometer, your range of motion in flexion and extension of the wrist joint while maintaining a firm fist. Repeat your observations while maintaining the metacarpal and interphalangeal joints in extension. How should the hand be held for greatest wrist flexion? for greatest wrist extension?

2. Abduct the index finger against resistance while palpating dorsal interossei 1. You should notice tension in the muscle. Continue to palpate as you make a firm fist, and again tension should be noted. Explain the activity of this muscle as it is involved in these two dissimilar movements.

3. Grasp the handle of a tennis racket, bat, or other such implement, and have a partner pull it from your grip in the direction of your thumb. Notice the comparative weakness of your grip against the pull. Generalize this to the releases taught in lifesaving and self-defense classes.

4. Use a grip dynamometer to determine your grip strength while holding the wrist in full extension. Repeat the observation while holding the wrist in linewith the forearm, and while maintaining full wrist flexion. Generalize your findings to explain the various grips used in industry.

5. The intrinsic muscles of the hand are difficult to study electromyographically because they are small and are frequently not superficial. The muscles comprising the superficial layer of the thenar and hypothenar eminences can be monitored, however, through the use of small electrodes. If appropriate electrodes are available, attach them to the midpoints of the two eminences and investigate the involvement of the various muscles during opposition, reposition, abduction, and flexion of the thumb and small finger.

THE SPINE AND PELVIC GIRDLE

6

THE SPINE

The spine is formed by thirty-three bones called vertebrae. The vertebrae are categorized, according to their locations, as cervical, thoracic, lumbar, sacral, and coccygeal. There are seven cervical, twelve thoracic, five lumbar, five sacral, and four coccygeal vertebrae (Fig. 6.1).

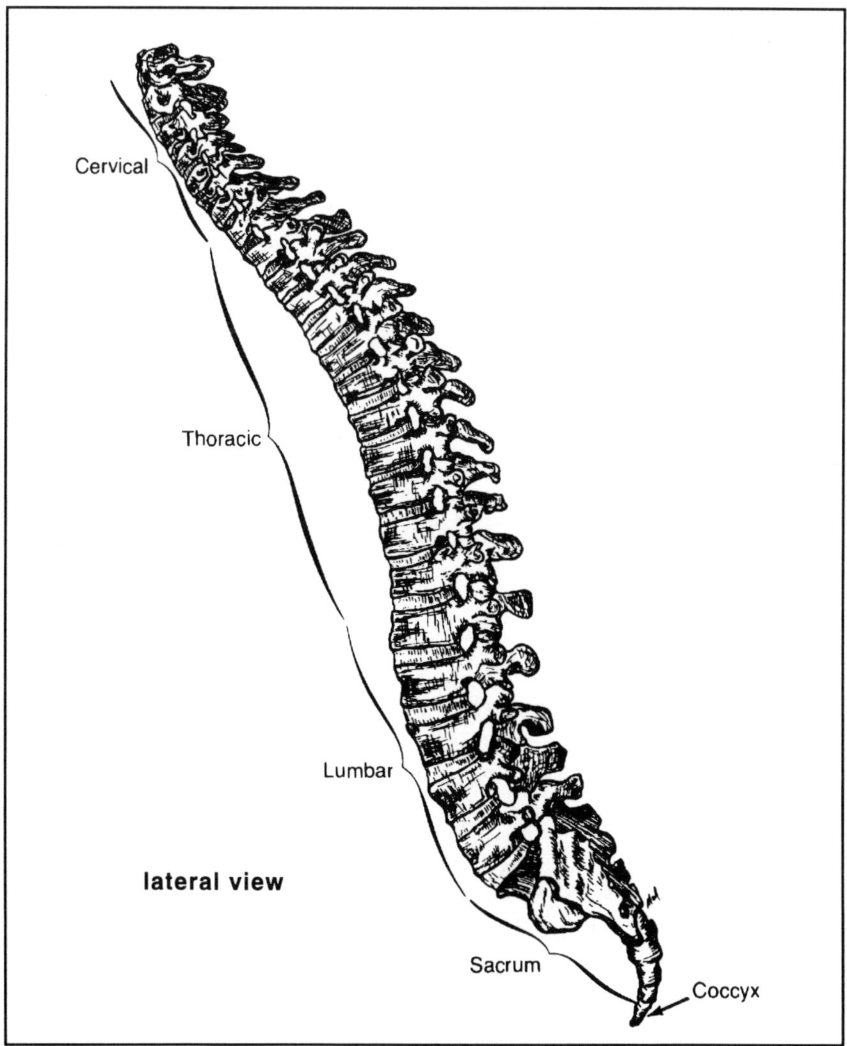

Fig. 6.1

The Spinal Column

THE VERTEBRAE

A vertebra is characterized generally by several parts (Fig. 6.2). The body is the largest of the parts and is cylindrical in shape. Intervertebral discs of fibrocartilage are attached to its superior and inferior surfaces through which each vertebra articulates with its neighbors.

A Typical Vertebra

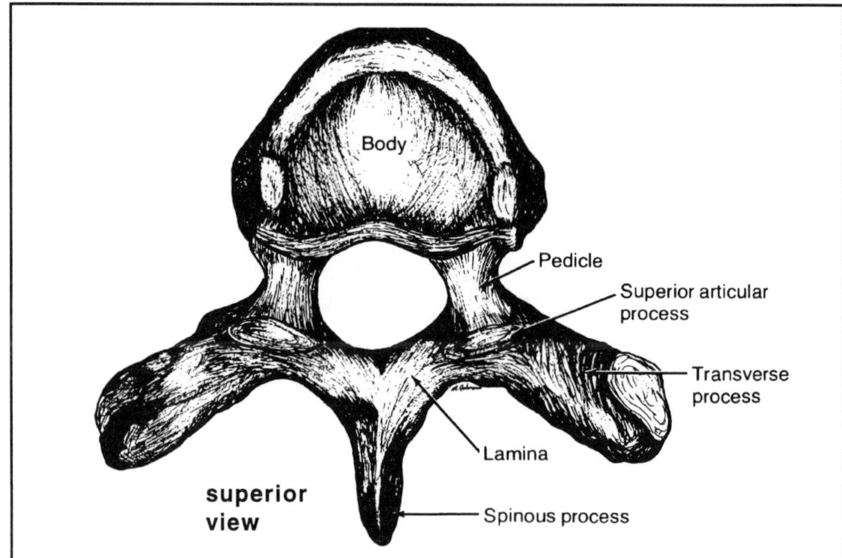

Fig. 6.2

Extending posteriorly from the body are the pedicles, and then to complete the vertebral foramen are the laminae. A spinous process extends posteriorly from the laminae and two transverse processes extend from the junctions between the laminae and pedicles. Two superior and two inferior articular processes extend upwardly and downwardly in the frontal plane (Fig. 6.3); just anterior to the inferior articulating processes and below the pedicles are the intervertebral notches through which nerves leave the spinal column. The pedicles and laminae, together with the processes they support, are referred to collectively as the vertebral arch.

A Lumbar Vertebra

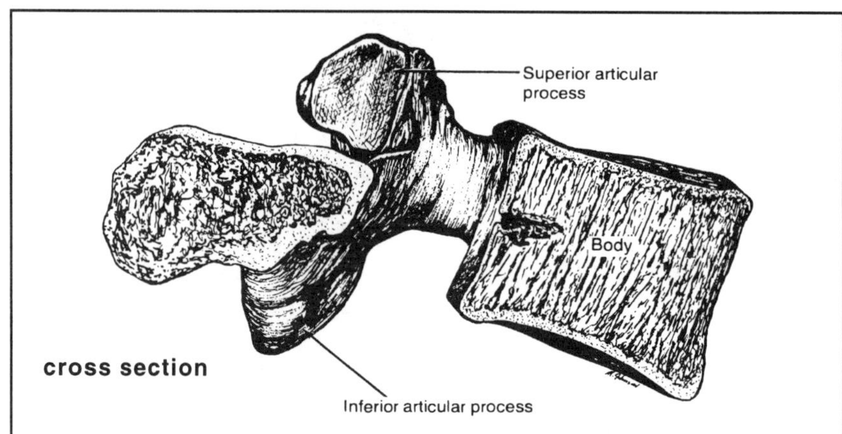

Fig. 6.3

Cervical Vertebrae

In the cervical area, three of the vertebrae, the first, second and seventh, exhibit certain peculiarities. The first cervical vertebra (Fig. 6.4), called the **atlas** because it supports the cranium, has no body but rather resembles a bony ring. Its spinous process is shortened but the transverse processes are long. On its superior surface are two large concavities which articulate with the occipital condyles of the skull to allow for flexion and extension around the frontal axis.

The First Cervical Vertebra (Atlas)

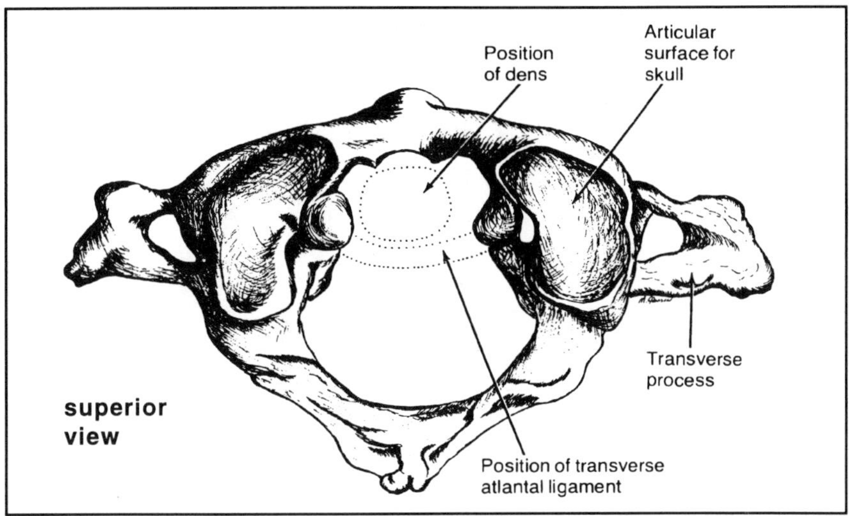

Fig. 6.4

The second cervical vertebra (Fig. 6.5) is called the **axis** because it is characterized by a short peg, the dens, which is the pivot around which the first vertebra, carrying the head, rotates. The dens extends into the vertebral foramen of the first vertebra where it is separated from the spinal cord by the large transverse atlantae ligament. This arrangement permits extensive range of movement around the vertical axis; as, for example, turning the head to look from side to side.

The Second Cervical Vertebra (Axis)

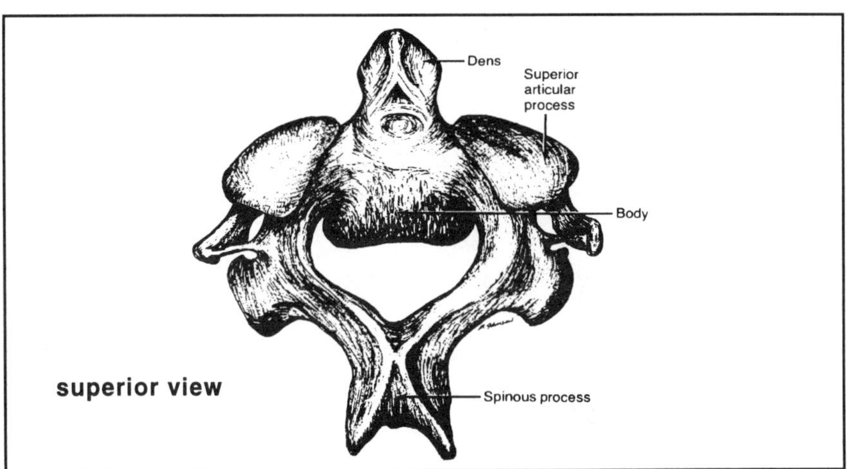

Fig. 6.5

The seventh cervical vertebra (Fig. 6.6) is distinguished by its unusually long spinous process. It is easily palpated on the posterior base of the neck and provides a convenient point of palpation between the cervical and thoracic regions of the spine.

The Seventh Cervical Vertebra

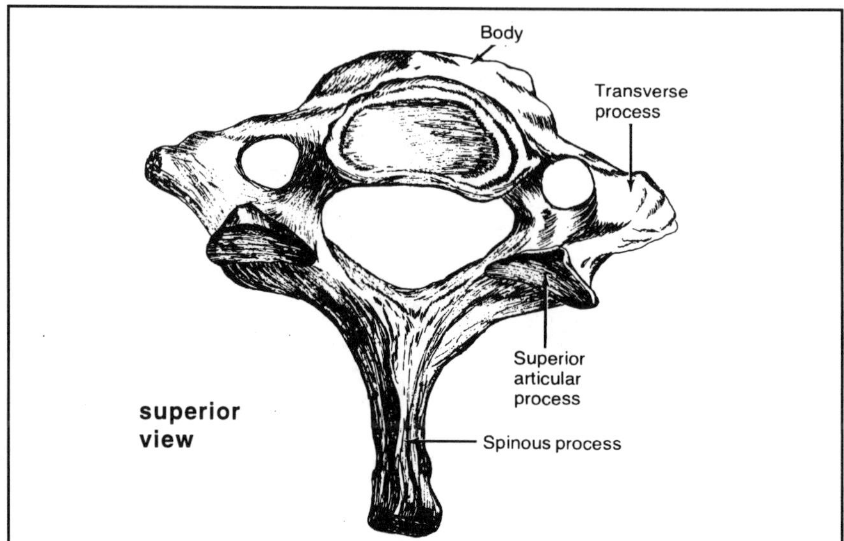

Fig. 6.6

Thoracic Vertebrae

Of the thoracic vertebrae, all exhibit four articular facets which are not to be found on the other vertebrae (Fig. 6.7). These facets form the articulations with the twelve ribs, to place an effective anatomical splint on the thoracic area. Resulting ranges of motion in flexion and lateral flexion are limited to the ability of the ribs to spread and close. An additional peculiarity of the thoracic vertebrae is that the spinous processes are projected downwardly, particularly in the second through the tenth vertebrae -- a characteristic which limits the ability of the thoracic spine to hyperextend.

A Thoracic Vertebra

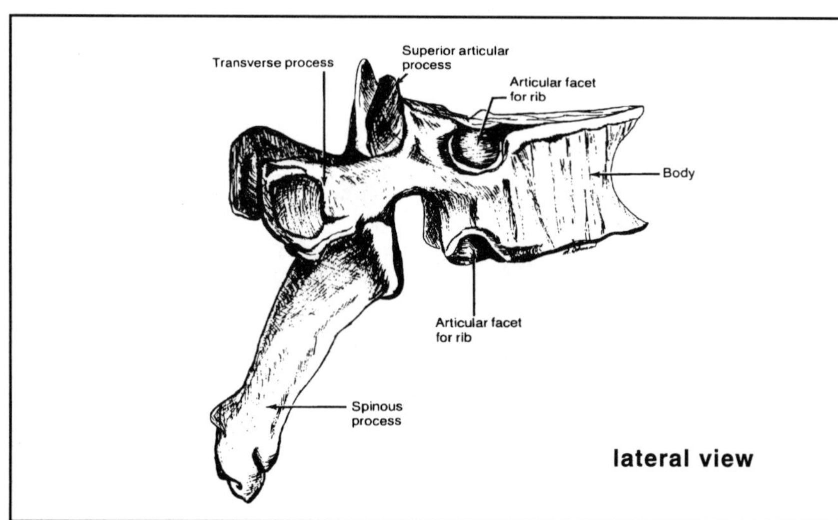

Fig. 6.7

Lumbar Vertebrae

The lumbar vertebrae (Fig. 6.8), being the largest of the movable vertebrae, must support the weight of the body above them. Their articular processes are more defined than in other vertebrae and provide more of an interlocking articulation which limits movement around the long axis. The fifth lumbar vertebrae deserves special comment in that it articulates distally with the sacrum through the lumbosacral junction. The range of movement is greater in this junction than elsewhere in the lumbar spine.

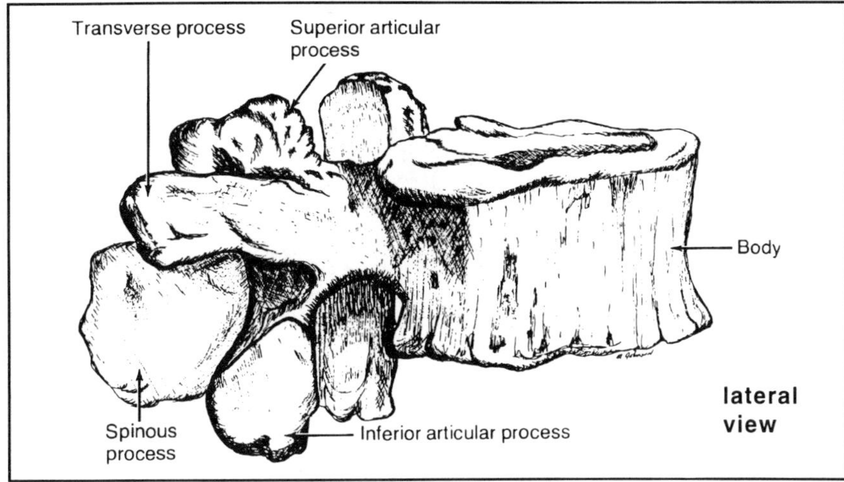

Fig. 6.8

A Lumbar Vertebra

Sacral Vertebrae

The sacrum (Fig. 6.9) represents the fusion of five sacral vertebrae to form a large triangular bone located like a wedge between the two hip bones. It articulates proximally with the last lumbar vertebra and distally with the coccyx. No movement is possible in this area of the spine.

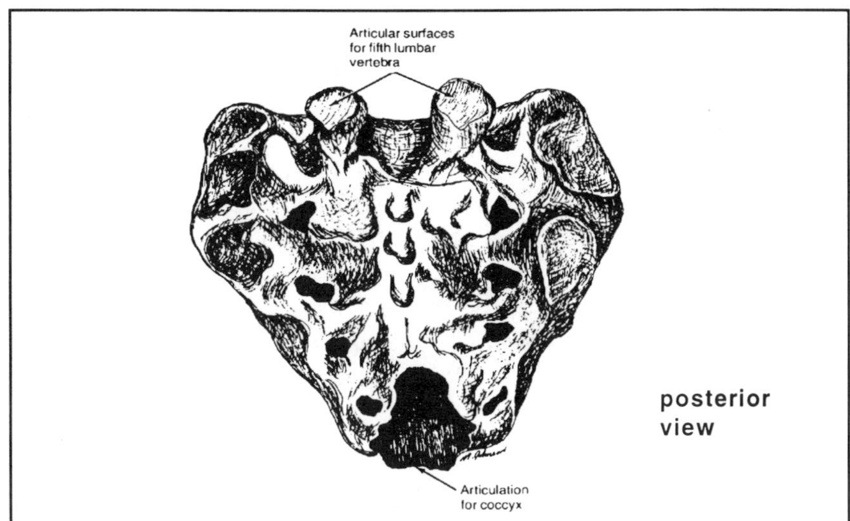

Fig. 6.9

The Sacrum

Coccygeal Vertebrae

The coccyx (Fig. 6.10) is formed of four rudimentary vertebrae, the last one of which is only a nodule of bone. No voluntary movement is possible.

The Coccyx

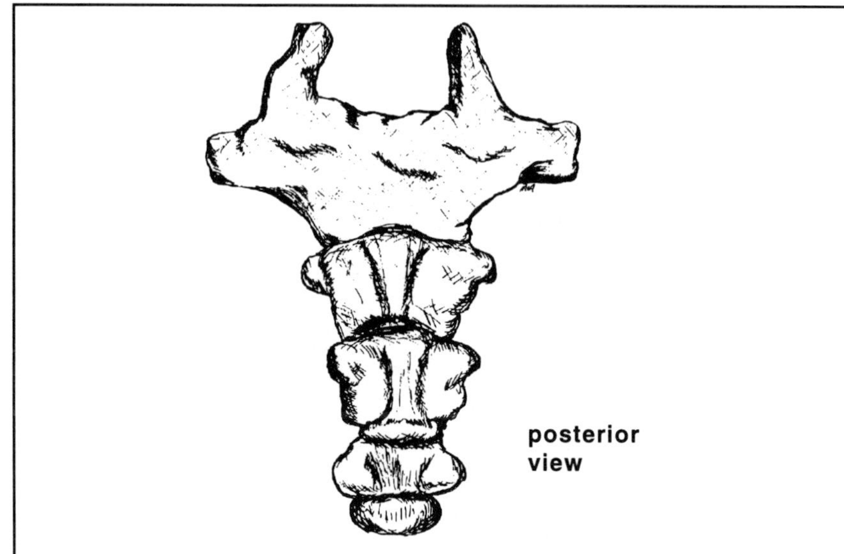

Fig. 6.10

Viewed laterally, the spinal column is seen to comprise four curves. Two of these, the curves of the thoracic and sacrococcygeal regions, are convex posteriorly whereas the remaining two curves, those of the cervical and lumbar regions are convex anteriorly. Since the former two curves existed before birth, they are referred to as **primary curves**. The cervical and lumbar curves develop during infancy and early childhood, and are called **secondary curves**.

LIGAMENTS OF THE SPINE

Seven ligaments of the spine will be discussed briefly. Two of these are ligaments of the vertebral bodies, and five are associated with the pedicles, laminae, and vertebral processes (the vertebral arches). The anterior longitudinal ligament (Fig. 6.11) extends from the inner surface of the occipital bone down the anterior surface of the vertebral bodies to the sacrum. It is thickest in the thoracic area. The posterior longitudinal ligament (Fig. 6.11) extends from the occipital bone down the posterior surface of the vertebral bodies to the coccyx. It is thickest in the thoracic area. The ligamenta flava (Fig. 6.11) connect the laminae of adjacent vertebrae. They are thickest in the lumbar region. The interspinous ligaments (Fig. 6.11) connect neighboring borders of the spinous processes. They are thin ligaments but are best developed in the lumbar region. The supraspinal ligament (Fig. 6.11) connects the posterior tips of the spinous processes. It extends from the seventh cervical vertebra to the sacrum and is thicker in the lumbar than in the thoracic region.

Ligaments of the Spine

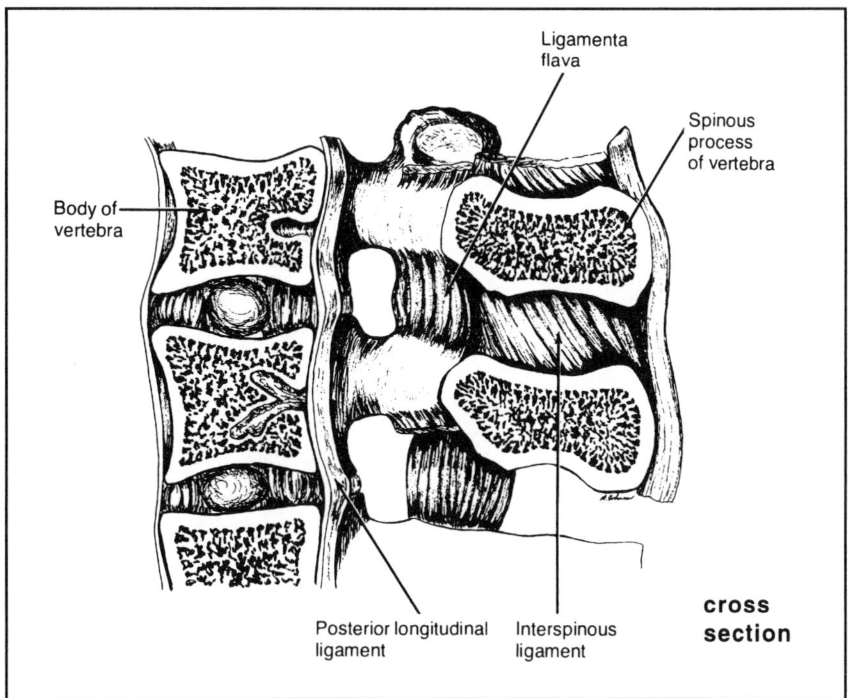

Fig. 6.11

The ligamentum nuchae (Fig. 6.12), or ligament of the neck, is an extension of the supraspinal ligament upwards from the seven cervical vertebrae to the occipital bone. It forms a division between the muscles on either side of the neck. The intertransversii ligaments are poorly developed ligaments which course between the transverse processes of adjacent vertebrae. They are best developed in the thoracic region.

Ligamentum Nuchae

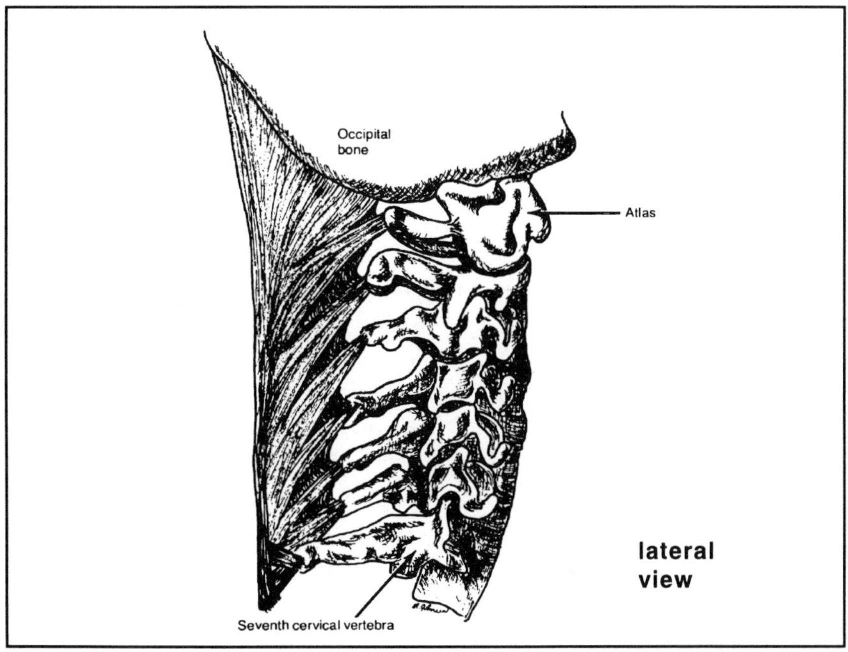

Fig. 6.12

MOVEMENTS OF THE SPINE

The movements of the spine are made possible by two types of articulations; those between the vertebral bodies, and those between the vertebral arches. With the exception of the joint between the first and second cervical vertebrae, the joints between the bodies are classified as cartilaginous because of the discs of fibrocartilage which occupy the intervertebral spaces. Each disc consists of an outer rim, the annulus fibrosis, and a pulpy nucleus, the nucleus pulposus (Fig. 6.13). The nucleus pulposus is firmly compacted material with elastic properties to permit compression in any direction around it.

Intervertebral Discs of Lumbar Spine

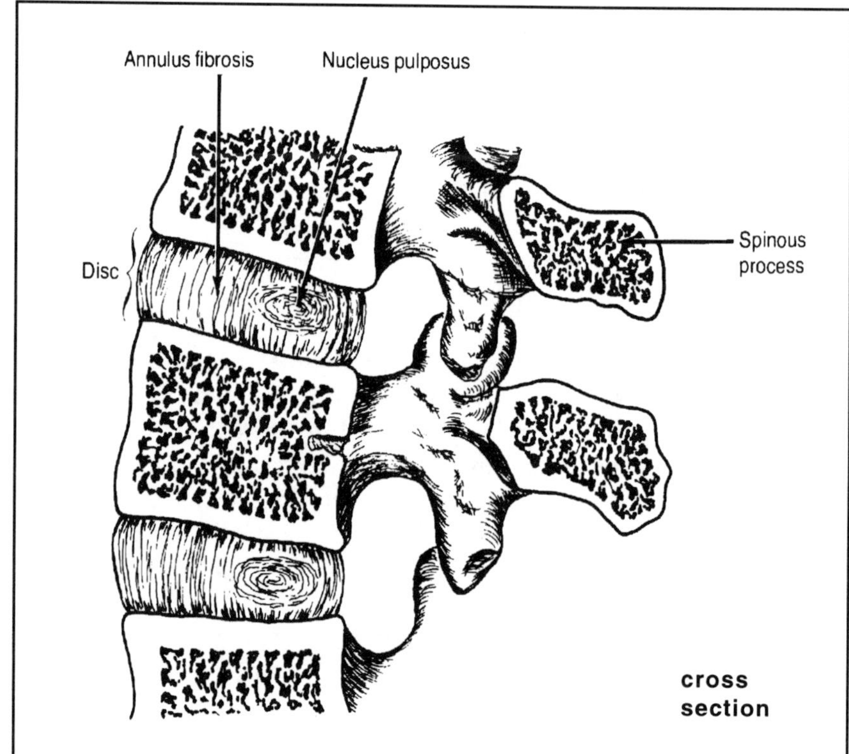

Fig. 6.13

Whereas no single disc can provide for more than slight compression, a cumulation of the compressive movement over several discs yields impressive ranges of motion not unlike those of a triaxial ball and socket joint (Fig. 6.14). Flexion, extension and hyperextension of the spine occur in the sagittal plane around multiple axes, each one passing from side to side through the nucleus pulposus of the compressing discs. Lateral flexion occurs in the frontal plane around sagittal axes passing, again, through the nucleus pulposus. Rotation of the spine, described as being either right or left, occurs in the transverse plane around a long axis passing downward from the top of the head through the discs to the sacral region. Circumduction combines the actions in the sagittal and frontal planes.

Movements of the Spine

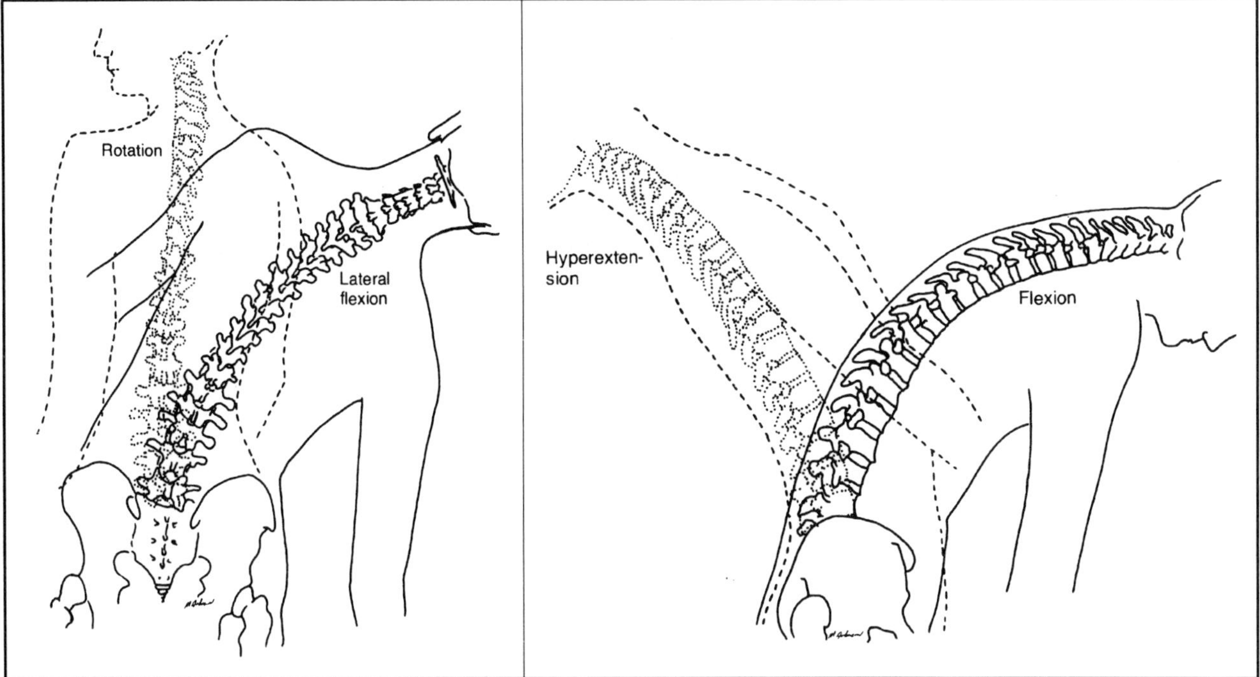

Fig. 6.14

The muscles acting on the spine can be categorized generally as anterior or posterior muscles. Anterior muscles function mainly to flex the spine; posterior muscles extend and hyperextend it. Lateral flexion is caused by either anterior or posterior muscles when only one side of each pair is contracted; rotation is caused by these muscles, also, but only if they do not lie parallel to the long axis.

It should be noted that the action of spinal rotation is always accompanied by a certain amount of lateral flexion to that side. Lateral flexion is, similarly, always accompanied by some rotation to the same side. This phenomenon explains the tendency of most individuals to exhibit a slight pelvic rotation when standing erect, or perhaps an asymmetrical projection of an upper rib. Because use of the preferred arm is so much greater than that of the nonpreferred arm, the musculature on the preferred side of the body is usually better developed, and pulls the spine into slight lateral flexion. The accompanying rotation can manifest itself in the thoracic region causing malalignment of the ribs, or in the lumbar area causing a right or left facing of the hips.

The articulation between the first and second cervical vertebrae, the atlantoaxial joint, has been discussed previously as being a pivot joint allowing only for rotation around the long axis. It should be remembered also that the occipitoatlantal articulation contributes to the overall flexion-extension-hyperextension movement of the spine.

The joints between the vertebral arches are nonaxial synovial joints which allow for a limited amount of gliding between the articulating surfaces. Such an arrangement permits the spinal column to change its shape in response to the temporary distortions of the intervertebral discs.

Figure 6.15 is presented to summarize the movements of the various regions of the spine. The spinal column is depicted in extension as it would be in upright posture, with notations regarding the type and extent of movements of which the several regions are capable. These notations are rather consistent regardless of whether the initial position of the spine is flexed, extended, or hyperextended, with this generalized exception: lateral flexion and rotation occur higher than usual when the starting position involves the flexed spine, and lower than usual when the spine is hyperextended.

Locations of Spinal Movements

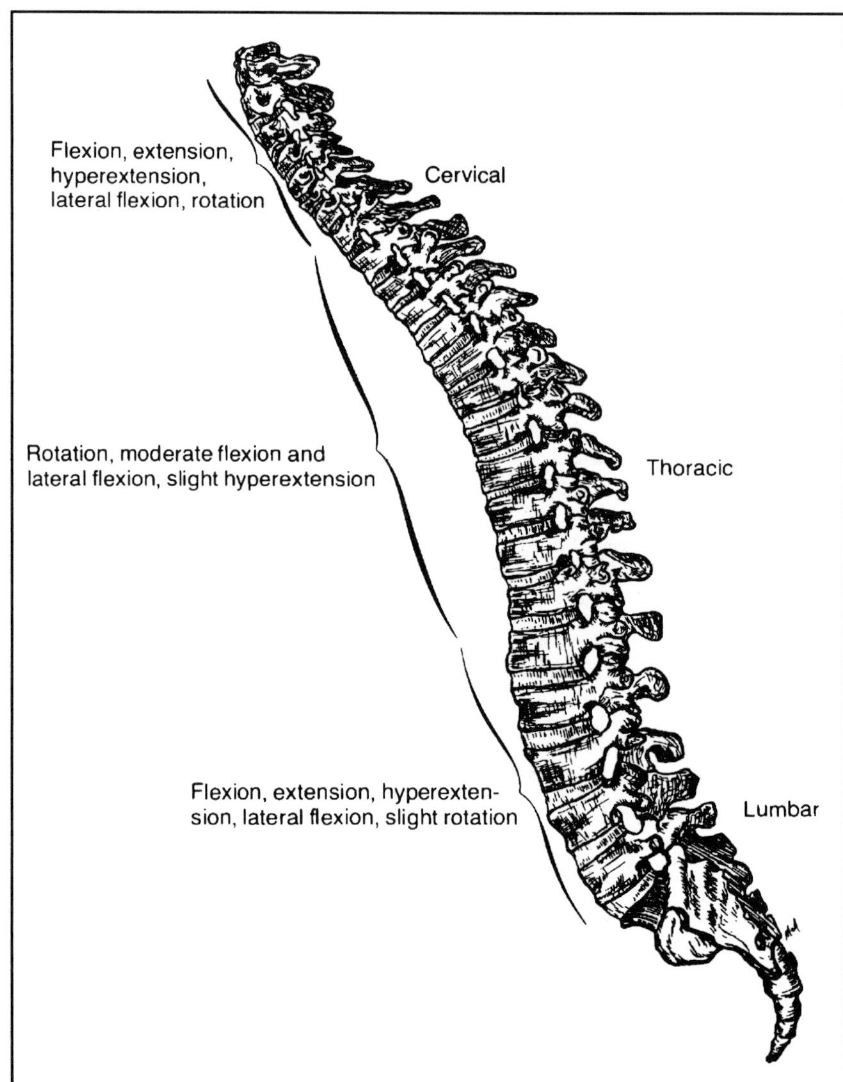

Fig. 6.15

THE PELVIC GIRDLE

The pelvic girdle (Fig. 6.16, 6.17) is comprised of two hip bones, each of which is formed by the fusion of the pubis, ilium, and ischium. The two hip bones themselves are joined around the sacrum, and then tied together at the symphysis to form a single unit.

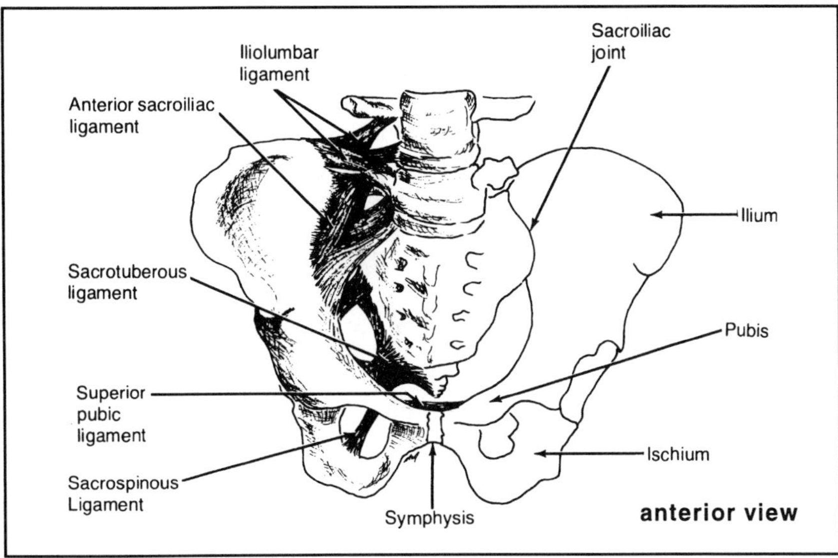

Fig. 6.16

The Pelvis

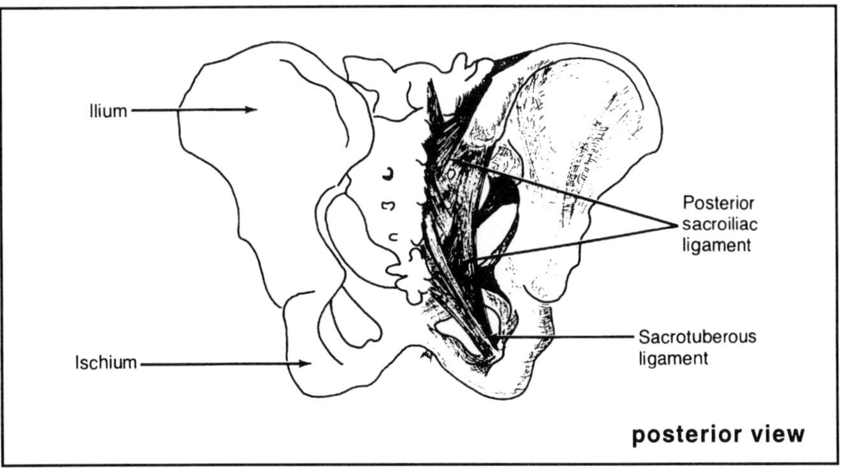

Fig. 6.17

The Pelvis

The sacroiliac articulation defies precise categorization. It presents characteristics of a nonaxial synovial joint in that a joint space containing synovial fluid is present in a portion of the articulation. Movement is extremely limited, however, and is never voluntary. The articulation also presents characteristics of a cartilaginous joint. There is an intervening plate of cartilage between the two bones which, together with the anterior and posterior sacroiliac ligaments and the interosseus ligament, is responsible for the near immobility of the joint.

The symphysis is a cartilaginous joint which joins the two pubes. The joint is only slightly movable, being reinforced heavily by the superior pubic and arcuate pubic ligaments.

The lumbosacral joint, discussed previously in this chapter, is the most important articulation to pelvic movement. All movements of the pelvic girdle occur around this joint.

Movements of the Pelvic Girdle

Forward Tilt	Hyperextension of the lumbosacral joint resulting in a downward and backward movement of the symphysis.
Backward Tilt	Reduction of hyperextension of the lumbosacral joint resulting in an upward and forward movement of the symphysis.
Lateral Tilt	Lateral flexion of the lumbosacral joint resulting in the raising or lowering of one iliac crest.
Rotation	Rotation to the right or left at the lumbosacral joint resulting in a pivotal movement of the hips around the long axis.

The muscles acting on the lumbosacral joint are those which move the spine and will be discussed in the following section. In general, muscles which cause forward and backward tilt will be those located on the posterior and anterior aspects of the spine, respectively. Lateral tilt and rotation will be caused by the contraction of only one side of paired muscles; rotation results specifically from contraction of those muscles which are not parallel to the long axis.

MUSCLES OF THE SPINE AND PELVIC GIRDLE

Most of the musculature of the spine can be conveniently organized into groups of two or more muscles with no consequential loss to the learning of the underlying concepts. It must be realized, however, that this approach necessitates the generalization of origins, insertions, innervations, and actions. Frequent referral to the illustrations and to a skeleton should clarify any confusion, but if more precision is required, one of the several classical texts of human anatomy may be consulted.

All of the muscle groups discussed in this section are paired, with one of each pair located on either side of the long axis. Their actions are, therefore, described according to whether both sides of the pair are contracting or only one side is active.

Reference will be made frequently to the axes around which the muscles act. It was noted earlier that there is no single sagittal or frontal or long axis of the spine. Rather, there are multiple axes passing through the discs between the compressing vertebrae. For practical purposes, however, it will suffice to refer to the three axes in the singular when describing the actions of the muscle groups.

Prevertebral Muscles

The prevertebral muscles (Fig. 6.18) are the rectus capitis anterior, rectus capitis lateralis, longus capitis, and longus colli (rec'tus cap'itis ante'rior, rec'tus cap'itis latera'lis, lon'gus cap'itis, and lon'gus col'li). They are deep muscles and cannot be palpated.

Prevertebral Muscles

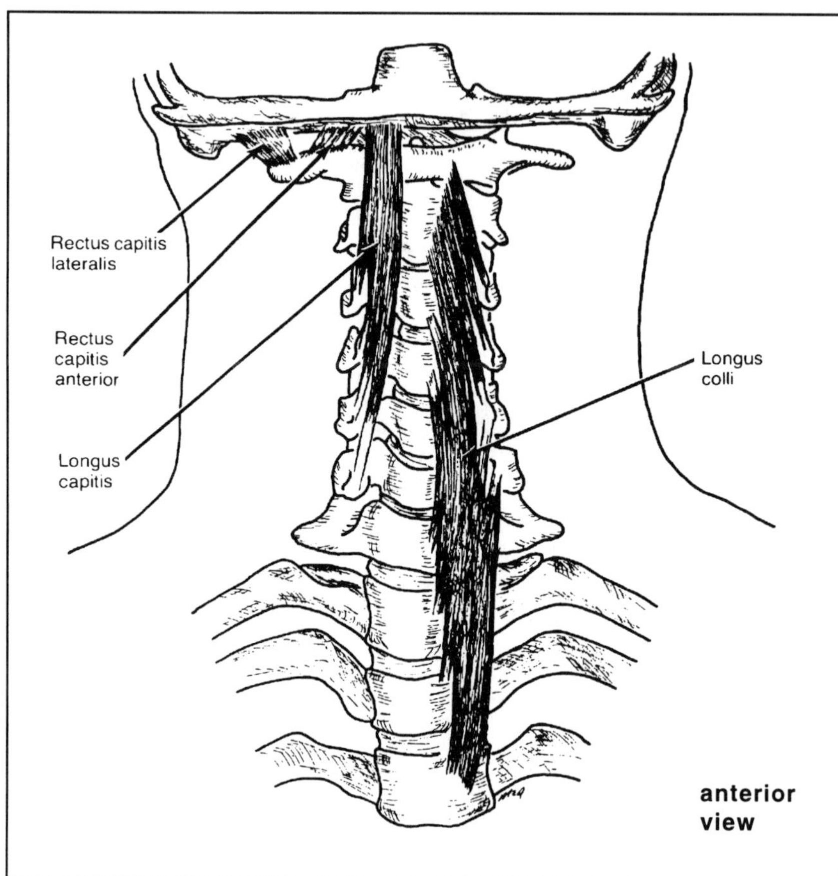

Fig. 6.18

Origin — Anterior surfaces of all cervical and first three thoracic vertebrae.
Insertion — Anterior aspect of the occipital bone and the cervical vertebrae.
Innervation — Cervical nerves.
Action — Both sides: Flexion of atlantooccipital joint and the cervical spine. One side: Lateral flexion of cervical spine.

The muscles of the prevertebral group are located anterior to the spine; however, with their attachments on the spine itself, they have short force arms. This, together with their small size, enables them to be only assistive in their actions.

The Scaleni

The scaleni (Fig. 6.19) are the scalenus anterior, scalenus posterior, and the scalenus medius (scale'nus ante'rior, scale'nus poste'rior, and scale'nus medius). They are located on the side of the neck between the sternocleidomastoid and Part 1 of the trapezius and are easily confused with those muscles during palpation.

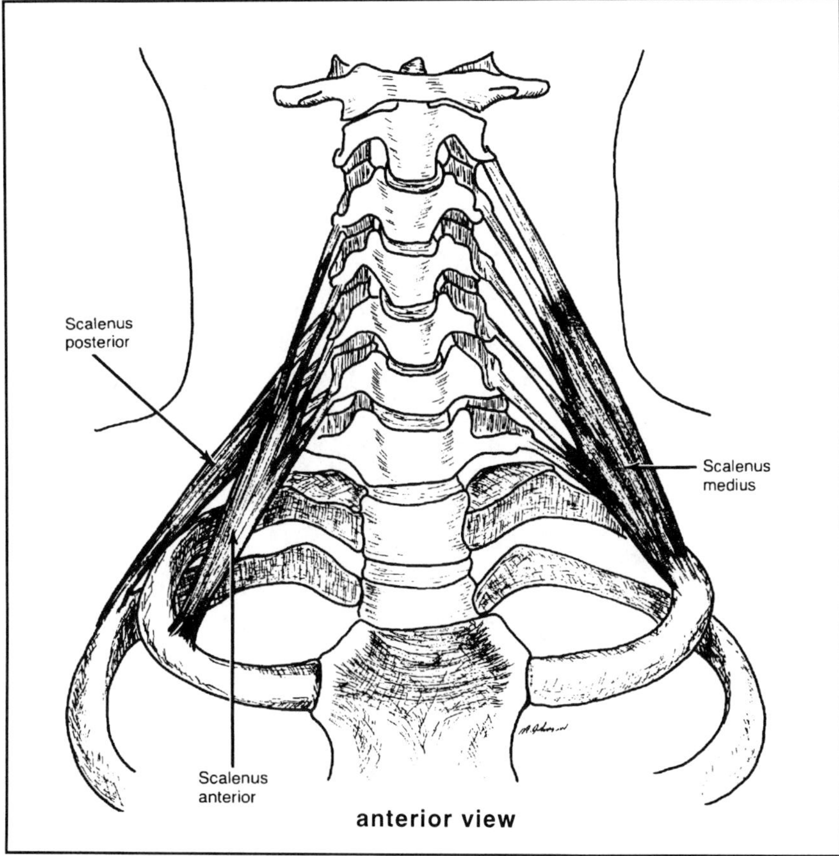

Fig. 6.19

The Scaleni Muscles

Origin — Upper two ribs
Insertion — Transverse processes of the cervical vertebrae.
Innervation — Second to seventh cervical nerves.
Action — Both sides: Flexion of cervical spine. One side: Lateral flexion of cervical spine.

The attachments of the scaleni locate the muscles only slightly anterior to the spine; hence, they are not capable of more than a weak contribution to flexion of the cervical spine. They are, however, well located for lateral flexion in that their attachments on the ribs serve to extend their force arms from the sagittal axis.

Sternocleidomastoid (ster'no cleid'o mas'toid)

The sternocleidomastoid (Fig. 6.20) is the large cord-like muscle located on each side of the neck. It may be palpated easily as the head is rotated to the opposite side.

Sternocleidomastoid of Both Sides of Neck

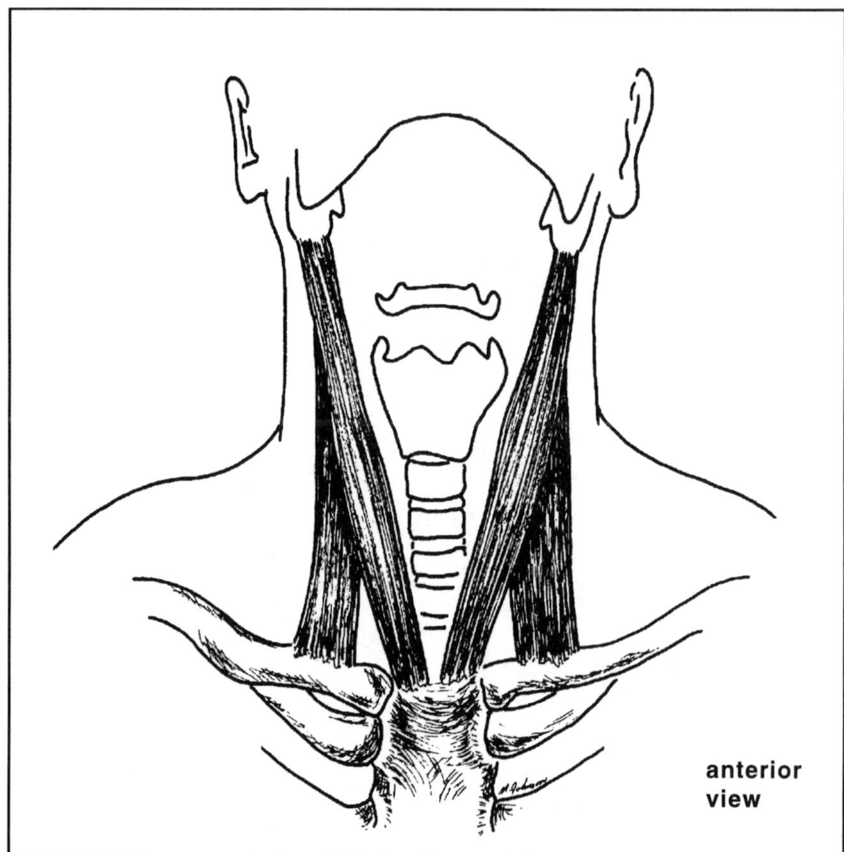

Fig. 6.20

Origin ——	By two heads, from the superior aspect of the sternum and the inner third of the clavicle.
Insertion ——	Mastoid process of the temporal bone.
Innervation —	Spinal assessory and second and third cervical nerves.
Action ——	Both sides: Flexion of atlantooccipital joint and by continued action, flexion of the cervical spine. One side: Lateral flexion of the cervical spine; rotation to opposite side of atlantoaxial joint and cervical spine.

The sternocleidomastoid is the largest of the anterior muscles acting on the head and neck. Its relatively long force arm to all three axes enables the muscle to exert a great deal of force in all of its actions.

Levator Scapulae (leva'tor scap'ulae)

The levator scapulae (Fig. 6.21) is located on the lateral and posterior aspect of the neck. It lies beneath Part 1 of the trapezius and cannot be palpated except through that muscle portion.

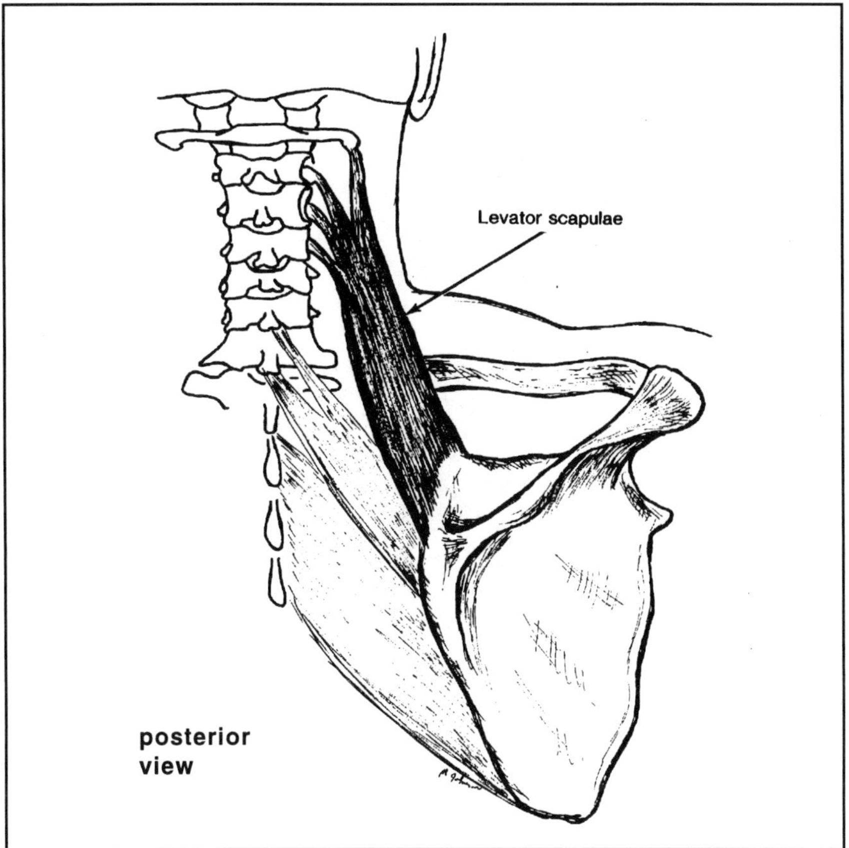

Levator Scapulae

Fig. 6.21

Origin	Vertebral border of the scapula, between the superior angle and the root of the scapular spine.
Insertion	Transverse processes of the first four cervical vertebrae.
Innervation	Dorsal scapular and third and fourth cervical nerves.
Action	Both sides: Stabilization of the cervical spine. One side: Lateral flexion of the cervical spine.

The primary function of the levator scapulae is to elevate the scapula; however, when the scapula is stabilized to provide an origin, the muscle, if only one side is contracted, will pull the cervical spine into lateral flexion. If both muscles are contracted, they neutralize each other's tendency to laterally flex, and cervical stability results.

Splenius Muscles

The splenius muscles (Fig. 6.22) are the splenius capitis and splenius cervicis (sple'nius cap'itis and sple'nius cer'vicis). The capitis is superficial between the sternocleidomastoid and trapezius, just below the skull.

Splenius Muscles

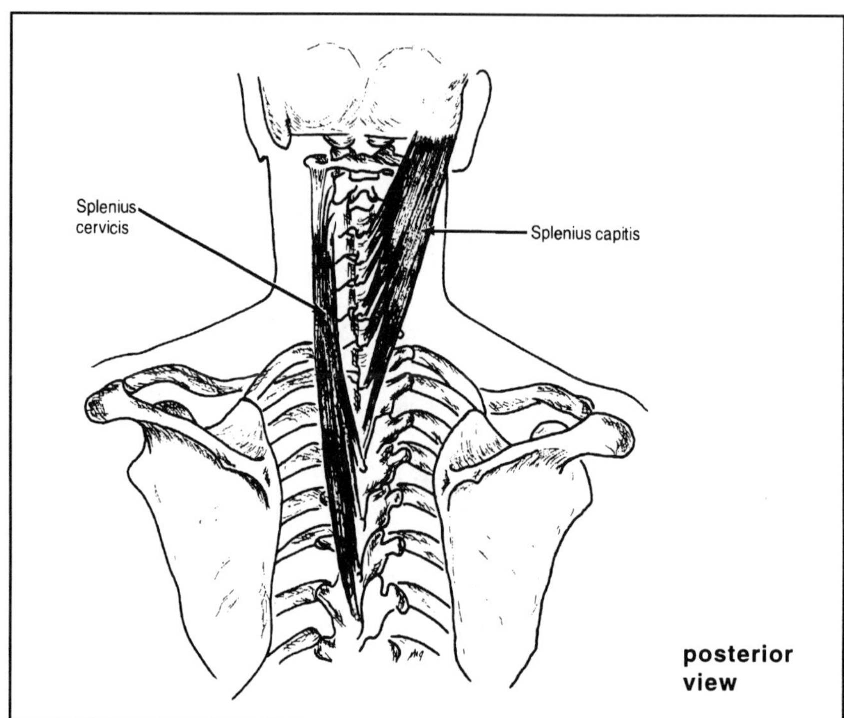

Fig. 6.22

Origin	Inferior half of ligamentum nuchae; spinous processes of last cervical and upper six thoracic muscles.
Insertion	Mastoid process of temporal bone; transverse processes of first three cervical vertebrae.
Innervation	Branches of the middle and lower cervical nerves.
Action	Both sides: Extension and hyperextension of atlantooccipital joint and cervical spine. One side: Lateral flexion and rotation to the same side of the cervical spine.

The splenius muscles are located posterior to the frontal axis, lateral to the sagittal axis, and by virtue of the attachment of the capitis on the mastoid process, are diagonal to the long axis. If both sides are contracted simultaneously, they neutralize their tendencies to rotate and laterally flex; the resultant action is a backward movement of the head and neck in the sagittal plane. If only one side is contracted, the muscles spend their action in lateral flexion and/ or rotation.

The Suboccipitals

The suboccipitals (Fig. 6.23) are the obliquus capitis superior, obliquus capitis inferior, rectus capitis posterior major, and rectus capitis posterior minor (obli'quus cap'itis supe'rior, obli'quus cap'itis infe'rior, rec'tus cap'itis poste'rior ma'jor, and rec'tus cap'itis poste'rior mi'nor). They lie deep below the skull and cannot be palpated.

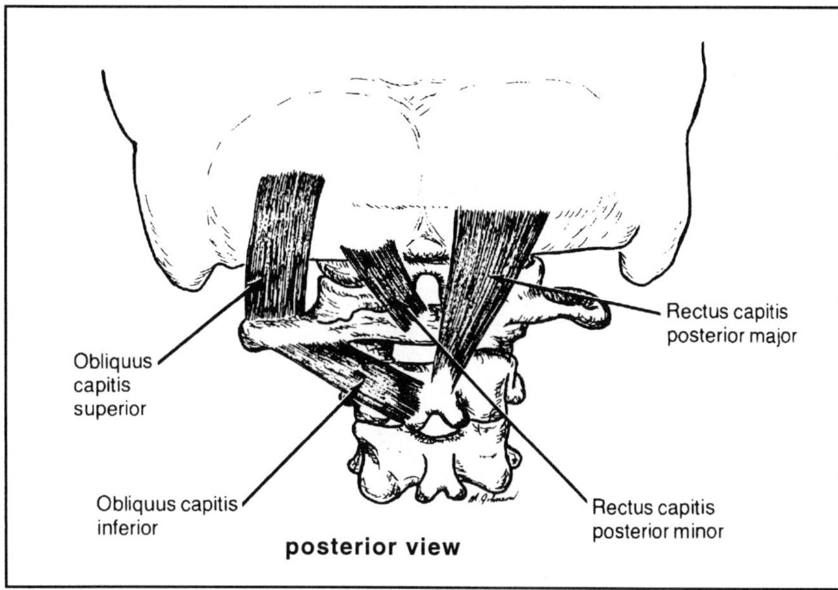

Fig. 6.23

The Suboccipital Muscles

Origin ——	Posterior surfaces of the first two cervical vertebrae (atlas and axis).
Insertion ——	Occipital bone and transverse process of the first cervical vertebra (atlas).
Innervation —	Suboccipital nerve.
Action ——	Both sides: Extension and hyperextension of the atlantooccipital joint. One side: Lateral flexion of the cervical spine and rotation to the same side.

The vertical line of pull of the two rectus muscles favors the extension/hyperextension function of the suboccipitals, whereas the two oblique muscles, with their diagonal lines of pull, favor rotation. None of the muscles is sufficiently large, however, to contribute more than assistively to any action.

Erector Spinae (erec'tor spi'nae)

The erector spinae (Fig. 6.24) is a massive muscle of the back consisting of the iliocostalis, longissimus, and spinalis (iliocosta'lis, longis'simus, and spina'lis) branches. Each branch is further subdivided according to its location as follows:

The Erector Spinae

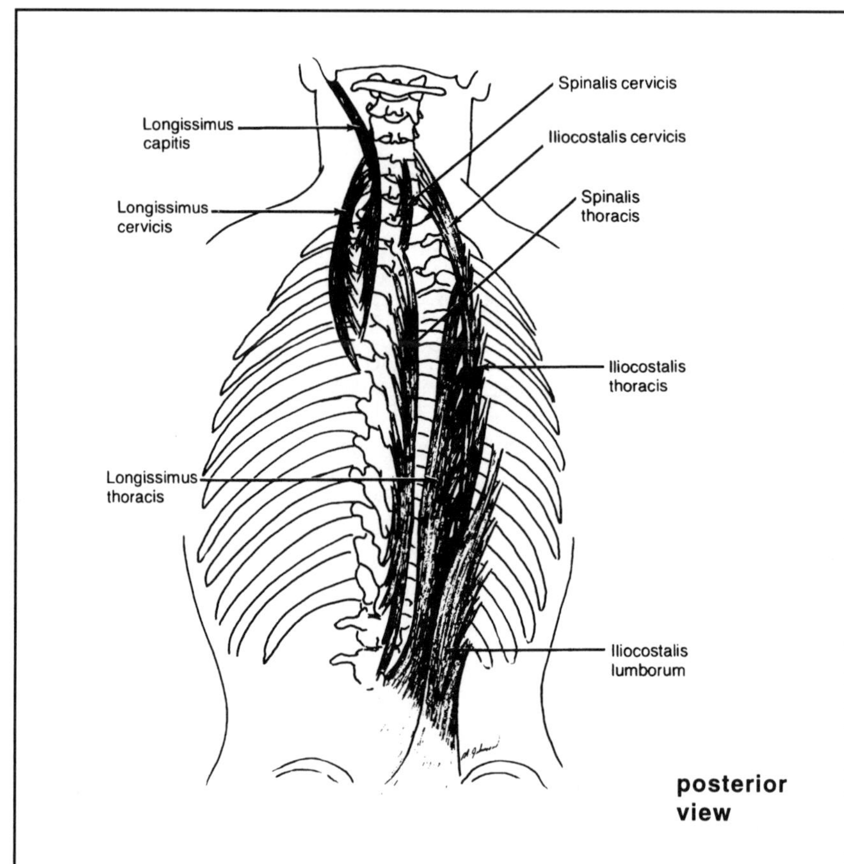

Fig. 6.24

Iliostalis —	Cervicis, thoracis, lumborum.
Longissimus —	Capitus, cervicis, thoracis.
Spinalis —	Cervicis, thoracis.
Origin —	Lower portion of ligamentum nuchae; posterior aspect of cervical, thoracic, and lumbar spine; angles of the lower nine ribs; iliac crest; posterior sacrum.
Insertion —	Mastoid process of temporal bone; posterior aspects of cervical, thoracic, and lumbar vertebrae; angles and adjacent portions of the twelve ribs.
Innervation —	Posterior branches of spinal nerves.
Action —	Both sides: Extension and hyperextension of atlantooccipital joint and entire spine. One side: Lateral flexion of entire spine and rotation to the same side.

The erector spinae is recruited completely during almost all movements of the spine; however, certain portions of the muscle will predominate according to whether the movement is in the sagittal, frontal, or transverse plane. In general, it might be said that the portions of the muscle closer to the spine favor extension and hyperextension, and those farther from the spine favor lateral flexion. Rotation is accomplished by those portions which have a diagonal rather than vertical line of pull with respect to the long axis of the spine.

The erector spinae is not only an important mover of the spine, it functions also to stabilize the spine by contracting eccentrically to control flexion and lateral flexion. For example, when the trunk is flexed from the anatomical reference position, the erector spinae becomes active in order to control the torso against the effects of gravity. Activity gradually ceases as full flexion is approached. At full flexion, the muscle is quiet, and the support of the trunk becomes the responsibility of the fasciae and posterior ligaments. Similarly, when the trunk is lifted through extension, the erector spinae does not resume activity until after the initial phase of the movement has been accomplished. The frequent warning, "lift with your legs, not your back," would appear to have validity if one is to avoid the dangers of overstressing the vertebral ligaments.

Semispinalis Muscles (semispina'lis)

The semispinalis muscles (Fig. 6.25) are the semispinalis capitis, semispinalis cervicis, and semispinalis thoracis (semispina'lis cap'itis, semispina'lis cer'vicis, semispina'lis thora'cis). The muscles lie in the neck and upper back; they cannot be palpated.

The Semispinalis Muscles

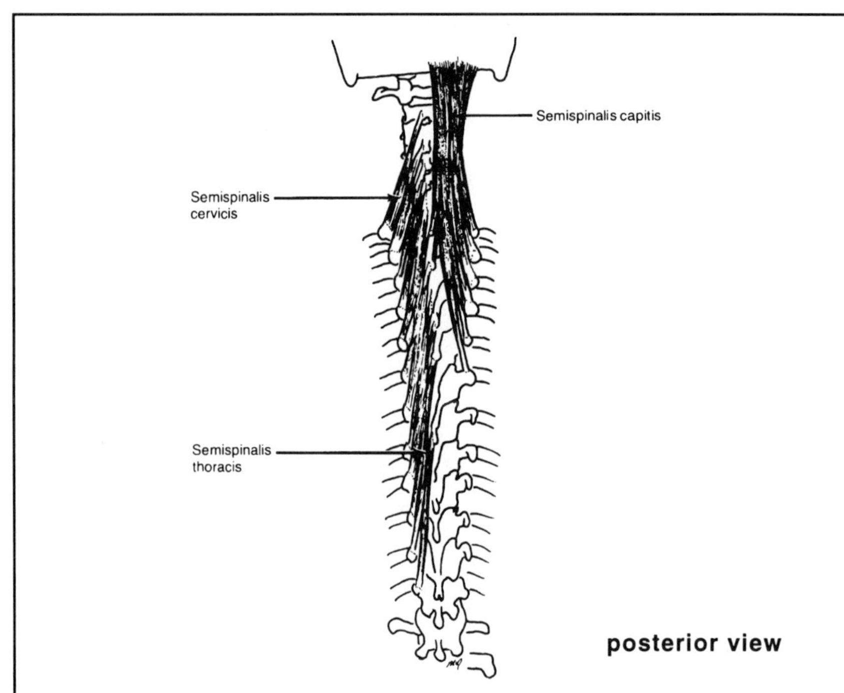

Fig. 6.25

Origin — Articular processes of the fourth through sixth cervical vertebrae; transverse processes of seventh cervical through tenth thoracic vertebrae.

Insertion — Occipital bone; spinous processes of second cervical through fourth thoracic vertebrae.

Innervation — Posterior branches of cervical and thoracic nerves.

Action — Both sides: Extension and hyperextension of atlantoocciptial joint and joints of cervical and thoracic spine. One side: Lateral flexion of cervical and thoracic spine; rotation of thoracic spine to opposite side.

The line of pull of the capitis portion of the semispinalis group is vertical, and whereas it is well-situated for extension, hyperextension and lateral flexion, it cannot contribute to rotation. The cervical and thoracic portions have a slightly diagonal direction and, in addition to moving the spine backwardly and laterally, can rotate it by pulling the spinous processes toward the transverse and articulating processes of the vertebrae below them. When the spinous processes are pulled in one direction, the resulting spinal rotation is in the opposite direction.

Deep Posterior Muscles

The deep posterior muscles of the spine (Fig. 6.26) are the rotatores, multifidus, interspinalis, intertransversii, and the levatores costarum (rotato'res, multif'idus, interspina'lis, intertransversa'rii, levato'res costa'rum). None of these muscles can be palpated.

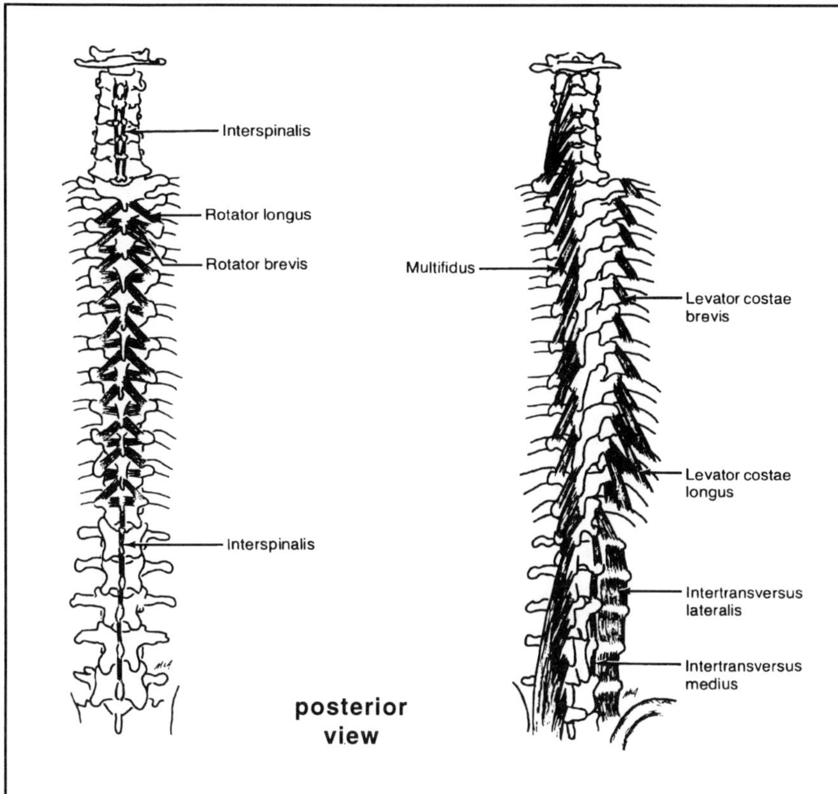

Deep Posterior Muscles

Fig. 6.26

Origin ——	Posterior processes of all vertebrae; posterior surface of sacrum.
Insertion ——	Spinous and transverse processes, and laminae of vertebrae above those on which the muscle portions originate.
Innervation —	Spinal and intercostal nerves, and eighth cervical nerve.
Action ——	Both sides: Extension and hyperextension of entire spine. One side: Lateral flexion of spine; rotation to opposite side.

These muscles are quite small, consisting of short slips which seldom span more than one vertebra from origin to insertion. The interspinalis and intertransversii lie parallel to the long axis and hence favor extension, hyperextension, and lateral flexion. The other portions lie diagonally to the long axis and thus are able to contribute the additional actions of rotation.

Quadratus Lumborum (quadra'tus lumbo'rum)

The quadratus lumborum (Fig. 6.27) is located on either side of the spine in the lumbar area. It is difficult to palpate because of the fatty tissue in the area.

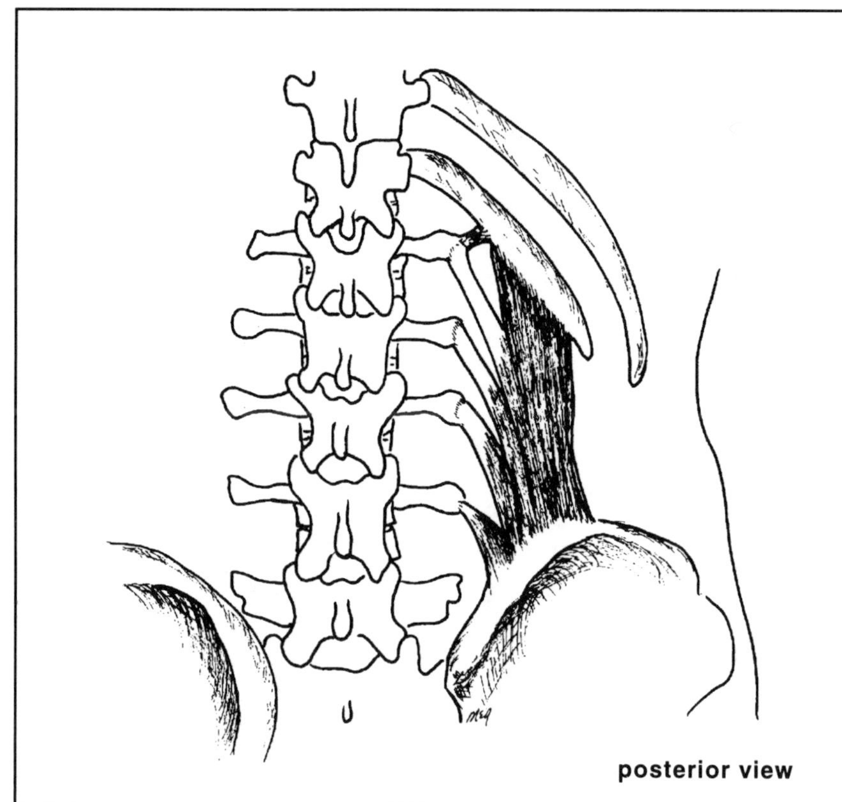

Fig. 6.27

Origin —	Iliolumbar ligament and adjacent portion of iliac crest.
Insertion —	Last rib; transverse processes of first four lumbar vertebrae.
Innervation —	Twelfth thoracic and first lumbar nerves.
Action —	Both sides: Stabilization of the lumbar spine. One side: Lateral flexion of the lumbar spine.

In addition to its importance as a stabilizer and lateral flexor, the quadratus lumborum is active in holding down the twelfth rib during periods of expiration.

Trapezius (trape'zius) **Part 1**

All parts of the trapezius are discussed under the shoulder joint. Part 1 (Fig. 6.28) is singled out for inclusion here because of its attachment to the cranium.

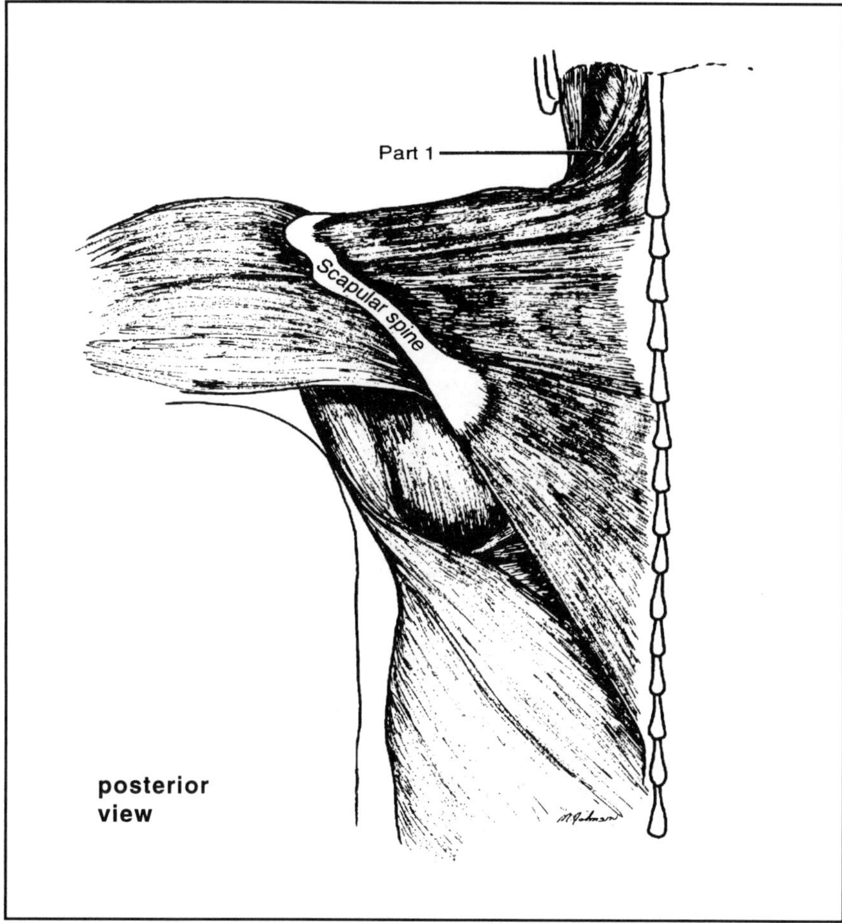

Trapezius

Fig. 6.28

Origin	Outer third of the clavicle.
Insertion	Base of the skull.
Innervation	Spinal assessory nerve.
Action	Both sides: Extension and hyperextension of the atlantooccipital joint. One side: Rotation of the atlantoaxial joint to the opposite side.

All parts of the trapezius are commonly known as scapula movers. When the scapula is stabilized, however, it forms an effective base from which Part 1 of the trapezius can pull backwardly against the head.

THE ABDOMINALS

The abdominal muscles are the rectus abdominis, external oblique, internal oblique, and transversalis abdominis. Because of their importance to the study of kinesiology, they will be considered separately, with the exception of the transversalis which is a respiratory muscle (see "Muscles of Respiration," Chapter 10).

Rectus Abdominis (rec'tus abdom'inus)

The rectus abdominis (Fig. 6.29) is the most superficial of the abdominal muscles. It can be palpated between the sternum and the pubis.

Rectus Abdominis

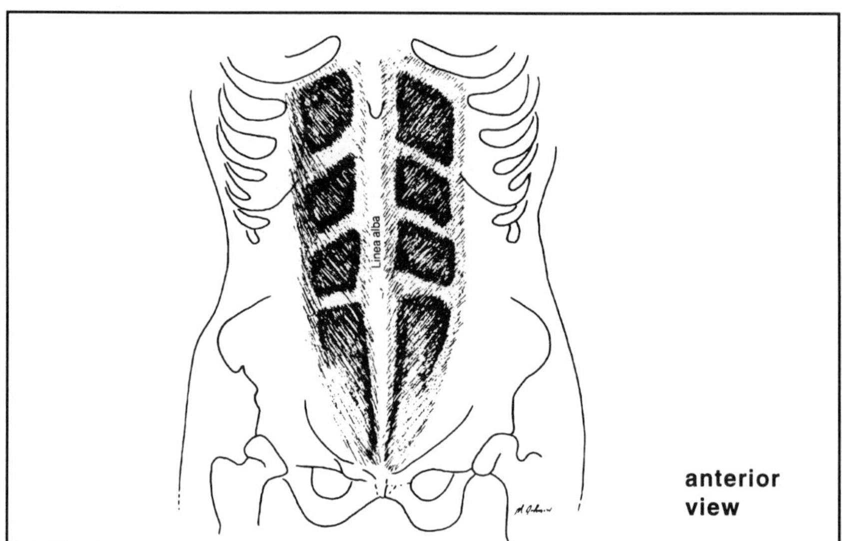

Fig. 6.29

Origin — Crest of the pubis.
Insertion — Cartilages of the fifth, sixth, and seventh ribs.
Innervation — Seventh to twelfth intercostal nerves.
Action — *Both sides:* Flexion of the spine.
One side: Lateral flexion of the spine.

The two sides of the rectus abdominis are separated by a broad tendinous band called the **linea alba**. This band, together with the horizontal tendinous inscriptions of the muscle, give the rectus a rippled appearance which is clearly visible in lean persons.

The primary action of the rectus abdominis is spinal flexion; it can contribute to lateral flexion but only in an assistive fashion because it is so near the sagittal axis. The muscle runs parallel to the long axis, and therefore cannot contribute to rotation.

External Oblique (exter'nal obli'que)

The external oblique (Fig. 6.30) is located on the front and side of the abdomen and is superficial in the area lateral to the rectus abdominis. It can be palpated by the finger tips when the hands are placed on the hips.

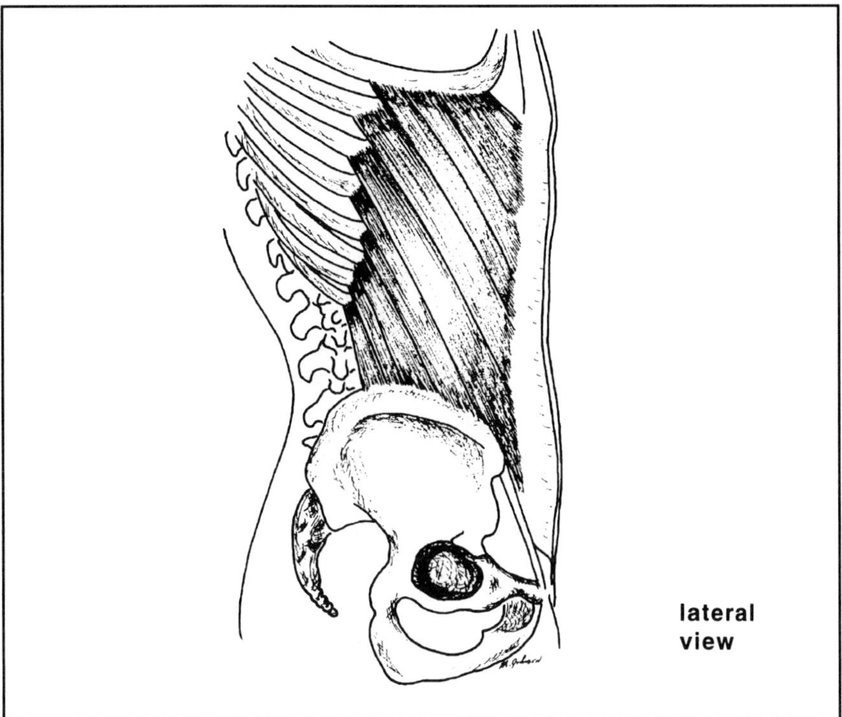

External Oblique

Fig. 6.30

Origin	Lower eight ribs by slips which interweave with those of serratus anterior.
Insertion	Anterior portion of iliac crest; crest of pubis via the linea alba.
Innervation	Iliohypogastric, ilioinguinal and eighth to twelfth intercostal nerves.
Action	Both sides: Flexion of the spine. One side: Lateral flexion of the spine and rotation to the opposite side.

The fibers of the external oblique are anterior and lateral to the frontal and sagittal axes, respectively, and course diagonally downward toward the linea alba to form a *V*. When both sides are contracted together, tendencies to laterally flex and rotate are neutralized and resultant action is that of spinal flexion. Contraction alone, each side of the muscle will laterally flex because of its relationship to the sagittal axis and/or will rotate the spine because of its diagonal line of pull. The action of rotation will be to the opposite side because the muscle's contraction will draw the ribs of the contracting side closer to the midline of the body.

Internal Oblique (inter'nal obli'que)

The internal oblique (Fig. 6.31) is located beneath the external oblique, and must be palpated through that muscle. The external oblique should first be relaxed on one side by rotating the spine to that side. The internal oblique can then be felt contracting beneath the relaxed external muscle.

Internal Oblique

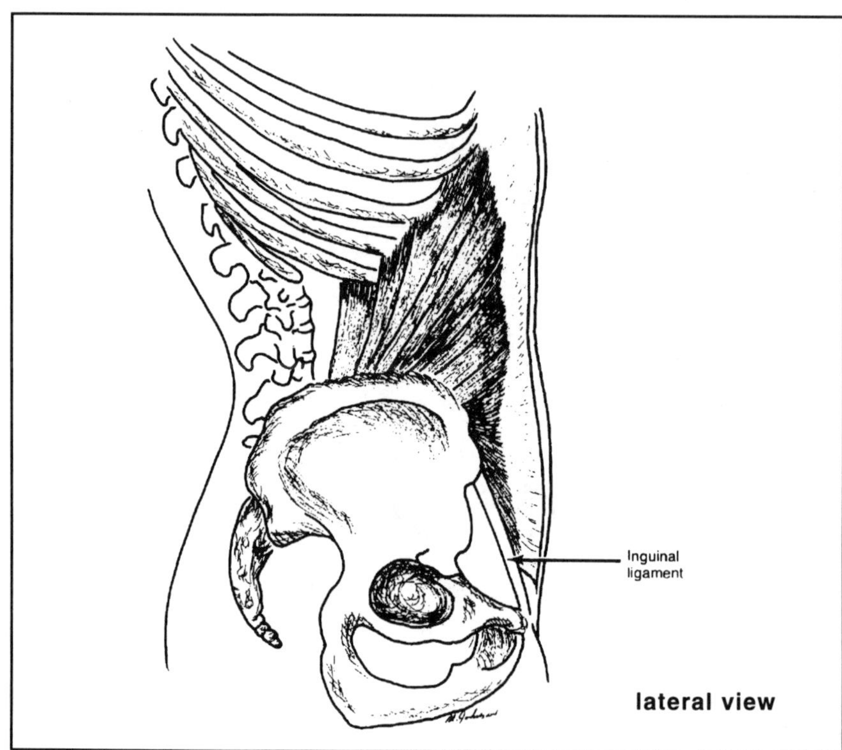

Fig. 6.31

Origin — Lateral half of inguinal ligament; crest of the ilium, thoracolumbar fascia
Insertion — Linea alba; cartilages of lower four ribs.
Innervation — Eighth to twelfth intercostal nerves; iliohypogastric and ilioinguinal nerves.
Action — Both sides: Flexion of the spine.
One side: Lateral flexion of the spine and rotation to the same side.

The actions of the internal oblique are accomplished in much the same manner as the external oblique. The direction of the fibers of the internal is opposite that of the external oblique, however, and as both sides of the muscle approach the linea alba, an inverted V is formed. In rotation, the ribs are pulled toward the iliac crest on that side, and the trunk is turned to that side. In flexion and lateral flexion, then, the two obliques are agonists; in the action rotation, they are antagonists.

Psoas Minor (pso'as mi'nor, "p" is silent)

The psoas minor (Fig. 6.32) lies deep in the abdominal cavity. It cannot be palpated.

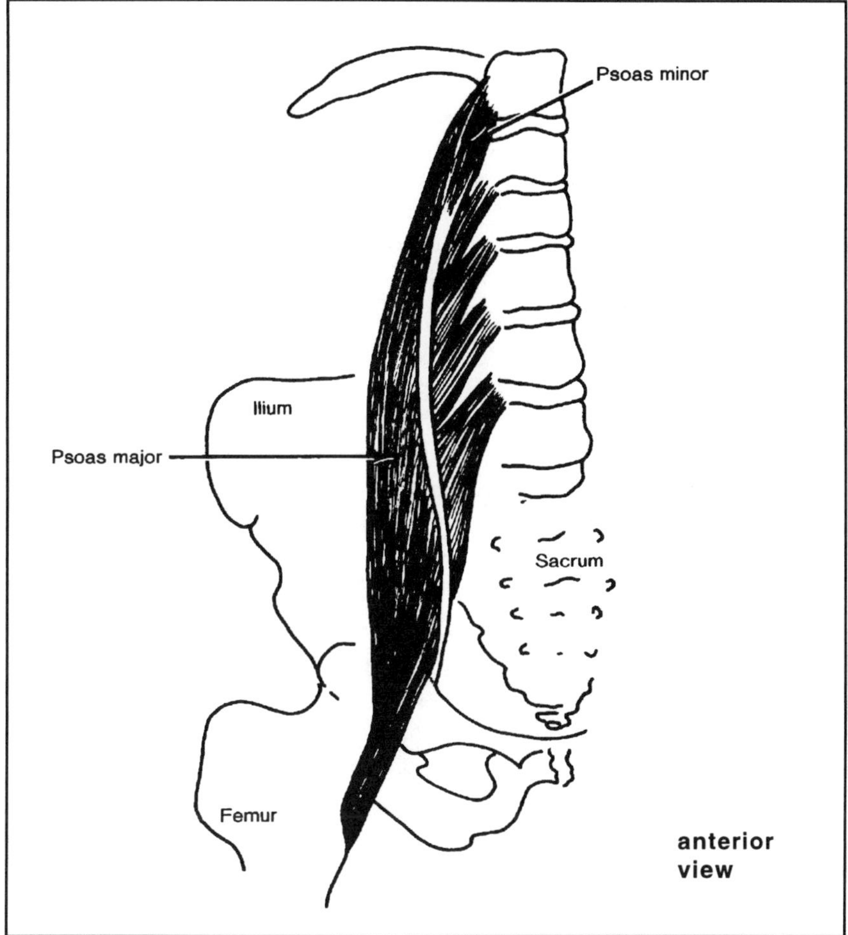

Fig. 6.32

Psoas Minor

Origin	Bodies of the last thoracic and first lumbar vertebrae.
Insertion	Pectineal line of the pubis.
Innervation	First lumbar nerve.
Action	Both sides: Stabilization of the lumbar spine. One side: Lateral flexion of the lumbar spine.

The psoas minor is frequently missing on one or both sides, but when present it is capable of contracting to such a degree that it can cause lumbar scoliosis. The muscle is usually more prone to contracture in the female because of her wide pelvis.

COMMENTS

The muscles of the spine and pelvic girdle are constantly at the mercy of the demands of upright posture. Poor body alignment, ill-conceived exercises, improper mechanics of lifting, pushing, and pulling can all contribute, to some degree, to their dysfunction. It would appear that every individual should maintain constant watch over these muscles, for nothing is more debilitating than acute back pain.

It is, perhaps, athletes who incorporate extreme ranges of spinal movement in their respective movement repertoires who are most susceptible to muscular discomfort. For instance, some activities in dance and gymnastics require hyperextension of the lumbosacral joint and hip (arabesques or backbends); if the hip is incapable of such flexibility, the performer compensates by overextending the lumbosacral joint. Pain or injury is inevitable.

Others are not immune to problems of the back. Mild scoliosis is quite common among those whose daily movement patterns result in overdevelopment of muscles on the preferred side of the body. Under the right (or wrong!) circumstances, a quick change of direction can cause painful spasm in the already shortened muscles.

It would be remiss, at this point, not to remind the reader that improper mechanics of force application are responsible for a high percentage of back problems. A generalization can be stated that may alleviate the problem: if the head is kept erect while lifting, pushing, and pulling, the muscular involvement will be safely delegated elsewhere. The erect head position will tend to keep the hips low and force the large and stronger muscles of the hip and knee to carry out the task.

Millions of Americans suffer from lower back pain. Common causes are strains of the muscles and ligaments surrounding the spine. These sprains can be the result of trauma such as an accident or improper lifting of an object. More often, however, they are caused by muscular imbalance, poor posture, sedentary habits, and overeating.

Frequently, simple changes in daily living habits can decrease back pain. When standing, position one foot ahead of the other and bend the knees slightly. Lean back while sitting and ensure that the knees are higher then the hips -- never allow the feet to dangle. Lying on the back will be more comfortable if the knees are bent to approximately 60 degrees or on a pillow. Avoid resting or sleeping in the prone position. Always bend the knees and keep the head higher than the hips when lifting.

When the back is hurting, a mild pain-killer followed by ice massage for 5 to 7 minutes will provide relief. Then, rehabilitation can begin.

Since poor muscular balance is a major cause of back pain, attention must be given to achieving and maintaining proper balance between the anterior and posterior muscles of the spine. Strengthening the abdominal muscles can both alleviate and prevent low back pain. Several beneficial exercises for this purpose are described below. Gradually increase the repetitions from 5 to 10, up to 15. If pain increases after 4 or 5 repetitions of an exercise, omit it from your regimen.

Anterior and Posterior Muscle Exercises

1. Lie supine and bring the knees, one at a time, to the chest. Hug the knees tightly while pressing the small of the back to the floor. Return the legs, again one at a time, to the extended position *maintaining floor contact with the small of the back.*

2. On hands and knees, allow back to sag toward the floor. Then, slowly bow the back (make a "cat back") by contracting the abdominals and gluteals.

3. Lie supine with knees bent and feet flat on the floor. Lift the head and then the shoulders until the hands can touch the patellas. Return slowly to the beginning position. This exercise is known as the "crunch" or modified sit-up.

As a final note, be attentive to the shoes being worn. Optimally, they should have flat heels as high heels often cause poor standing and walking postures.

A quiz for this material can be found in the back of this book on page 291.

LABORATORY EXERCISES

1. Have a partner lie supine on a table with hands on shoulders and hips and knees extended. Palpate the small of the back to detect whether it is contacting the table or whether it is arched upwardly. Ask the partner to press the small of the back to the table and palpate the abdominals. Which muscles are acting as agonists and which as antagonists, as this is done? Assume your partner is unable to press the back to the table. Which muscles should be strengthened and which should be stretched?

2. Having completed Experience 1 above, have your partner bend the knees so the feet can be placed flat on the table. Palpate the small of the back and notice that it is easily touching the table. Which muscles have been slackened by placing the legs in this new position?

3. Finally, following the two experiences above, ask your partner to straighten the legs and raise them briefly a few inches off the table. What happens to the small of the back? Why?

4. Place electrodes on the rectus abdominis of a partner and monitor the action potentials while such exercises as the cat back (on hands and knees while alternately hyperextending and flexing the spine), bent-knee situp, head-raising while supine lying, and the baskethang (bring knees to chin while hanging from a horizontal bar). Rank the exercises so they present a logical progression for the development of strength in the rectus abdominis.

5. Place electrodes on the superficial portion of the erector spinae of a partner. Have the partner begin in anatomical position and, slowly, touch the toes, return to the reference position, hyperextend the spine, and return to the reference position. When is the erector spinae active during these movements? What muscles, ligaments, and so on, are active when the erector spinae is silent?

Note. It is difficult to explore fully the involvement of the abdominals without including the powerful hip flexors known as the iliopsoas. It is suggested that the student gain familiarity with the muscle complex (see Chapter 7) so that the laboratory experiences will be more meaningful.

THE HIP

STRUCTURE AND MOVEMENTS OF THE HIP JOINT

As was noted in Chapter 2, the hip joint represents the most striking example of the ball and socket joint in the body (Fig. 7.1). The globe-shaped head of the femur fits deeply into the acetabulum and is grasped tightly in place by a ring of fibrocartilage, the labrum, situated along the rim of the socket. The acetabulum is formed by the fusion of the pubis, the ischium, and the ilium.

The Hip Joint

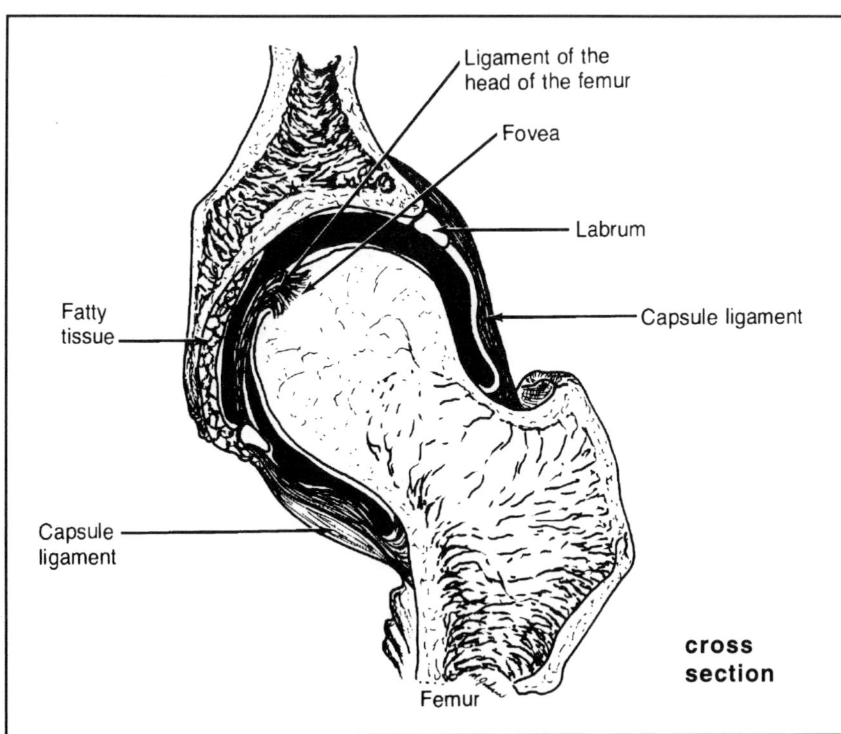

Fig. 7.1

Cartilaginous tissue completely covers the head of the femur except for a small interruption at the top of the head called the fovea. A large horseshoe-shaped portion of the acetabulum is also covered with cartilage, and is broadest along its upper part where it receives the greatest pressure from the femur during upright posture. These two sets of cartilage are intended to provide smooth articulating surfaces which can withstand wear and also provide some shock absorption.

The synovial capsule encloses the entire joint and is formed of a heavy fibrous material which is thickened in some of its portions to form ligamentous bands (Figs. 7.2). These bands, although seldom discernible from the rest of the capsule, are identified kinesiologically as ligaments and are named according to the bone from which they originate -- the pubo-femoral, ischio-femoral, and ilio-femoral (*Y*) ligaments. All of the ligaments become taut when the hip is hyperextended; the pubo-femoral aids, additionally, in checking extreme abduction.

Ligaments of the Hip Joint

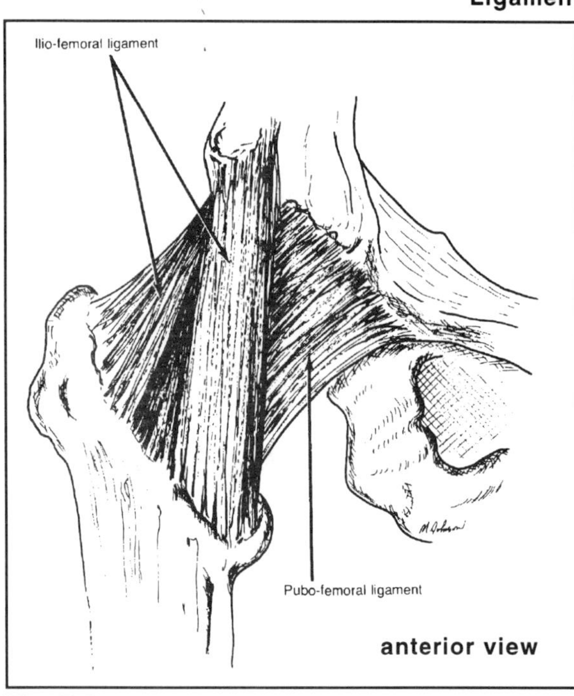

Fig. 7.2a

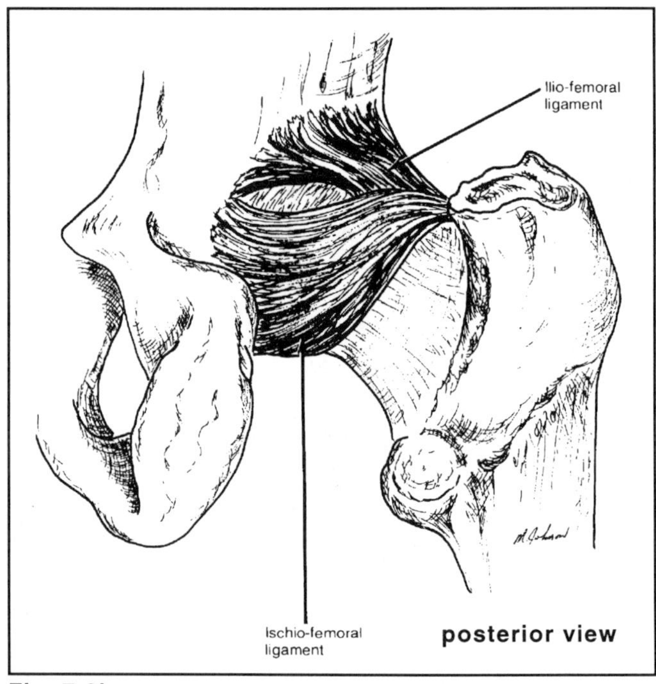

Fig. 7.2b

It has been mentioned that the fovea, a small portion of the head of the femur, is not covered with cartilage; rather, the fovea is the point of insertion of the ligament of the head of the femur. Its origin is along the floor of the acetabulum, and as it courses around the head of the femur, it carries blood supply to the area of the fovea. The tissues of this so-called ligament are too weak to provide the usual ligamentous function of joint stabilization, and therefore its true function in joint stabilization is uncertain.

The actions of the hip joint are those expected of a triaxial joint and are shown in Fig. 7.3. A forward swinging of the femur around the frontal axis is known as flexion; backward swinging to the reference position is extension; and continued backward swing is hyperextension. Sideward movements of the femur around the sagittal axis are referred to as abduction if they are away from the body and adduction if they are toward the body. Twisting movements around the long axis are called internal and external rotation.

Movements of the Hip Joint

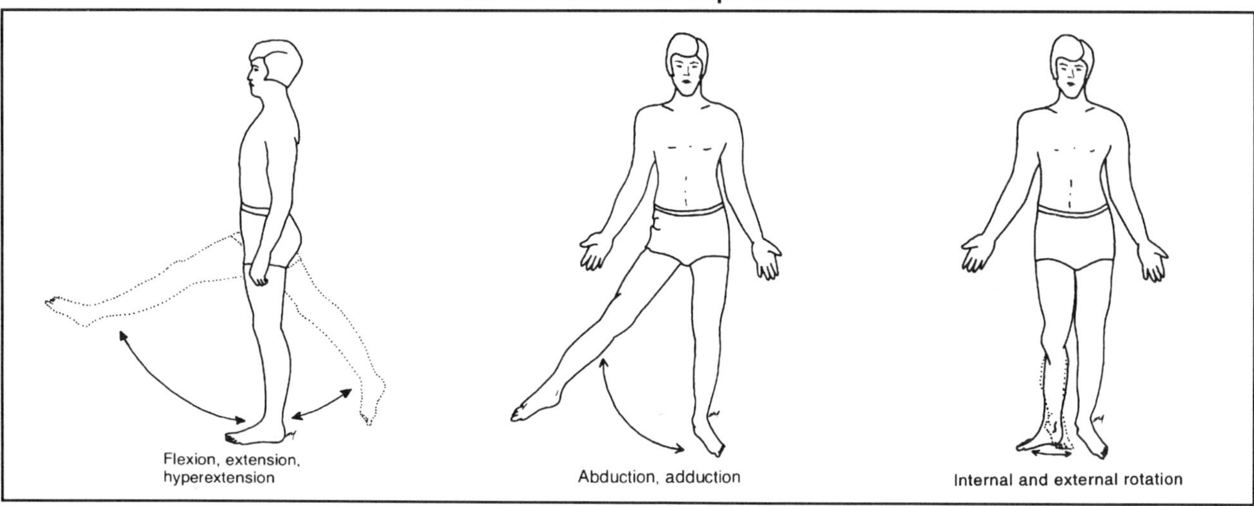

Fig. 7.3

The hip joint is capable of performing an action in which the femur is placed in the transverse plane and moved around the long axis (Fig. 7.4). These movements are called horizontal abduction and horizontal adduction, and, as was the case with the shoulder joint, are not pure movements since they cannot be performed from the reference position without some preliminary movement such as flexion or abduction.

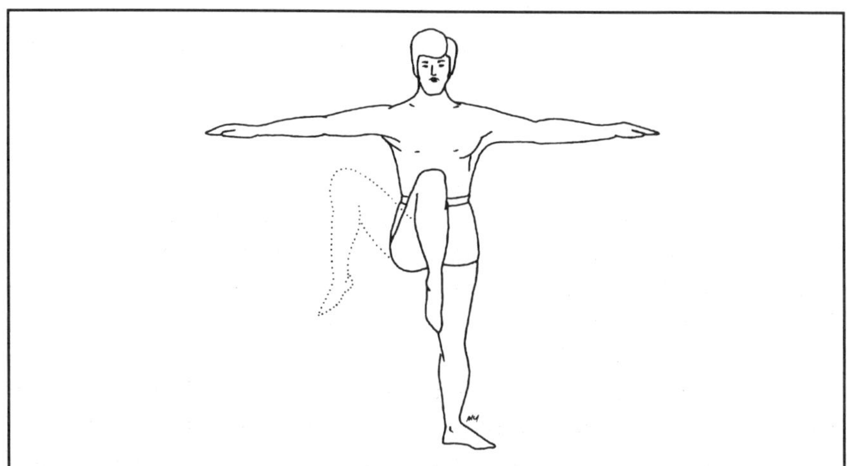

Horizontal Abduction and Horizontal Adduction of the Hip Joint

Fig. 7.4

BONE MARKINGS

Anatomical landmarks pertinent to discussion of muscles of the hip are presented in Figure 7.5. The reader is urged to use them in conjunction with a skeleton.

Bones of the Pelvis and Upper Leg

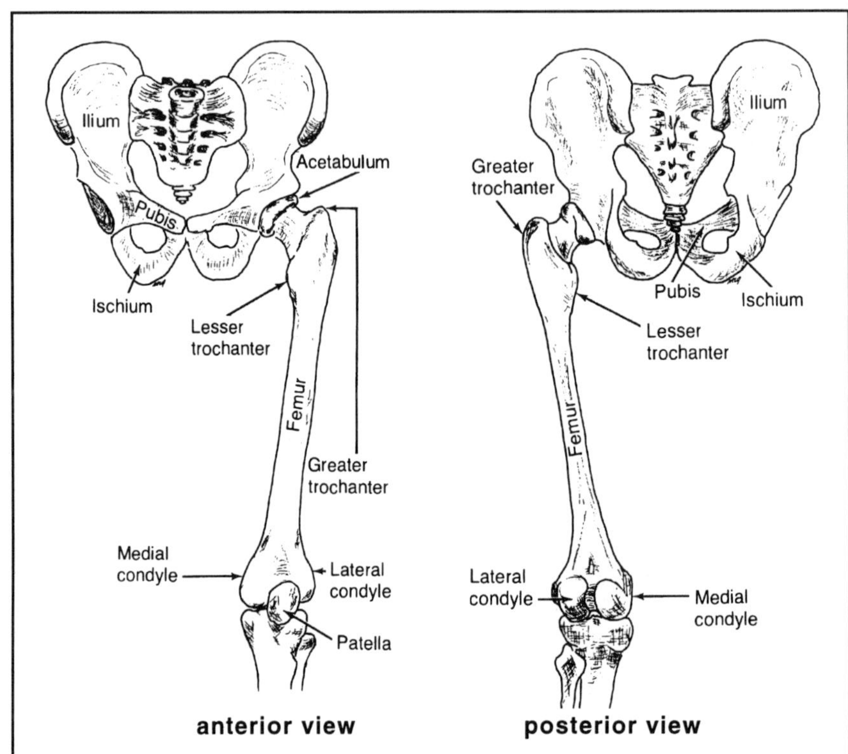

Fig. 7.5

MUSCULATURE

The twenty-two muscles acting on the hip joint derive their various actions from their positions relative to the three axes of the joint. Muscles which pass anterior or posterior to the frontal axis will flex or extend (or hyperextend) the joint, whereas those which pass lateral or medial to the sagittal axis will abduct or adduct, respectively. Internal and external rotation will be accomplished by muscles which originate on the pelvis and, as they course to their insertions on the femur, pass the long axis. Muscles which contract to cause horizontal abduction and horizontal adduction will be those which cause abduction and adduction, since those are the muscles that will pass in front or in back of the long axis when the femur is in the transverse plane. Because all abductors are also horizontal abductors, and all adductors are also horizontal adductors, it has become practice to omit reference to horizontal abduction/adduction as a specific action and rather to infer it from stated abduction/adduction functions.

Psoas (pso'as)

The psoas (Fig. 7.6), often described as two portions called the psoas major and psoas minor, lies deep in the abdominal cavity and cannot be palpated. The psoas major is a hip flexor and the psoas minor is a spinal muscle. The discussion that follows relates to the psoas major.

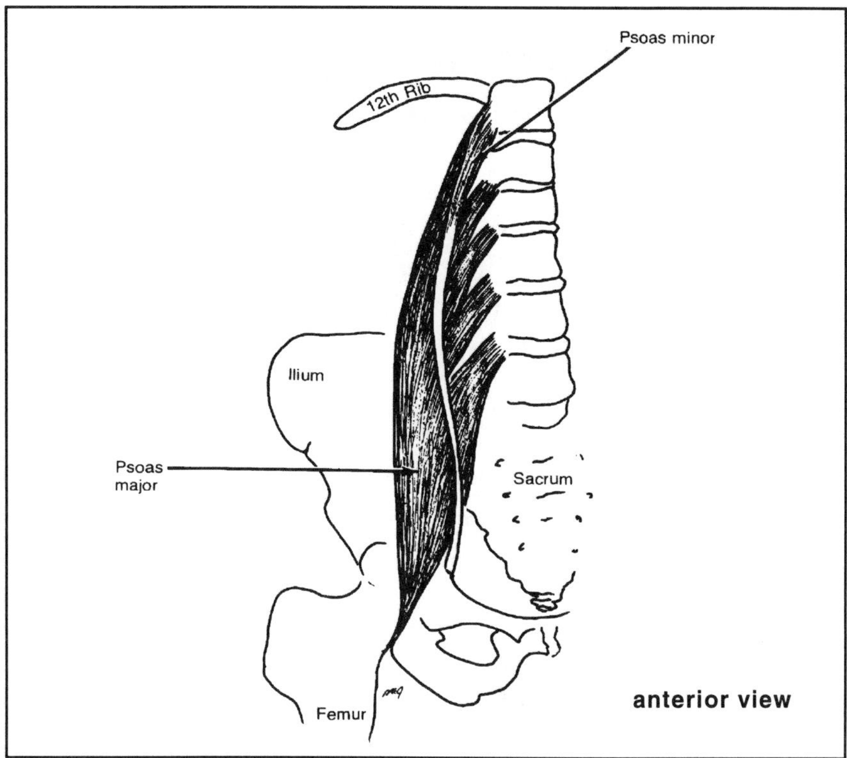

Fig. 7.6

The Psoas

Origin ——	Sides of the twelfth thoracic and all lumbar vertebrae and their intervertebral cartilages.
Insertion ——	Lesser trochanter of the femur.
Innervation —	Femoral nerve.
Action ——	Flexion of the hip.

The psoas major is particularly effective during the initial part of hip flexion since the muscle is then long. As hip flexion progresses through the full range, the psoas becomes increasingly shorter and less effective. This is the basis for the reasoning which led to the bent-knee situp and eventually to the "crunch". Bending the knees while lying supine must be accompanied by hip flexion and thus the psoas, in shortened state, is made to be ineffective. The situp must now be performed by the abdominals as they flex the spine.

Iliacus (ili'acus)

The iliacus (Fig. 7.7) lies along the anterior surface of the ilium, the bone for which it is named. It cannot be palpated.

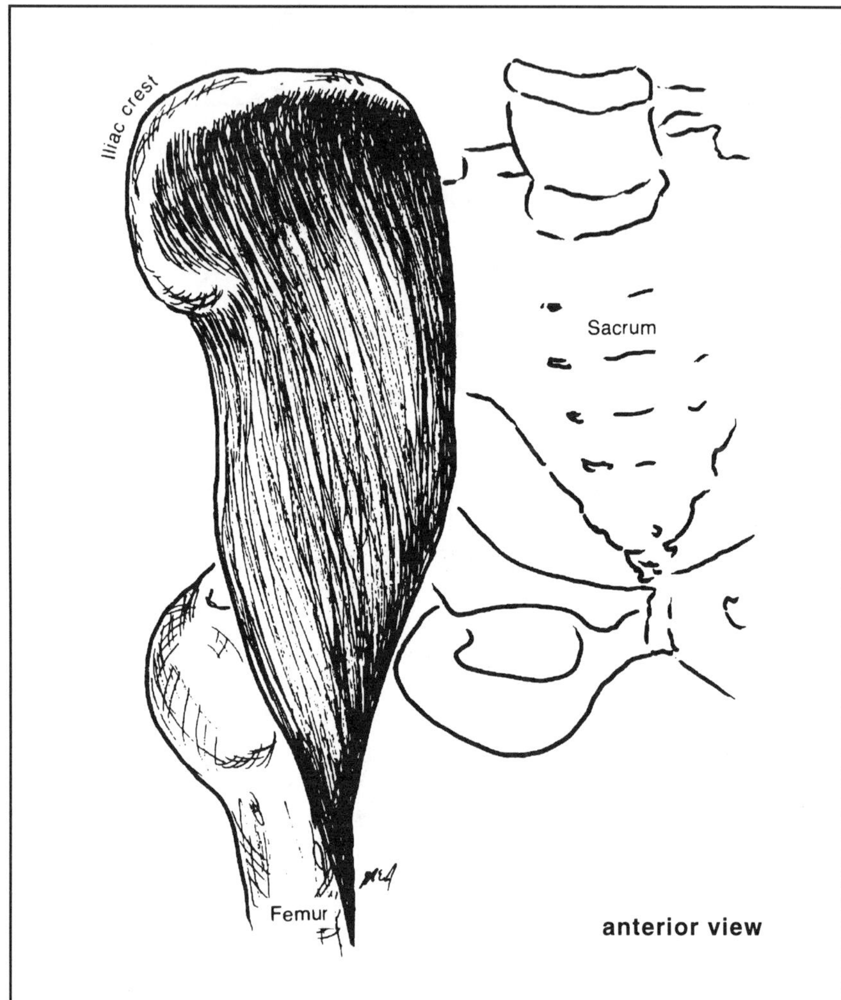

Fig. 7.7

Origin — Anterior surface of the ilium and adjacent border of sacrum.
Insertion — The tendon of the psoas superior to its attachment on the lesser trochanter.
Innervation — Femoral nerve.
Action — Hip flexion.

The iliacus and psoas major are frequently regarded by kinesiologists as a single muscle, the iliopsoas. Together, the two muscles are capable of exerting great strength to flex the hip, and are of considerable importance in activities such as kicking and jumping during which the hip must be forcefully and quickly flexed.

Rectus Femoris (rec'tus fem'oris)

The rectus femoris (Fig. 7.8) lies on the anterior aspect of the thigh. It is a penniform muscle and is palpable midway between the hip and knee joints.

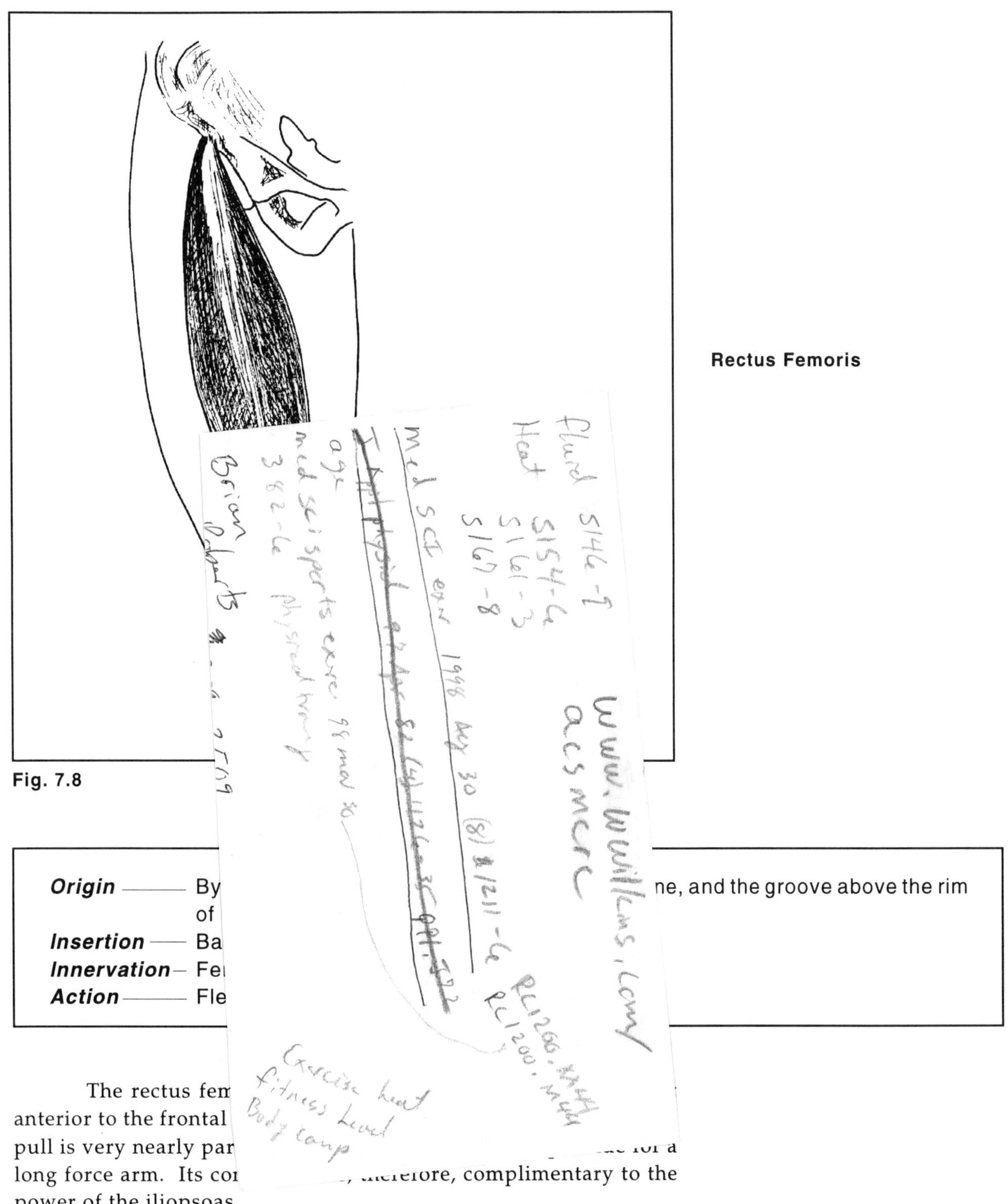

Fig. 7.8

Origin	By ... ne, and the groove above the rim of
Insertion	Ba
Innervation	Fe
Action	Fle

The rectus fem ... anterior to the frontal ... pull is very nearly par ... for a long force arm. Its co ... therefore, complimentary to the power of the iliopsoas.

Pectineus (pectin'eus)

The pectineus (Fig. 7.9) is located just below the groin and is almost completely covered by the rectus femoris and sartorius. Palpation is difficult if not impossible because the muscle is easily confused with those muscles which cover or surround it.

Pectineus

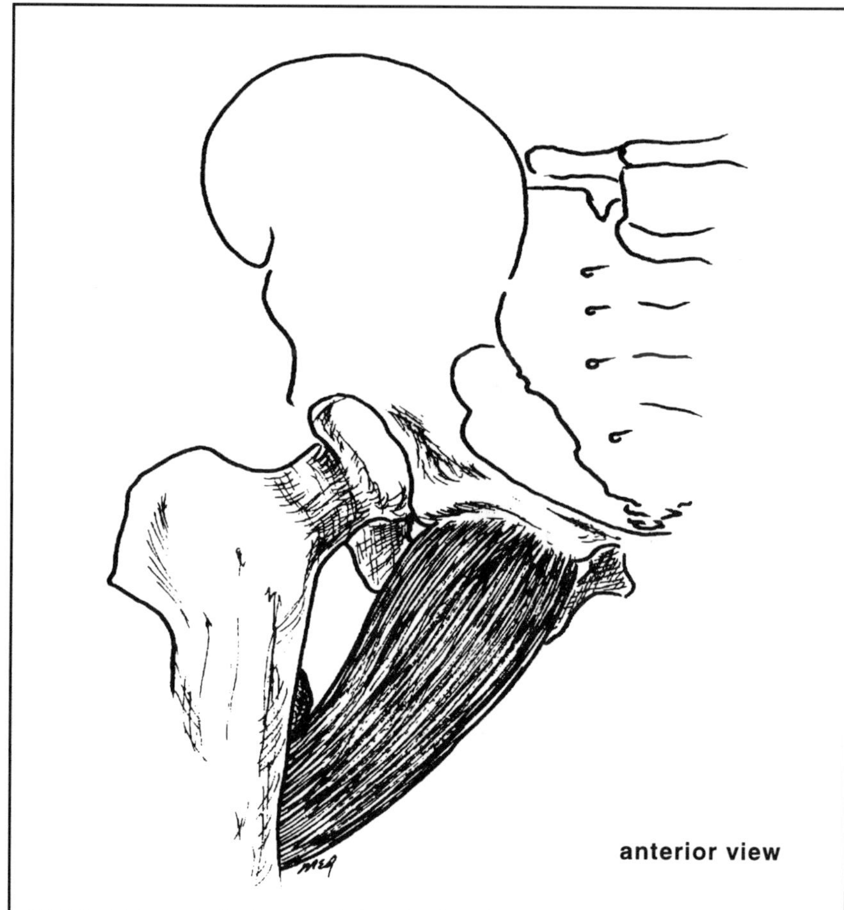

Fig. 7.9

Origin ———	On the pubis between the iliopectineal eminence and the pubic tubercle.
Insertion ——	On the medial aspect of the femur between the lesser trochanter and the linea aspera.
Innervation–	Femoral nerve.
Action ———	Flexion and adduction of the hip joint.

The pectineus crosses the hip joint anterior to the frontal axis and inferior to the sagittal axis. It enjoys a relatively long force arm to both axes as well as an advantageous angle of insertion. The muscle is, therefore, quite powerful in both flexion and adduction.

Sartorius (sarto'rius)

The sartorius (Fig. 7.10) is the longest muscle in the body. It is superficial as it courses diagonally medialward across the front of the thigh, but is difficult to palpate except in the area of its tendon of origin. Palpation can be accomplished during resisted flexion of the hip when the femur has been placed in a position of external rotation as in the crosslegged sit. The superior portion of the muscle can be felt and observed just below the superior iliac spine. A dimple-like depression will be noted just lateral to the sartorius which separates it from the tensor fasciae latae.

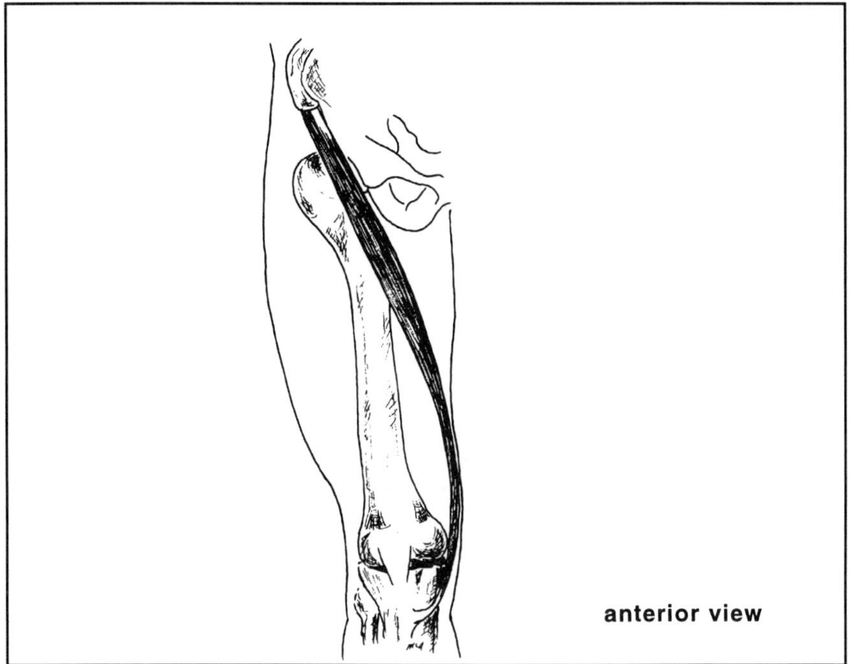

Sartorius

Fig. 7.10

Origin —— Anterior superior iliac spine and the adjacent portion of the notch distal to the spine.
Insertion —— Upper and medial aspect of the tibia.
Innervation — Femoral nerve.
Action —— Flexion, abduction, and external rotation of the hip joint.

The sartorius is a narrow band of muscle capable of great ability to shorten. It is more effective as a hip flexor than an abductor or outward rotator because its force arm is longest to the frontal axis. Its force arm is quite short to the sagittal axis rendering it a weak abductor at best. The external rotation function is similarly limited, and cannot be performed unless the knee is held in full extension, for otherwise the contraction of the muscle would be spent in moving the tibia.

Tensor Fasciae Latae (ten'sor fas'ciae la'tae)

The tensor fasciae latae (Fig. 7.11) is a small muscle located superficially on the anterior and lateral aspect of the upper thigh. It can be palpated lateral to the sartorius when the hip joint is flexed and externally rotated (see sartorius).

Tensor Fasciae Latae

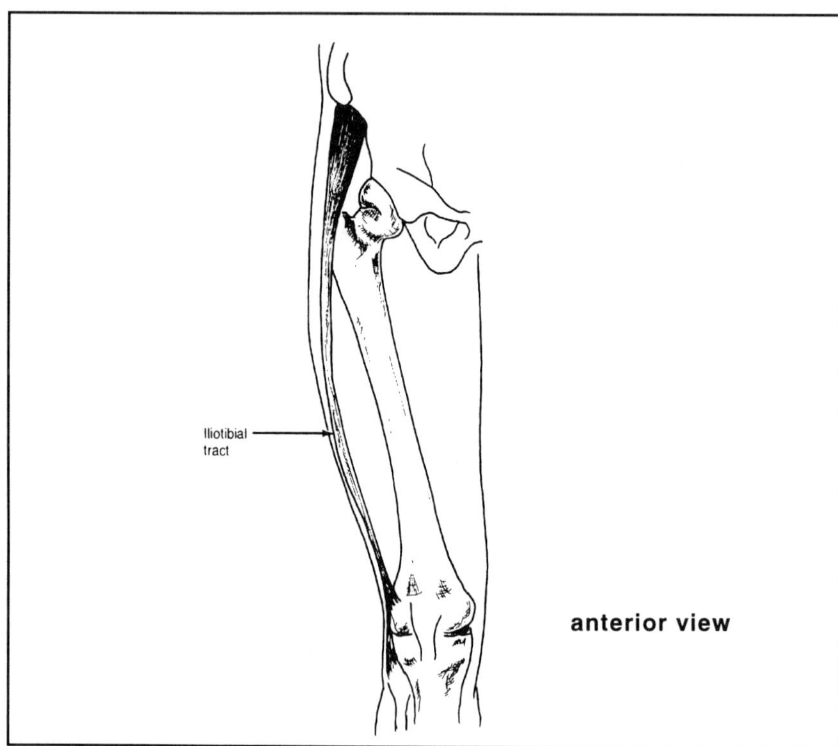

Fig. 7.11

Origin — The crest of the ilium near the anterior superior iliac spine.
Insertion — The iliotibial tract of the fascia lata.
Innervation — Superior gluteal nerve.
Action — Tenses the fascia lata; through the fascia lata, the muscle flexes, abducts, and internally rotates the hip joint.

The tensor fasciae latae does not have a bony insertion; however, since the fascia lata extends down the lateral aspect of the thigh to attach to the tibia, the muscle is able to extend its action from tightening the fascia to moving the hip joint. The tensor passes to the anterior side of the frontal axis and to the lateral side of the sagittal axis, to become a flexor and abductor, respectively. Its internal rotation function is weak and even debatable, since it and the fascia are nearly parallel to the femur as they course between the ilium and tibia. The muscle's ability to rotate internally would therefore be enhanced if the femur were already in a position of external rotation.

Gluteus Maximus (glu'teus max'imus)

The gluteus maximus (Fig. 7.12) is a large buttocks muscle on the posterior aspect of the hip. It is easily observed and palpated.

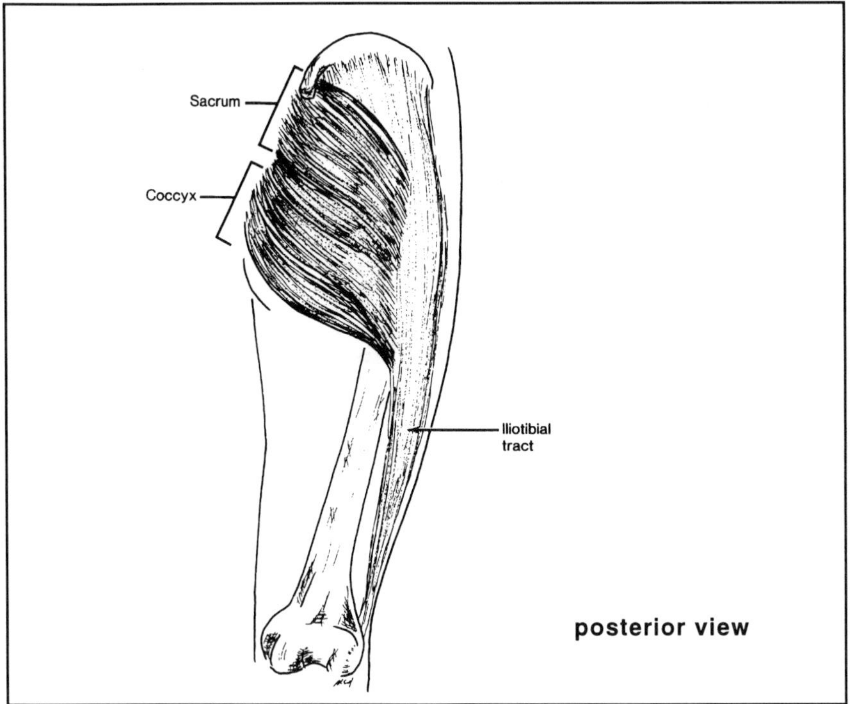

Gluteus Maximus

Fig. 7.12

Origin —	Posterior gluteal line of the ilium and the adjacent portion of the iliac crest; posterior and inferior surface of the sacrum; and the side of the coccyx.
Insertion —	Posterior aspect of femur below the greater trochanter; iliotibial tract of the fascia lata.
Innervation —	Inferior gluteal nerve.
Action —	Extension, hyperextension, and external rotation of the hip joint.

The gluteus maximus is notoriously lazy during activities associated with daily living. It is perhaps for this reason that the muscle so easily loses its firmness and attracts fat deposits. The only prevention for such conditions appears to be through planned exercises which incorporate hyperextension and/or external rotation of the hip. It should be noted however, that excessive contraction of the maximus may lead to unwanted bulk. **Turn-out**, dancers' term for external rotation, has been named as the cause of such hypertrophy of the maximus that range of motion can become restricted. In addition to turn-out, however, the muscle "set" of the gluteus practiced by the dancer is probably equally responsible for the hypertrophy.

Gluteus Medius (glu'teus me'dius)

The gluteus medius (Fig. 7.13) is partially covered by the gluteus maximus and the tensor fasciae latae; it is superficial, just inferior to the iliac crest, and may be palpated there as the hip joint is abducted to raise the foot from the floor.

Gluteus Medius

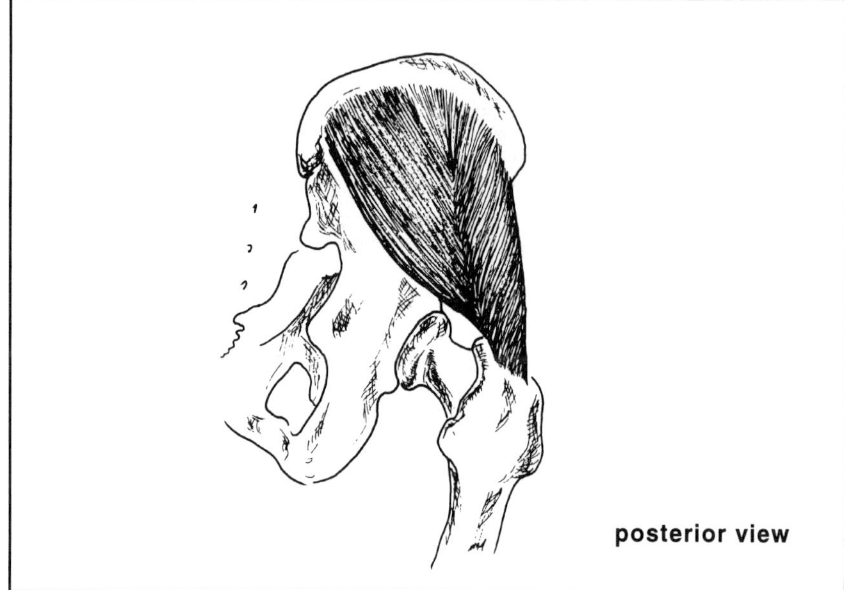

Fig. 7.13

Origin —	Posterior surface of the ilium in the region bounded by the iliac crest and the posterior and anterior gluteal lines.
Insertion —	Oblique ridge on the lateral aspect of the greater trochanter.
Innervation —	Superior gluteal nerve.
Action —	Abduction of the hip joint; anterior fibers flex and internally rotate; posterior fibers extend and externally rotate.

Since all of the fibers of the gluteus medius pass the sagittal axis of the hip joint to the lateral side, the muscle is an excellent abductor. In addition, the angle of attachment of the medius on the greater trochanter approximates 90 degrees, affording superior mechanical advantage.

When the medius is viewed with respect to the frontal and long axes, it is seen that the middle portion of the muscle passes directly over these axes and is, therefore, nonfunctional in either frontal or transverse plane movements of the femur. The anterior and posterior portions are, however, able to contribute to flexion/extension and internal/external rotation since, by virtue of the size of the muscle, they are removed from the frontal and long axes. The gluteus medius and the deltoid are similar in their placement around the three axes of their respective ball-and-socket joints.

Gluteus Minimus (glu'teus min'imus)

The gluteus minimus (Fig. 7.14) is the smallest of the gluteal group and is covered by the gluteus medius. It cannot be palpated.

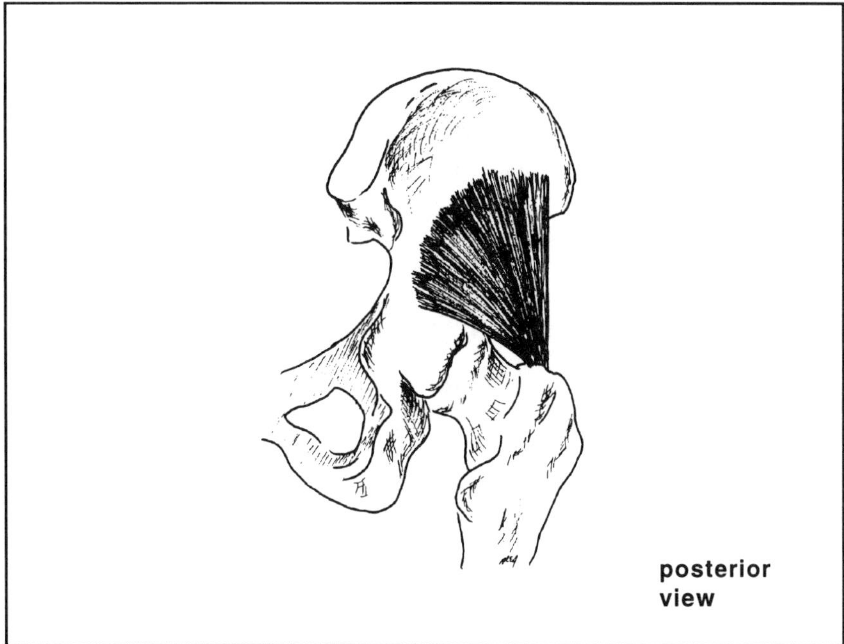

Gluteus Minimus

Fig. 7.14

Origin —— Posterior surface of ilium between the anterior and inferior gluteal line, and from the edge of the greater sciatic notch.
Insertion —— Anterior border of the greater trochanter.
Innervation — Superior gluteal nerve.
Action —— Abduction of the hip joint; anterior fibers aid in internal rotation and flexion; posterior fibers aid in external rotation and extension.

The gluteus minimus and medius have similar relationships to the three axes of the hip joint and have, therefore, equivalent actions. The minimus, being smaller, is less powerful.

Adductor Magnus (adduc'tor mag'nus)

The adductor magnus (Fig. 7.15) is the largest of the adductor muscles and is located on the medial aspect of the thigh. It is difficult to palpate because of surrounding musculature; however, it may be isolated just medial to the gracilis at mid-thigh.

Adductor Magnus

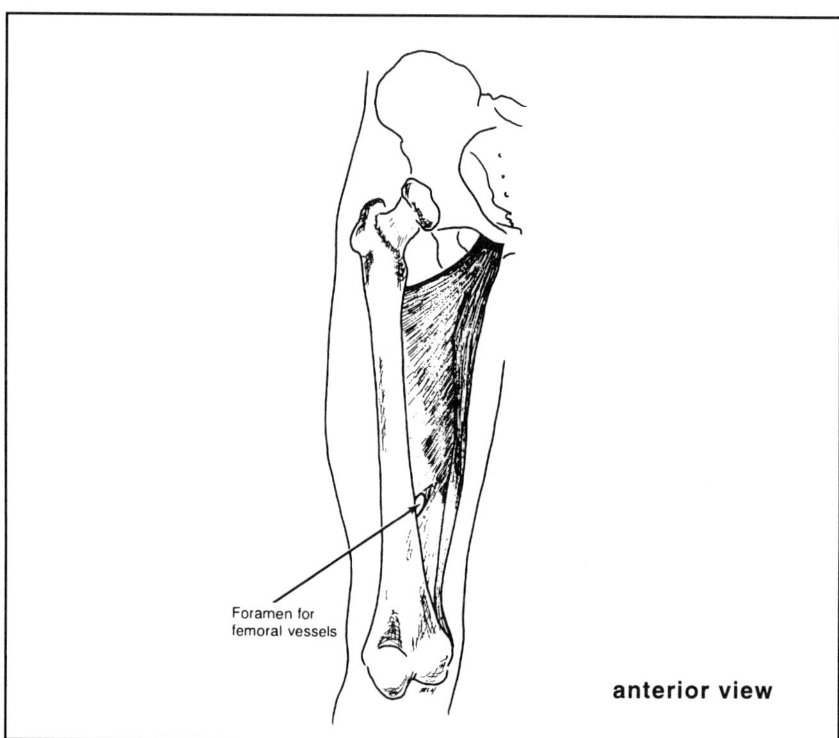

Fig. 7.15

Origin	Inferior ramus of the pubis and ischium, and inferior part of the ischial tuberosity.
Insertion	Entire length of linea aspera, and supracondylar ridge, and adductor tubercle of the femur.
Innervation	Obturator and sciatic nerves.
Action	Adduction of the hip joint; upper portion aids in internal rotation and flexion; lower portion aids in external rotation and extension.

The adductor magnus, like the other adductors, fluctuates in its action on the femur according to postural states. For example, the magnus is active during internal rotation from a position of external rotation. The muscle has little if any ability to internally rotate from the anatomical or fundamental reference position. Similarly, the ability of the upper magnus to flex the hip joint is enhanced if the femur is in positions of hyperextension or extension; and ability of the lower portion to extend is best when the hip joint has already been flexed. Regardless of posture, however, the magnus is well-placed to adduct, but is recruited to this action only when resistance is met.

Adductor Longus (adduc'tor lon'gus)

The adductor longus (Fig. 7.16) lies just medial to the pectineus and can be palpated at the medial aspect of the groin.

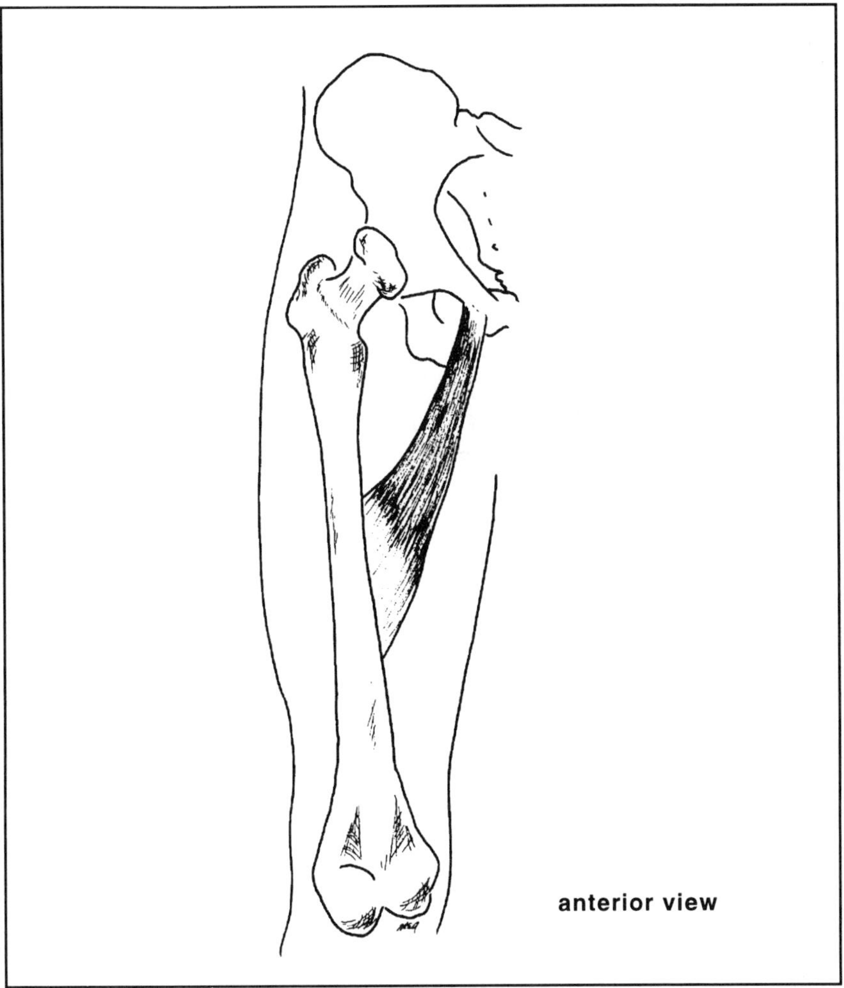

Adductor Longus

Fig. 7.16

Origin —— Anterior surface of the pubis just below the crest.
Insertion —— Middle one-half of the linea aspera.
Innervation — Anterior obturator nerve.
Action —— Adduction of the hip joint; aids in flexion and internal rotation.

The adductor longus is active in all stages of adduction regardless of whether the leg is resisted or unresisted. The ability of the muscle to flex or internally rotate is increased if the hip joint has previously been extended (or hyperextended) or externally rotated, respectively.

Adductor Brevis (adduc'tor bre'vis)

The adductor brevis (Fig. 7.17) is the smallest of the adductors. It lies beneath the adductor magnus and adductor longus and cannot be palpated.

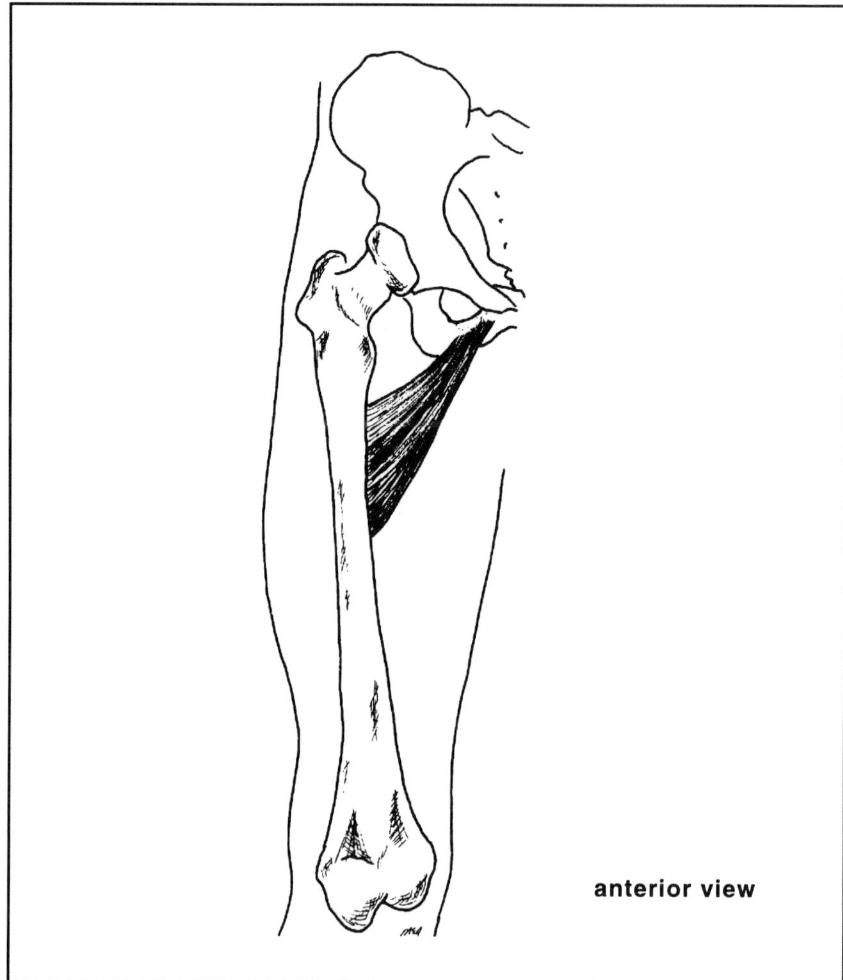

Fig. 7.17

Origin	Outer surface of pubis, on the inferior ramus.
Insertion	Line from the lesser trochanter to the linea aspera including the upper portion of the linea aspera.
Innervation	Anterior obturator nerve.
Action	Adduction of the hip joint; aids in flexion and internal rotation.

The adductor brevis has a line of pull which is similar to that of the adductor longus and, therefore, responds in like fashion to positions of the femur.

Gracilis (gra'cilis)

The gracilis (Fig. 7.18) is a long and slender muscle located superficially along the inner thigh. It is difficult to palpate because it is easily confused with surrounding muscles; however, its tendon of insertion can usually be felt. Begin the palpation in the middle of the posterior aspect of the knee, then move the fingers medially until the large tendon of the semitendinosus is encountered. If the fingers are moved slightly medially, the smaller tendon of the semimembranosus will be felt. The tendon of the gracilis lies just medial to the semimembranosus. Palpation may be facilitated by internally rotating the tibia against resistance.

Origin — Inferior half of the symphysis and the superior half of the arch of the pubis.
Insertion — Medial aspect of the tibia just below the condyle.
Innervation — Anterior division of the obturator nerve.
Action — Adduction of the hip joint; aids in flexion and internal rotation.

The gracilis is well located to be an adductor since it crosses the hip joint to the medial side of the sagittal axis. The muscle can be a weak flexor of the hip joint also, but only through the part of the flexion range in which the muscle courses anterior to the frontal axis. Study of a skeleton will indicate that when the femur reaches a point at which it is approximately perpendicular to the trunk, the gracilis is no longer anterior to the axis but rather in line with it. If the femur is raised even higher, the gracilis will course posterior to the axis and will become an extensor.

That the gracilis will be an internal rotator is questionable since the two attachments of the muscle are aligned in parallel fashion with the femur regardless of the position of the thigh. If the gracilis does make a contribution to internal rotation, it would be under conditions of an externally rotated hip joint and an extended knee.

Gracilis

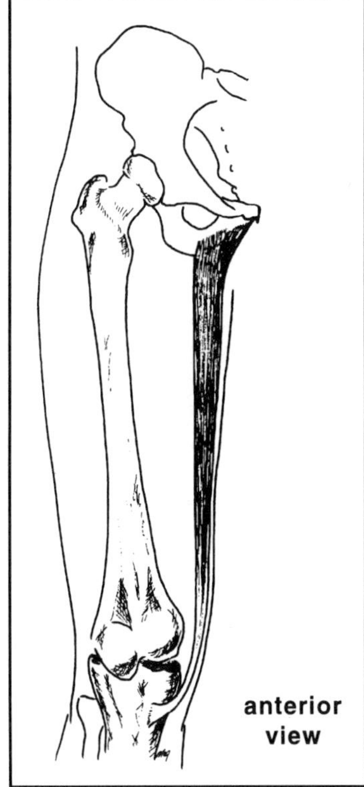

Fig. 7.18

Semitendinosus (semitendino'sus)

The semitendinosus (Fig. 7.19) is one of the hamstring muscles and is located superficially along the medial and posterior aspect of the thigh. It is most easily palpated in the area of its tendon of insertion as described under the gracilis.

Semitendinosus

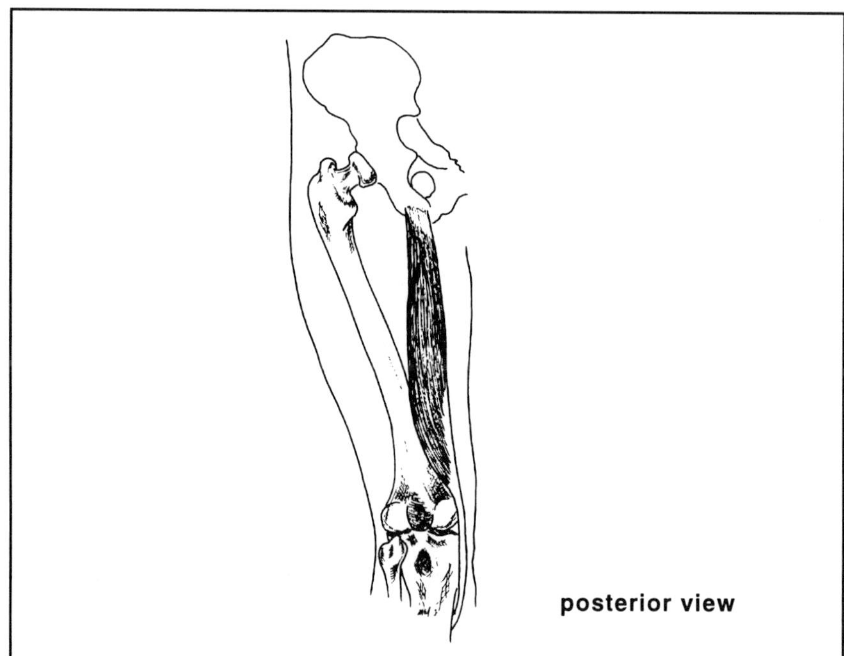

Fig. 7.19

Origin ——	Medial facet of the ischial tuberosity by a common tendon with the long head of the biceps femoris
Insertion ——	Medial-anterior surface of the tibia just distal to the insertion of the gracilis.
Innervation —	Tibial portion of sciatic nerve.
Action ——	Extension and hyperextension of the hip joint; aids in internal rotation and adduction.

The semitendinosus crosses the hip joint posterior to the frontal axis and, because of the tuberosity of the ischium, attaches at angles which afford it good mechanical advantage, especially through the range of extension.

The internal rotation function of the muscle follows from the fact that it wraps partially around the tibia as it inserts. If the knee is held extended, contraction of the muscle will assist the entire leg to rotate internally.

Comparison of the location of the semitendinosus with that of the sagittal axis of the hip joint will indicate that the muscle is an adductor. Its contribution is only assistive because of its short force arm to the sagittal axis.

Semimembranosus (semimembrano'sus)

The semimembranosus (Fig. 7.20), a hamstring muscle, lies on the posterior aspect of the thigh. It is best palpated along its tendon of insertion as described under the gracilis.

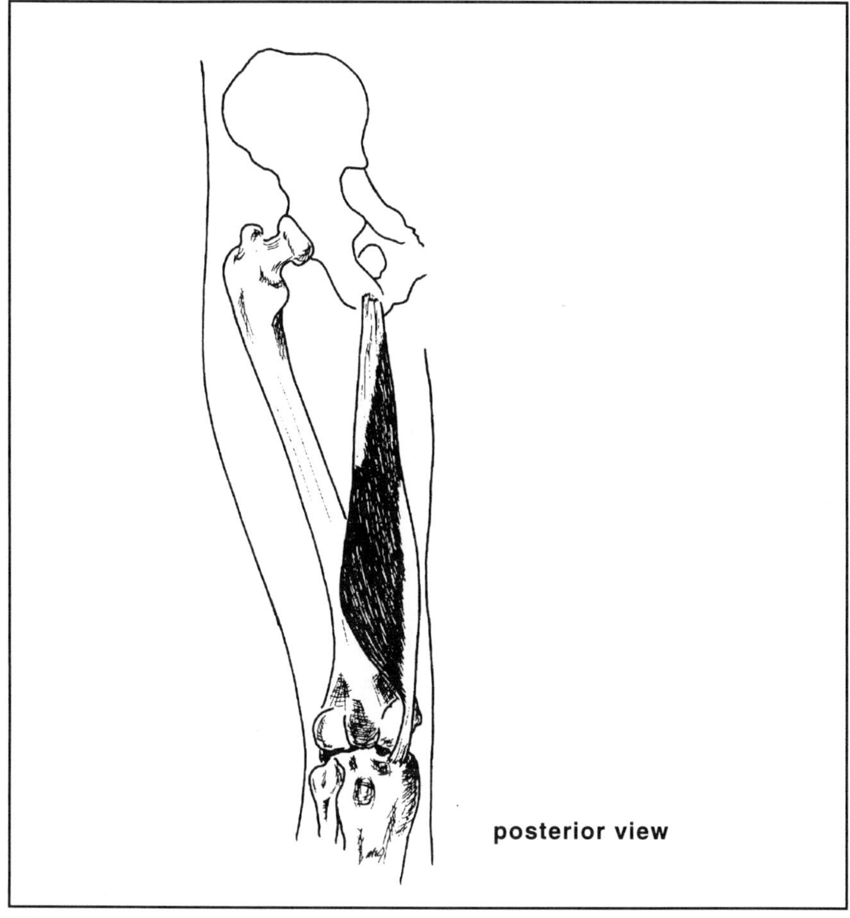

Semimembranosus

Fig. 7.20

Origin —— Lateral facet of the ischial tuberosity.
Insertion —— The medial and posterior aspect of the medial condyle of the tibia.
Innervation— Tibial portion of the sciatic nerve.
Action —— Extension and hyperextension of the hip joint; aids in internal rotation and adduction.

The line of pull of the semimembranosus is very similar to that of the semitendinosus, with one exception -- the origin of the semimembranosus is somewhat more lateral than that of the semitendinosus. The semimembranosus is thus placed diagonally with respect to the long axis to aid in internal rotation.

Biceps Femoris (long head) (bi'ceps fem'oris)

The long head of the biceps femoris (Fig. 7.21) is located superficially on the lateral and posterior aspect of the thigh. It is best palpated in the region of its tendon of insertion as it crosses behind the knee on the lateral side. The biceps femoris is one of the three hamstring muscles.

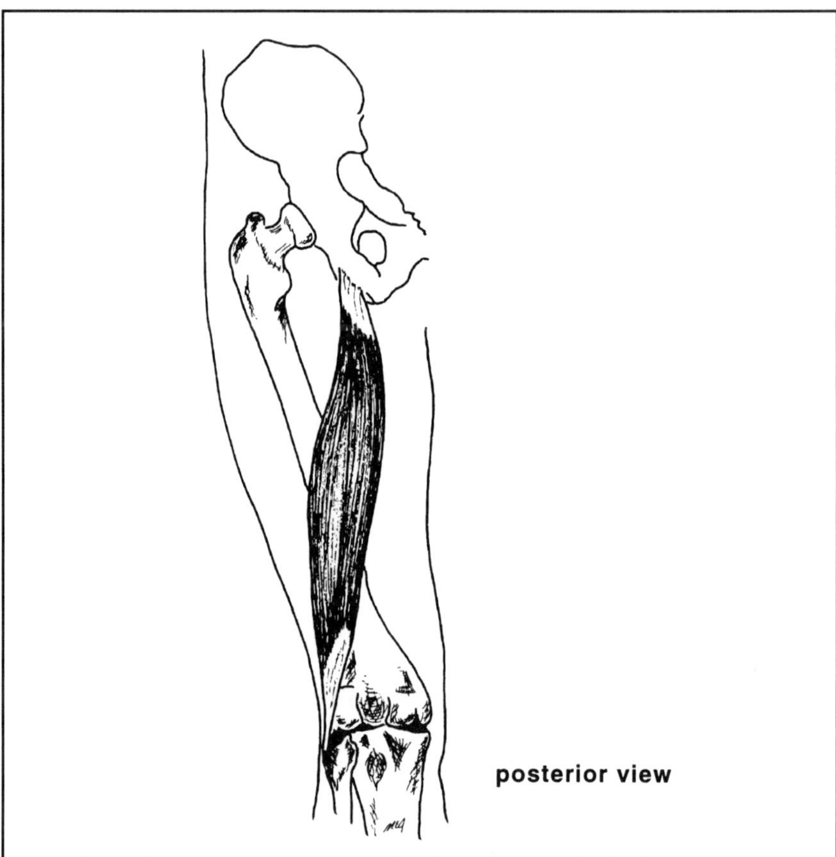

Fig. 7.21

Origin ——— Medial facet of the ischial tuberosity.
Insertion —— Lateral condyle of the tibia and head of the fibula.
Innervation— Tibial portion of sciatic nerve.
Action ——— Extension and hyperextension of the hip joint; aids in external rotation.

All of the hamstrings -- the semitendinosus, semimembranosus, and biceps femoris -- have essentially the same mechanical advantage in moving the femur through the range of extension and hyperextension. The biceps differs from the other hamstrings in its ability to rotate the hip joint because it crosses the long axis from inside to out, or from medial to lateral, and is therefore an external rotator rather than an internal rotator.

The Outward Rotators

Six muscles (Fig. 7.22) lying deep in the pelvis have, as their primary action, the ability to rotate the hip joint outwardly. Although each is a specific muscle, it has become practice, in the study of kinesiology, to group them.

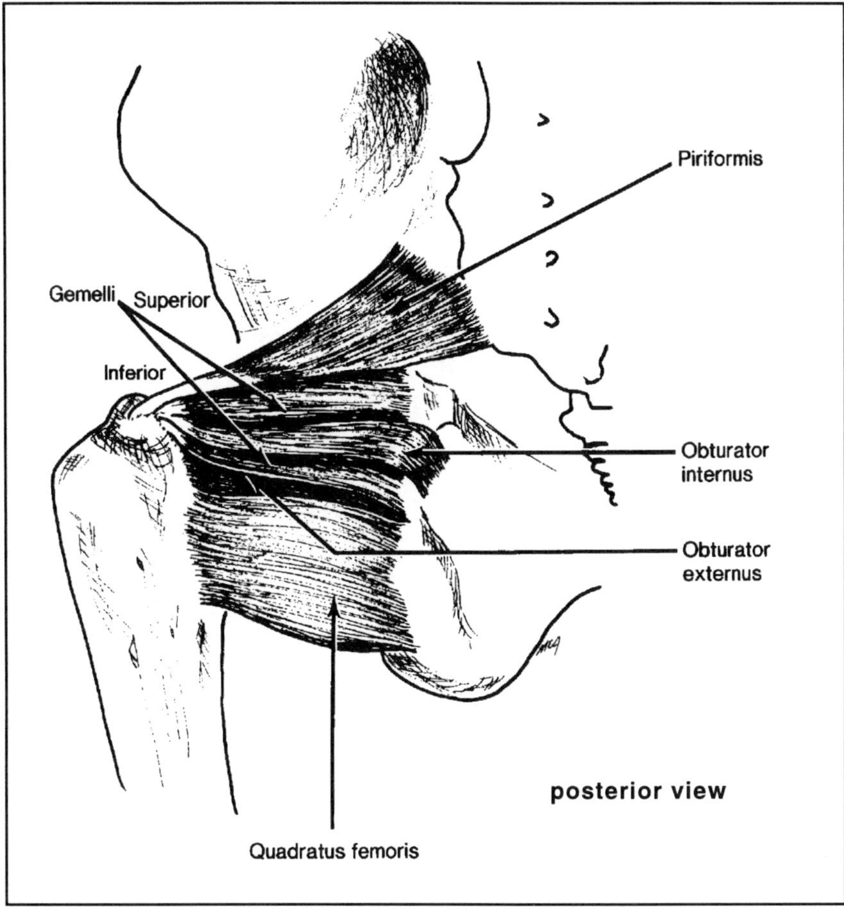

Fig. 7.22

The Outward Rotators

Origin —	Anterior and posterior surfaces of sacrum, and of the pelvis around the obturator foramen.
Insertion —	Greater trochanter of the femur.
Innervation —	Piriformis: First and second sacral nerves. Obturator internus: First and second sacral and fifth lumbar nerves. Obturator externus: Obturator nerve. Quadratus femoris: First sacral, and fourth and fifth lumbar nerves. Gamellus superior: A branch of the nerve to the obturator internus. Gamellus inferior: A branch of the nerve to the quadratus femoris.
Action —	External rotation of the hip joint; if the hip joint has been flexed, they act to horizontally abduct the joint.

COMMENTS

The twenty-two muscles of the hip comprise the largest muscle mass of the body. Their strength is required not only because of their function in weight-bearing but also because they must move the long, heavy third class lever represented by the lower leg. Most of the muscles are of the spurt type; those that cross the knee joint are shunt muscles and provide valuable stabilizing force at the hip joint. By this arrangement, they can, in addition, contribute to movement at two joints rather than one.

The two-joint function of the rectus femoris and hamstrings is an interesting one to consider. When the hip is flexed, the rectus is an agonist and the hamstrings are antagonists. During hip extension, the muscles reverse roles; the hamstrings become the agonists and the rectus functions as an antagonist. Flexion and extension of the knee involves like responsibilities of these muscles; for example, during knee flexion, the hamstrings are agonists and the rectus is an antagonist, and during extension, their muscle roles reverse. If both hip and knee movement are performed simultaneously, however, muscular responsibilities are more complicated. A place kick in soccer involves hip flexion and knee extension. The rectus must contract to flex the hip as well as extend the knee, and the hamstrings must relax to allow the leg to move as required. If the hamstrings lack the needed extensibility, they will limit the range of the leg, and their tension will be transferred to their origin, the ischial tuberosity. In response, the pelvic girdle will be pulled into backward tilt which will result in a hyperextension of the pelvis on the femur of the supporting leg. The iliofemoral or *Y* ligament checks this movement sharply and forcefully, and, in some instances, will actually pull the supporting leg off the ground.

Simultaneous execution of hip and knee flexion or hip and knee extension requires that both the hamstrings and rectus femoris be agonists at one joint and antagonists at the other. This would appear to be a contradictory situation since it is known that muscles, when they contract, tend to act as agonists at all joints they cross. The expected result is that the contracting rectus and hamstrings will neutralize each other at both joints and no motion will occur. Yet, that the muscles are apparently able to function cooperatively is demonstrated commonly in the execution of the vertical jump. Both muscle components contract sharply to project the body from the floor. The resulting actions of simultaneous hip and knee extension indicate that the hamstrings can exert more force than the rectus at the hip, but the rectus is the more forceful of the two muscles at the knee. Study of the force arms of the muscles at the two joints will confirm the conclusion; the force arm of the hamstrings is longer at the hip than that of the rectus, whereas the force arm of the rectus is the longer of the two at the knee.

A quiz for this material can be found in the back of this book on page 293.

LABORATORY EXPERIENCES

1. Stand with the feet spread side-to-side at approximately shoulder width. Shift the bulk of the weight to the left foot and, while holding this position, note the range of movement of the hips during their rotation to the left. Stand with the bulk of the weight on the right foot and, again, note the range of left rotation of the hips. You should find that the range is greater when the weight is on the right foot. The degree to which the hips can be rotated in the transverse plane is highly related to success in imparting force to the respective sports objects. Can you make a generalization regarding the timing of weight shift and the rotation of the hips?

2. Place electrodes on the gluteus maximus of a partner. Have your partner lie across a table while keeping the feet on the floor. Monitor the activity of the gluteus maximus as the leg is raised, with extended knee, to horizontal and then into hyperextension of the hip joint. During which portion of the movement is the gluteus maximus more active?

3. Have your partner place the foot back on the floor (see Experience #2) and apply resistance to the back of the ankle as the leg is raised. How does the activity of the gluteus maximus compare with that found during the movement performed in Experience #2?

4. Monitor the electrical activity of the gluteus maximus as your partner pedals a bicycle which has touring handle bars, and one which has dropped handle bars. Do you note any difference in the two electromyograms?

5. Perform the palpations described in this chapter. After each, indicate an exercise or movement which will (1) strengthen the muscle involved, and (2) stretch the muscle.

THE KNEE

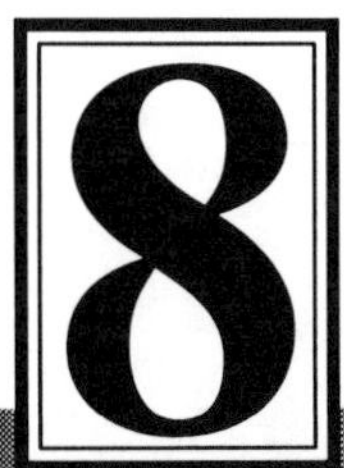

THE STRUCTURE AND MOVEMENTS OF THE JOINT

The knee is the largest joint in the body and is actually comprised of three subjoints; two biaxial condyloid joints between the femur and tibia, and the nonaxial joint between the patella and the femur.

The two condyloid joints articulate the medial and lateral condyles of the femur with the medial and lateral condyles of the tibia (Fig. 8.1). The menisci, crescent shaped discs of fibrocartilage, serve to deepen the tibial articulation with the condyles of the femur.

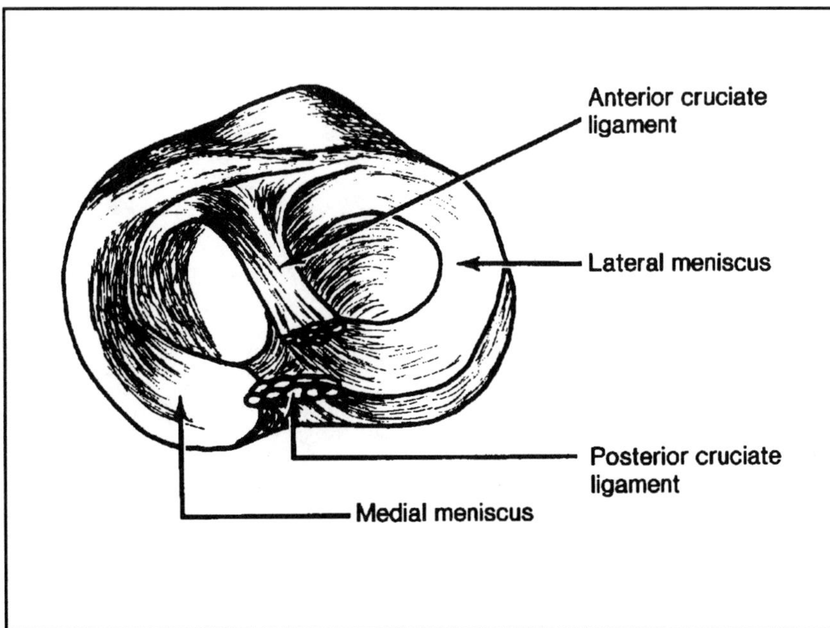

Articulating Surface of Head of Right Tibia

Fig. 8.1

The synovial capsule of the knee is a strong and extensive membrane strengthened throughout by bands of tendons which cross the knee and by the fascia lata. The capsule is lined with a synovial membrane which begins at the proximal edge of the patella and extends distally to beneath the patellar ligament and the infrapatellar fat pad, then projects into the interior of the joint both superior and inferior to the menisci, and finally courses posteriorly to a position beneath the tendon of the popliteus. The cruciate ligaments are not included within the capsule.

Numerous bursae surround the knee joint. Some communicate with the joint capsule while others do not. Each bursa is located between tissues which would otherwise wear from friction.

The ligaments of the knee are the popliteals, collaterals, cruciates, coronary, transverse, and patellar (Fig. 8.2). The popliteal ligaments, called the **oblique popliteal** and the **arcuate popliteal ligaments**, course between the posterior aspects of the femur and tibia, and between the lateral condyle of the femur and the articular capsule. The collateral ligaments, called the **medial** and **lateral collaterals** (or the tibial and fibular collaterals) join the medial condyles of tibia and femur, and lateral condyle of the femur with the head of the fibula, respectively. In the interior of the joint, the anterior and posterior cruciate joins the anterior intercondylar portion of the tibia with the posterior part of the intercondylar fossa of the femur, and the posterior cruciate runs between the posterior intercondylar region of the tibia with the anterior aspect of the intercondylar fossa of the femur.

Superficial Tissues of Right Knee

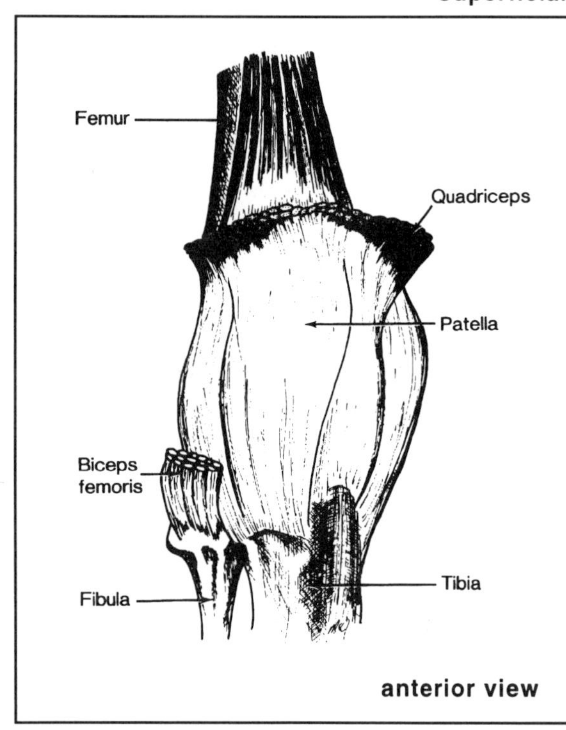

Fig. 8.2a

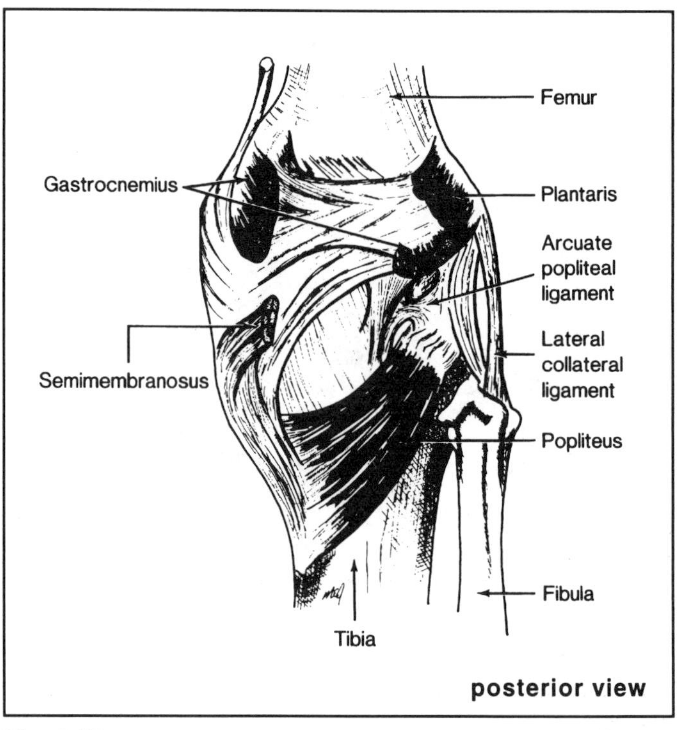

Fig. 8.2b

Deep Tissues of Right Knee

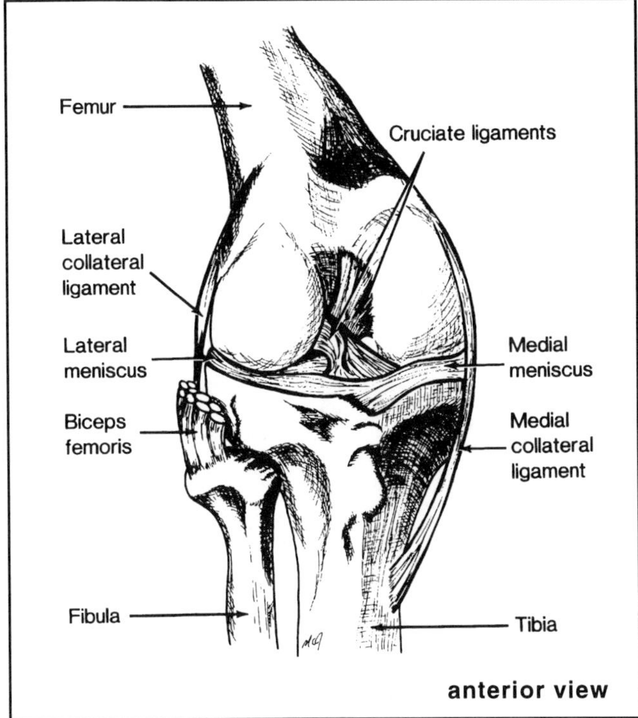

Fig. 8.2c

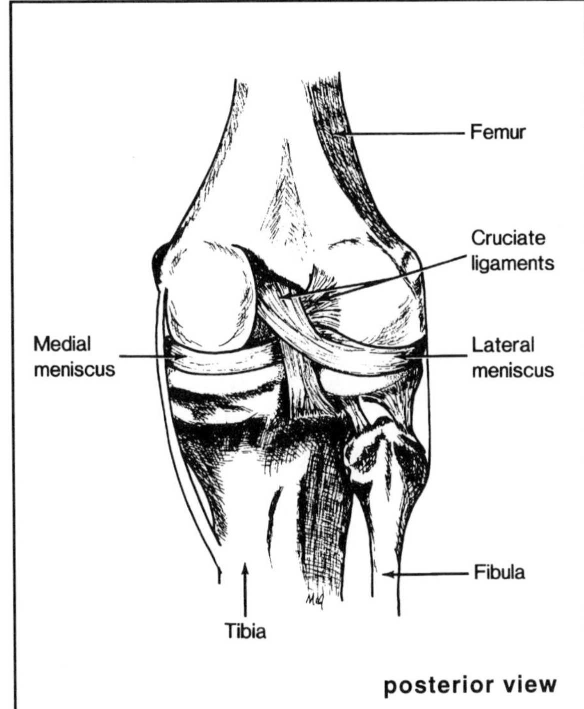

Fig. 8.2d

The coronary ligaments connect the rims of the medial meniscus and lateral meniscus to the head of the tibia. The transverse ligament courses anteriorly between the two menisci, connecting their forward edges. It is sometimes absent. The patellar ligament is the mid-portion of the quadriceps femoris tendon which is extended from the patella to the tibial tuberosity.

Movements of the tibia around the femur are biaxial. Flexion and extension occur around the frontal axis and are caused by muscles which cross the joint posterior or anterior to that axis. Internal and external rotation occur around the long axis and will be performed by muscles which insert on the medial and lateral aspect of the tibia.

The joint between the patella and the femur is essentially of the gliding type, although the articulating surfaces of the joint do not match exactly. The articulation is further complicated by the presence of seven facets on the inner surface of the patella which are brought into contact with the femur as the knee joint is moved through its range of flexion/extension and internal/external rotation.

BONE MARKINGS

The bone markings pertinent to the origins of the muscles of the knee joint have been presented in the preceding chapter. Figure 8.3 displays only those markings concerned with the insertions of the several muscles.

Proximal Portion of the Tibia and Fibula

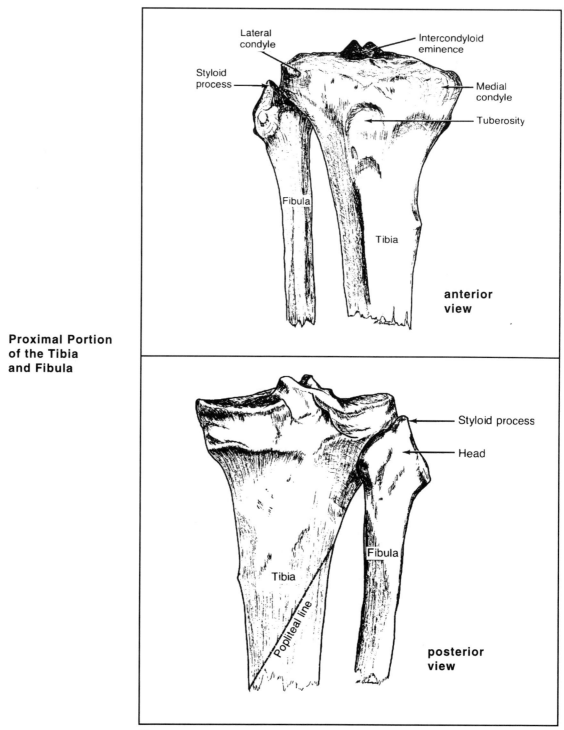

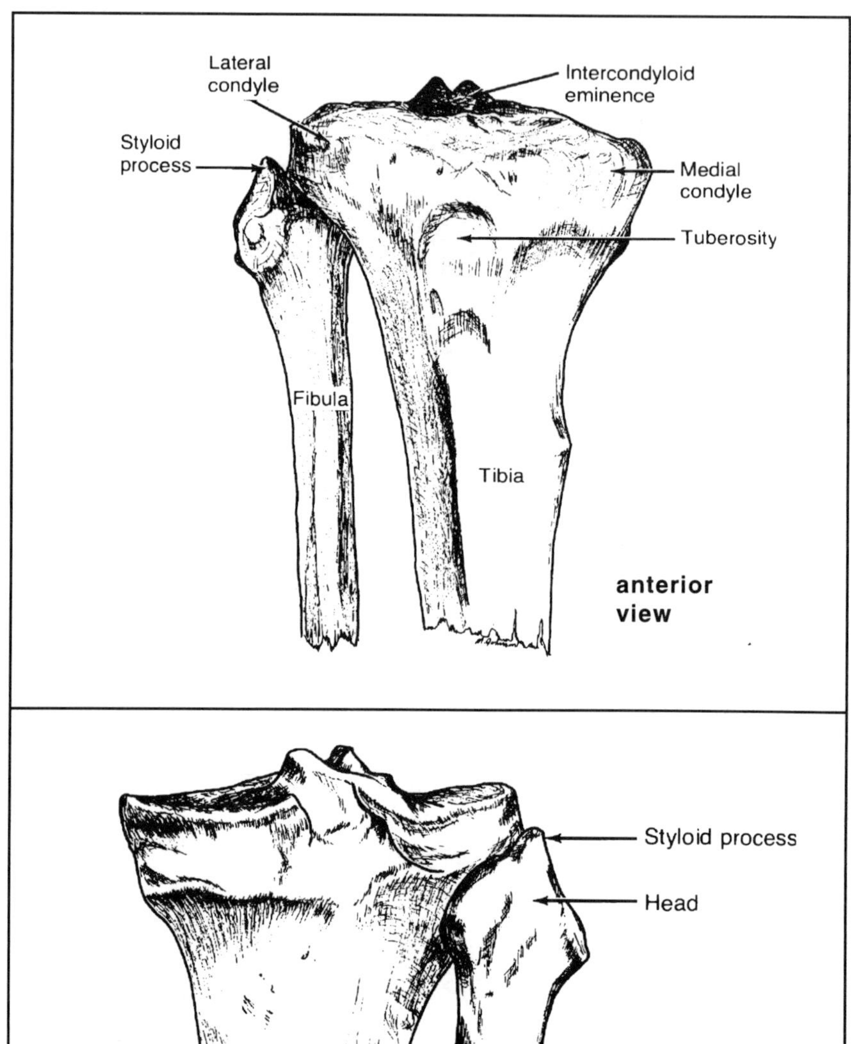

Fig. 8.3

MUSCULATURE

Rectus Femoris (rec'tus fem'oris)

The rectus femoris (Fig. 8.4) lies on the anterior aspect of the thigh. It is a penniform muscle and is palpable midway between the hip and knee joints.

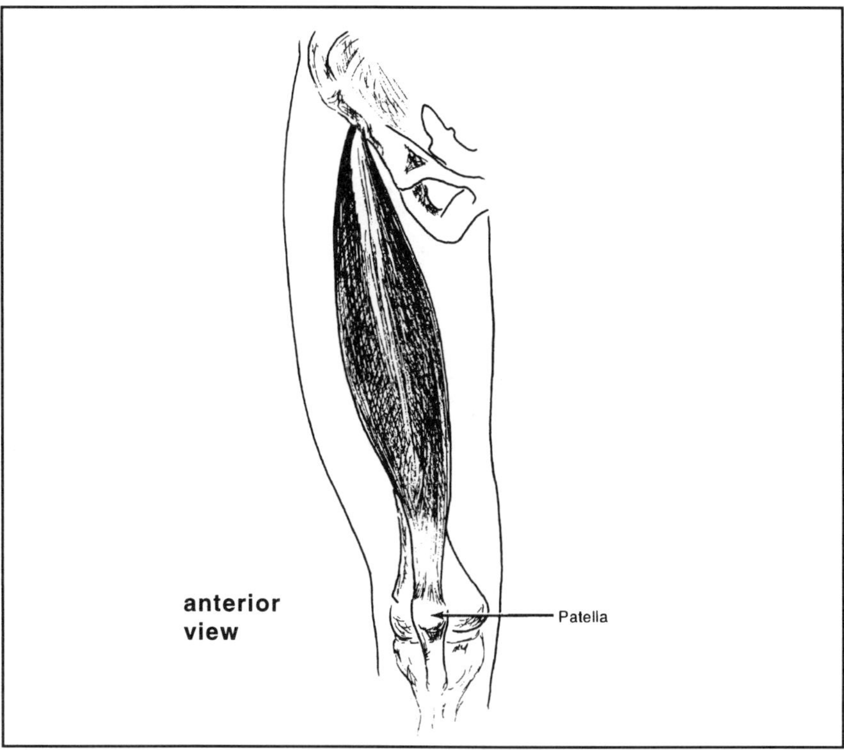

Rectus Femoris

Fig. 8.4

Origin ——	By two heads, from the anterior inferior iliac spine, and the groove above the rim of the acetabulum.
Insertion ——	Base of the patella.
Innervation —	Femoral nerve.
Action ——	Extension of the knee joint.

Whereas the rectus femoris is a forceful mover of the hip joint, it is also an effective knee extensor. When both hip flexion and knee extension comprise an activity -- as in the case with kicking -- the muscle contribution is second to none. When its power as a hip flexor is coupled with its force as a knee extensor, it is capable of generating great momentum in the foot. One only need recall the pain associated with "stubbing" the toe to appreciate the momentum of the lower leg that is generated by the rectus femoris.

The Vasti

The vasti (Fig. 8.5) are three muscles located on the front and sides of the thigh. They are the vastus lateralis, vastus medialis, and vastus intermedius (vas'tus latera'lis, vas'tus media'lis, and vas'tus interme'dius) which, together with the rectus femoris, form the muscle group known as the quadriceps femoris. The lateralis may be palpated at mid-thigh to the lateral side of the rectus femoris. The medialis is best palpated proximal and medial to the patella when the knee is held in extension. The intermedius lies beneath the rectus femoris and cannot be palpated.

The Vasti Muscles

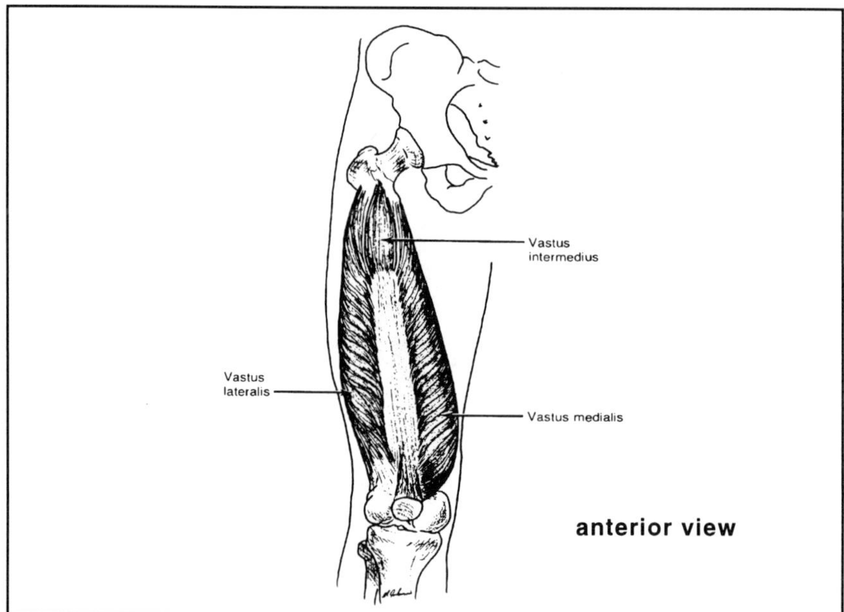

Fig. 8.5

Origin	Vastus lateralis: Lateral aspect of the femur extending from just below the greater trochanter to and including the upper half of the linea aspera of the femur. Vastus medialis: Entire length of the linea aspera and supracondylar line of the femur. Vastus intermedius: Proximal two-thirds of the femur from its anterior and lateral surfaces.
Insertion	All three vasti muscles insert on the patella through the tendon of the quadriceps femoris.
Innervation	Femoral nerve.
Action	All of the vasti extend the knee joint.

The lateralis and medius approach the patella and the tendon of the quadriceps femoris diagonally. Each requires the balancing pull of the other if a straight line of pull against the patella is to result. Since the intermedius is centered along the front of the thigh, it requires no neutralization. Its entire line of pull is directed optimally for knee extension.

Semitendinosus (semitendino'sus)

The semitendinosus (Fig. 8.6) is one of the hamstring muscles and is located superficially along the medial and posterior aspect of the thigh. It is most easily palpated in the area of its tendon of insertion as described under the gracilis (Chapter 7).

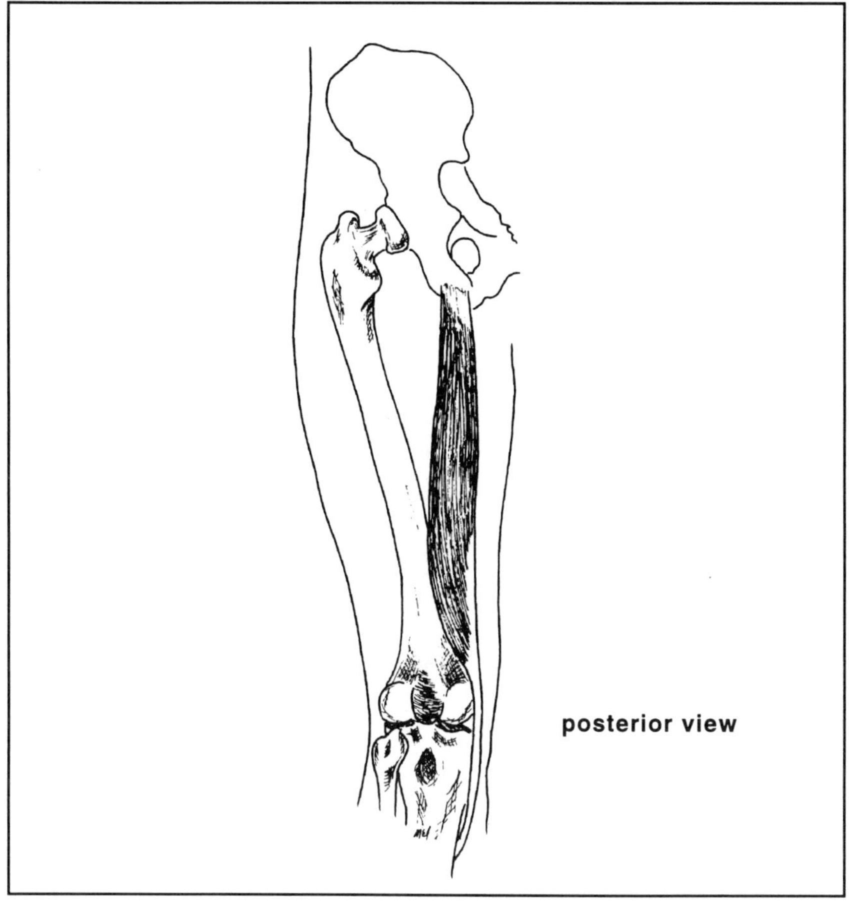

Semitendinosus

Fig. 8.6

Origin	Medial facet of the ischial tuberosity by a common tendon with the long head of the biceps femoris.
Insertion	Medial-anterior surface of the tibia just distal to the insertion of the gracilis.
Innervation	Tibial portion of sciatic nerve.
Action	Flexion and internal rotation of the knee.

The semitendinosus is not only posterior to the frontal axis as it crosses the knee joint but is also medial to the long axis. It is, therefore, a dual action muscle at the knee, performing both flexion and internal rotation. Its tendon of insertion with those of the sartorius and gracilis forms part of a broad tendinous structure called the pes anserinus.

Semimembranosus (semimembrano'sus)

The semimembranosus (Fig. 8.7), a hamstring muscle, lies on the posterior aspect of the thigh. It is best palpated along its tendon of insertion under the gracilis as described in Chapter 7.

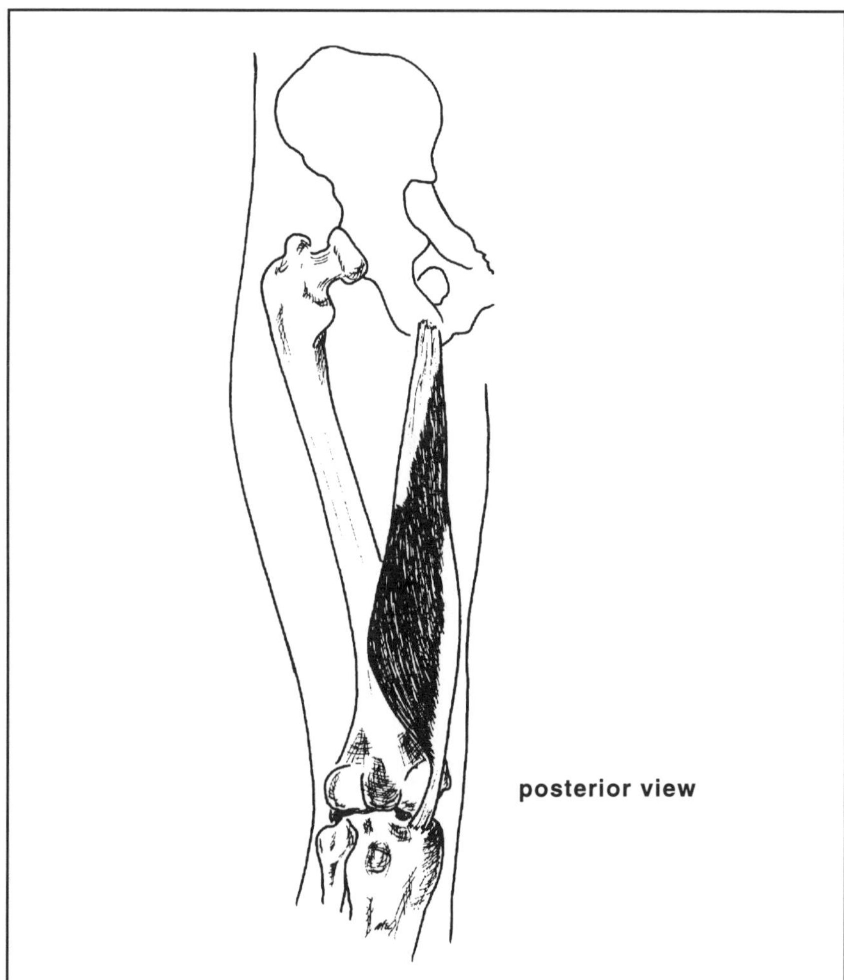

Fig. 8.7

Origin —— Lateral facet of the ischial tuberosity.
Insertion —— The medial and posterior aspect of the medial condyle of the tibia.
Innervation — Tibial portion of the sciatic nerve.
Action —— Flexion and internal rotation of the knee joint.

As one of the medial hamstring muscles, the semimembranosus crosses the knee joint posterior to the frontal axis and medial to the long axis. The resulting actions of the muscle are flexion and internal rotation, respectively.

Biceps Femoris (bi'ceps fem'oris)

The biceps femoris (Fig. 8.8) is comprised of a long head which crosses both the hip and the knee joints, and a short head which crosses the knee joint only. The muscle is the lateral hamstring and may be palpated on the posterior and lateral aspect of the thigh.

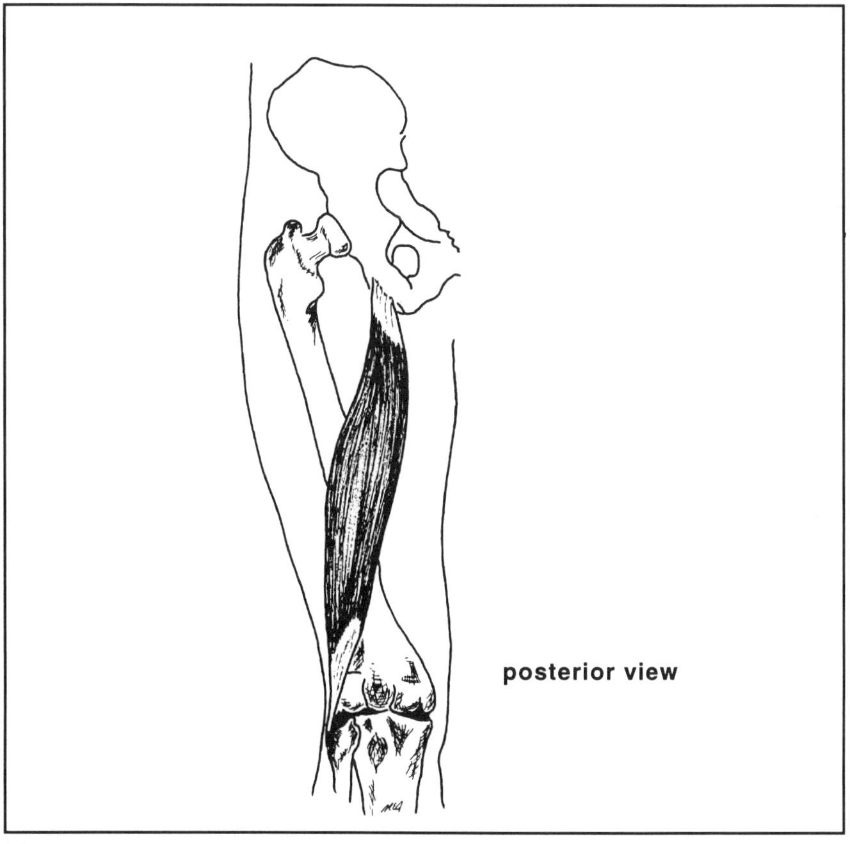

Biceps Femoris

Fig. 8.8

Origin ——	Long head: Posterior aspect of ischial tuberosity. Short head: Lateral ridge of the linea aspera.
Insertion ——	Both heads: Head of fibula and lateral condyle of tibia.
Innervation —	Long head: Tibial portion of sciatic nerve. Short head: Peroneal portion of sciatic nerve.
Action ——	Flexion and external rotation of the knee joint.

The biceps femoris is the lateral hamstring and crosses the knee joint posterior to the frontal axis and lateral to the long axis. It joins the other hamstrings in knee flexion, but is one of the few muscles responsible for external rotation of the tibia. In this latter action, the biceps femoris is extremely important to the integrity of the knee joint since it is the major muscle which will neutralize the internal rotation tendencies of the other knee flexors.

Sartorius (sarto'rius)

The sartorius (Fig. 8.9) is the longest muscle in the body. It is superficial as it courses diagonally medialward across the front of the thigh, but is difficult to palpate except in the area of its tendon of origin. Palpation can be accomplished during resisted flexion of the hip when the femur has been placed in a position of external rotation. The superior portion of the muscle can be felt and observed just below the superior iliac spine. A dimple-like depression will be noted just lateral to the sartorius which separates it from the tensor fasciae latae.

Sartorius

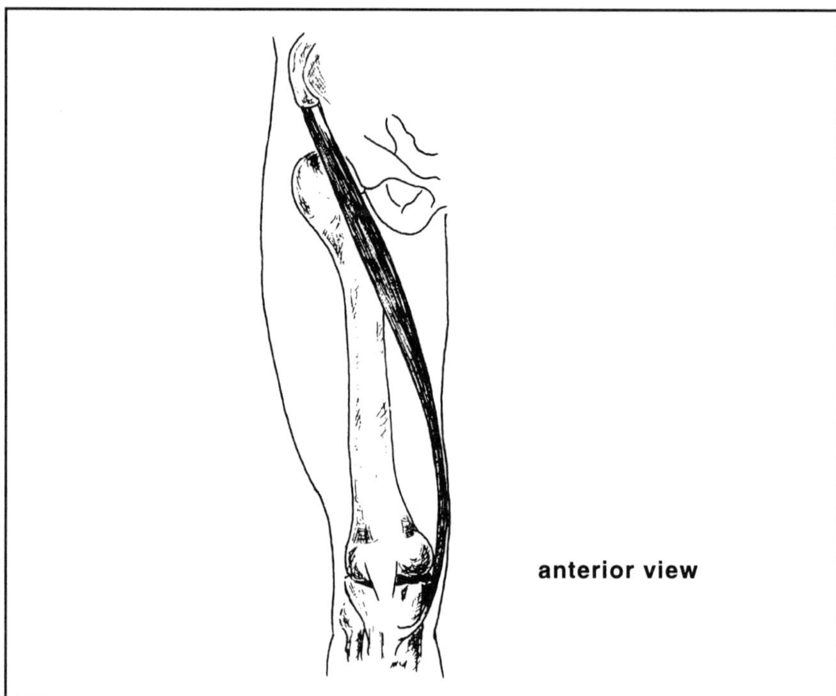

Fig. 8.9

Origin — Anterior superior iliac spine and the adjacent portion of the notch distal to the spine.
Insertion — Upper and medial aspect of the tibia.
Innervation — Femoral nerve.
Action — Flexion and internal rotation of the knee joint.

The tendon of insertion of the sartorius wraps around the medial aspect of the upper tibia to attach nearly as far forward as the anterior crest. In addition to its ability to flex the knee, it is well located to internally rotate by executing its unwrapping motion on the tibia. It should be noted that the muscle crosses anterior to the knee joint in a few individuals, and in such cases acts to extend the knee.

Gracilis (gra'cilis)

The gracilis (Fig. 8.10) is a long and slender muscle located superficially along the inner thigh. It is difficult to palpate because it is easily confused with surrounding muscles; however, its tendon of insertion can usually be felt clearly. Begin the palpation in the middle of the posterior aspect of the knee, then move the fingers medially until the large tendon of the semitendinosus is encountered. If the fingers are moved slightly medially, the smaller tendon of the semimembranosus will be felt. The tendon of the gracilis lies just medial to the semimembranosus. Palpation may be facilitated by internally rotating the tibia against resistance.

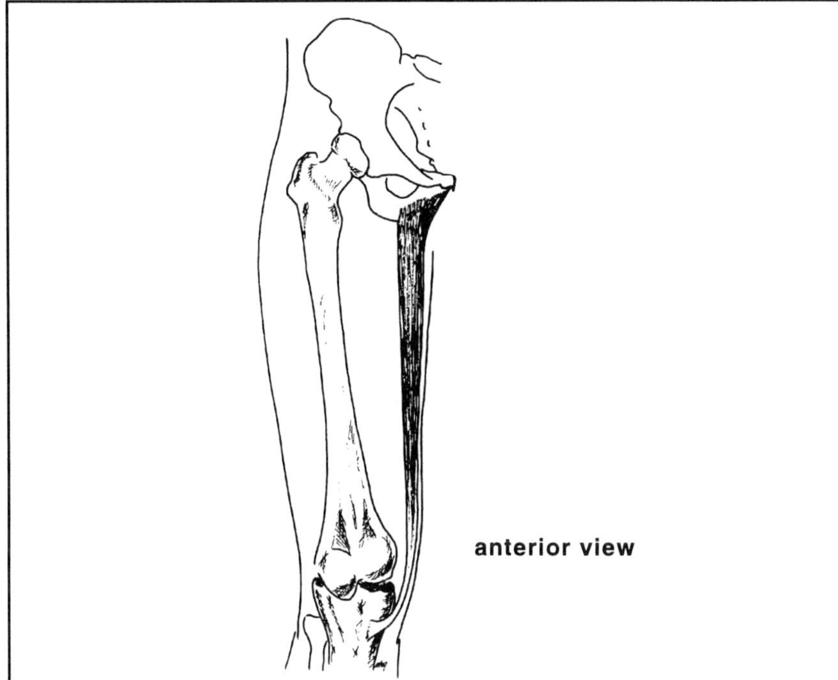

Gracilis

Fig. 8.10

Origin	Inferior half of the symphysis and the superior half of the arch of the pubis.
Insertion	Medial aspect of the tibia just below the condyle.
Innervation	Anterior division of the obturator nerve.
Action	Flexion and internal rotation of the knee joint.

The tendon of insertion of the gracilis passes posterior to the medial condyle of the femur, then curves around the medial condyle of the tibia to attach to the proximal tibia on its medial surface. At its insertion, it is above the tendon of the semitendinosus and below that of the sartorius; these three tendons of insertion form the structure known as the pes anserinus.

Popliteus (poplite'us)

The popliteus (Fig. 8.11) is a small muscle located deep on the posterior surface of the knee. It cannot be palpated.

Popliteus

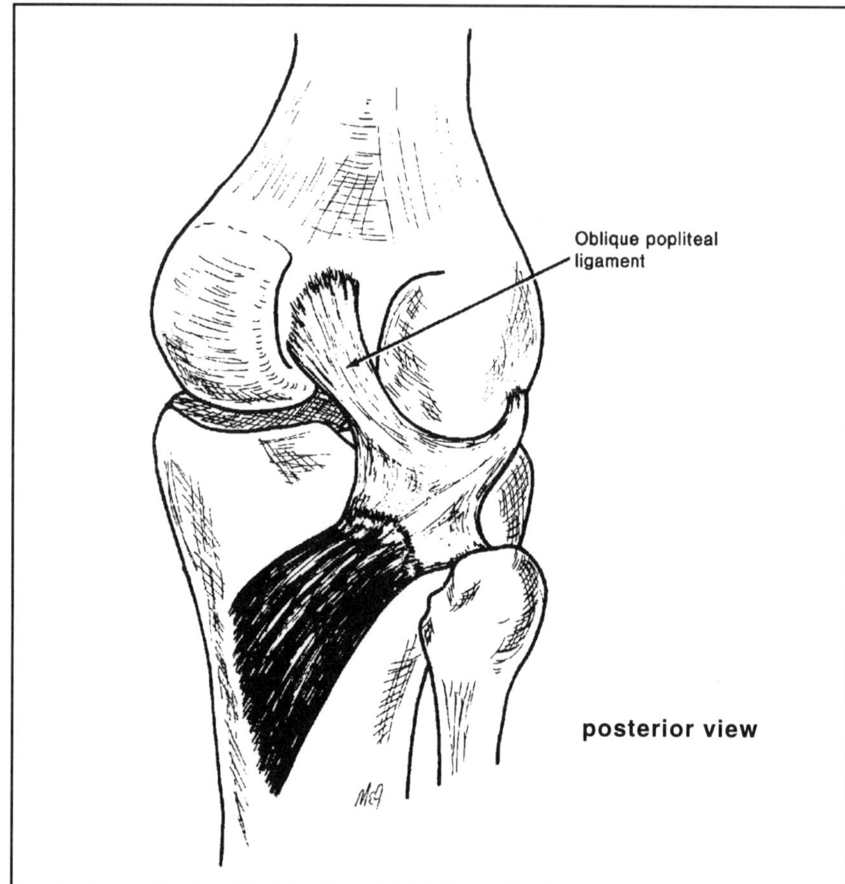

Fig. 8.11

Origin ——	Anterior and lateral portion of the lateral condyle of the femur; head of fibula; lateral meniscus; and oblique popliteal ligament.
Insertion ——	Posterior surface of the tibia, proximal to the popliteal line.
Innervation —	Tibial nerve.
Action ——	Flexion and internal rotation of tibia.

Resolution of the line of pull of the popliteus yields a vertical or flexion component, and a horizontal or rotational component. If the tibia is free to move, contraction of the popliteus will flex and internally rotate the knee joint by moving the tibia. If the tibia is held stationary, as it would be while standing, contraction of the muscle will pull against the femur and lateral meniscus to initiate the unlocking action of the knee which must occur at the beginning of flexion.

Gastrocnemius (gastrocne'mius)

The gastrocnemius (Fig. 8.12) is the large superficial muscle located on the posterior aspect of the lower leg. It may be palpated and observed easily as the ankle is moved through dorsi- and plantar flexion.

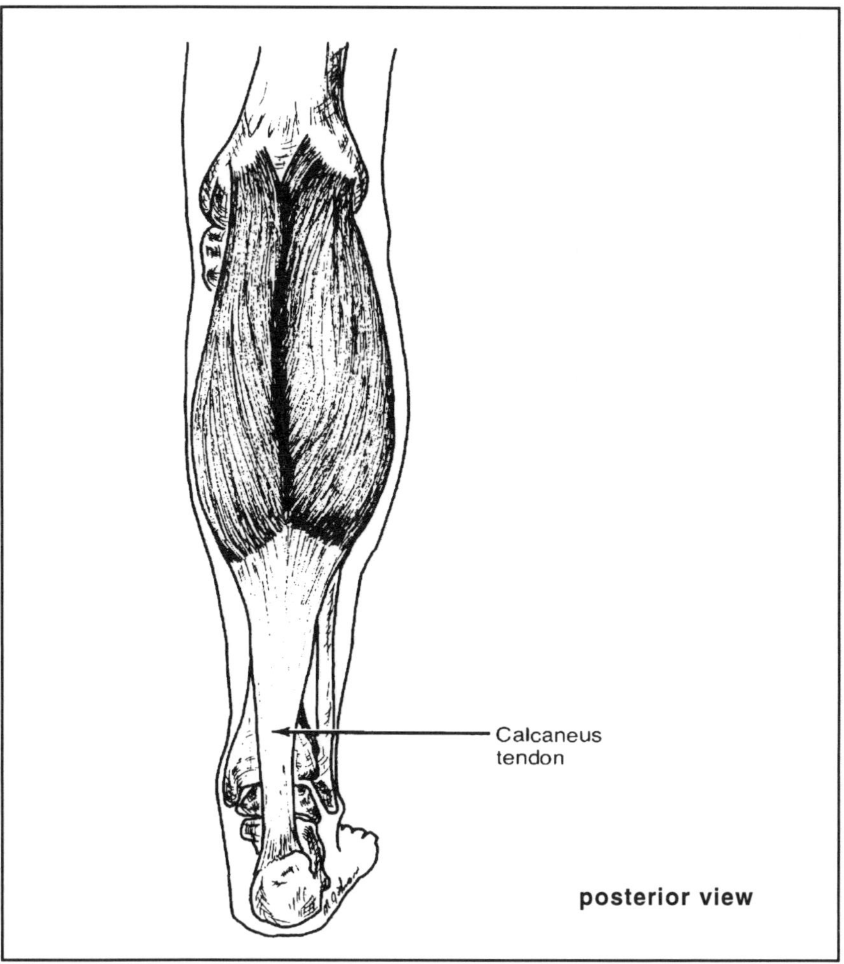

Gastrocnemius

Fig. 8.12

Origin —— By two heads, from the posterior surfaces of the two femoral condyles.
Insertion —— Posterior aspect of calcaneus through the calcaneal (Achilles) tendon.
Innervation — Tibial nerve.
Action —— Aids in flexion of the knee joint.

The contribution of the gastrocnemius to knee flexion is only assistive because, despite the fact that it does cross the knee posterior to the frontal axis, it is rather close to it and does not exhibit a long force arm.

Plantaris (planta'ris)

The plantaris (Fig. 8.13) is poorly developed in man and is missing in some. The muscle lies between the gastrocnemius and the soleus. It cannot be palpated.

Plantaris

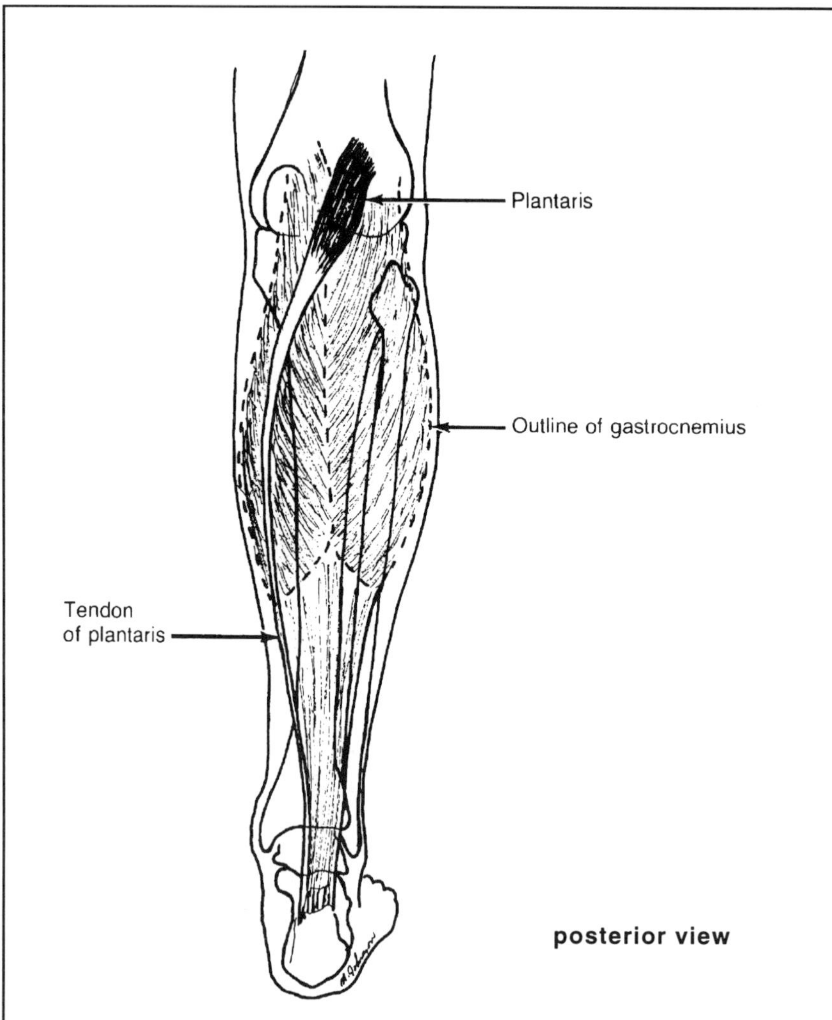

Fig. 8.13

Origin ——	Distal portion of the linea aspera of the femur; oblique popliteal ligament of the knee joint.
Insertion ——	Posterior surface of calcaneus.
Innervation —	Tibial nerve.
Action ——	Weak assistant for knee flexion.

COMMENTS

The knee joint has become a major topic of conversation. The high incidence of injury has focused attention of the injured, and their physicians on the joint and, as a result, innumerable conceptions -- and misconceptions -- have flourished and spread. Most of these have not been verified by research, so it becomes of extreme importance to learn the anatomical and mechanical aspects of the knee joint in order to form a sound and practical basis for prevention of injury.

Consideration of the composite actions of the joint should be the initial step. When the knee is flexed, the ligaments are lax, and the tibia is allowed to rotate around its long axis; when it is extended, the ligaments and the bony structure of the joint prohibit tibial rotation. Since, in many movements the knee is in the flexed position far more often than it is in extension, it follows that an effort should be made to ensure that the musculature of the knee, its last line of defense, be maintained at peak strength so that it can act to check excessive and injurious twisting of the tibia. The task of selecting appropriate exercises is a simple one; all of the muscles which cross the joint are either flexors or extensors; they may have added abilities to rotate the tibia, but all will be involved in moving the lower leg around the frontal axis. One needs only to ensure therefore, that strength-gaining exercises be performed during both flexion and extension. Care must be taken, however, not to overly strengthen either set of muscles. A ratio of four to three, or four to two, of extensor strength to flexor strength, is satisfactory. It is noted, additionally, that the musculature of the knee should be held in contraction if there is possibility of an impending blow to the knee. For example, individuals involved in contact-type activities (i.e., football) must be taught to maintain tension in the thigh muscles after the tackle until they are sure that no late hits will occur.

Joint action between the patella and femur is also important to this discussion. The vastus medialis and lateralis exert opposite forces on the patella. If one muscle is stronger that the other, the patella will be pulled off-center when the quadriceps are contracted. Comparable strength in the two muscles can be achieved by exercising the knee joint through its full range of extension.

As a second step toward the prevention of injury, one must consider normal ranges of motion of the knee joint. The reader is urged to determine the maximum amount of flexion, extension, internal and external rotation of which the joint is capable when it is unencumbered by the body weight. Use of these ranges as guidelines when body weight is superimposed will result in conservative but preventative allowances. For instance, when the knee is fully flexed by drawing the foot from the floor toward the buttocks, the angle between the upper and lower leg will be approximately 30 degrees. During full knee bends, however, the knee is forced, by the body weight, to flex to the point at which the femur and tibia are almost parallel; surely, the possibility of overstretching the ligaments is a real one. If the knee bends are performed only to the 30-degree point, however, possibility of causing trauma will be largely negated. Similarly, it can be established that the joint can hyperextend only minimally from muscular contraction alone. Assumption of positions of upright posture which require the knee to hyperextend farther than this point can carry the risk of injury.

COMMENTS ON TWO-JOINT MUSCLES

There are several muscles of the human body that cross two or even more joints as they course between their origins and insertions. Many of these are found in the lower arm and leg and are discussed in those chapters. Such muscles are typically arranged in order to cause the same action at all the joints they cross. For example, the flexor digitorum profundus crosses four major joints, causing all of them to flex. The extensor digitorum longus crosses some five joints, causing extension of each. The basic mechanics of these muscles reside in their domino-like action of moving the most distal bony segment first followed, in turn, by the next most distal segment, and so on. Because of the sameness of their actions at the joints they cross, they can easily be overstretched or overshortened and will, therefore, be compromised in attaining certain positions demanding strength.

Coordinaton of the Hamstrings and Rectus Femoris

The two-joint muscles of the upper leg deserve special attention in that they cause opposite movements of the joints they cross. The hamstrings (biceps femoris, semitendinosus, semimembranosus) are active as hip extensors and knee flexors. The rectus femoris, antagonistic to the hamstrings, causes hip flexion and knee extension. The cooperation of these muscles must be quite precise during locomotor movements as well as during any movement that requires motion at the hip and/or the knee.

These muscles have been the focus of numerous kinesiological and biomechanical studies. Their cooperative activities during gait, running, squatting, and other such movements have been explored and, whereas each investigator has supplied us with more information than we had previously, we have been unable to unlock the secret of success.

Emerging from the research that has been done are some conclusions and postulates that are of interest to performers and coaches alike. The first regards the discomfort of contracting these muscles when they are at their shortest lengths. Knee extension accompanied by hip flexion places the rectus femoris at its shortest length. If the muscle is contracted strongly while the leg is in this position, a heavy, painful cramp will often occur. A rather common situation in which these conditions are found is on a so-called "quadriceps bench" on which a person sits and lifts weights with one or both legs. Overly heavy weights held at full extension of the knee can easily cause the onset of a cramp, especially if the trunk is inclined forward.

A similar condition can be seen in the hamstrings when the knee is flexed and hip extended. One need only to stand on one foot and attempt to touch the buttocks with the opposite foot while pressing down against it with the hand. Verification will be both immediate and vivid.

Just as these muscles can be shortened by selective placements of the hip and knee joints, they can also be lengthened. The rectus femoris reaches its most extreme length during knee flexion with hip hyperextension -- that position in which runners find themselves after "toe-off" of each stride. Running with maximum effort early in the season is accompanied all too frequently by tears of the rectus femoris. One should be cautious, also, about changing from smooth-soled shoes to cleated shoes. Cleated shoes provide for more ground friction; however, they also require more effort to remove them from the ground -- an effort provided by the hamstrings. Increased contraction of the hamstrings after toe-off causes, in turn, increased knee flexion and hip hyperextension. Unless a gradual change to the new footwear is made, chances for a tear in the rectus femoris are very good indeed.

Muscle Tear: Too Much or Too Little Lean?

The hamstrings are placed at their greatest length when the knee is extended with the hip flexed. Such a position is reached during the "sit and reach" exercise -- an exercise that is performed for the purpose of stretching the hamstrings. Although this extreme position is not reached during all sport and dance techniques, it is approximated by long jumpers, hurdlers, and runners, to name a few. Since hamstring tears occur so often during these activities, it would only seem logical to maintain these muscles at a length that will accommodate such stresses. Exercise programs do not appear to solve the total problem, however. Athletes can work diligently to achieve extreme flexibility of the hip joint only to be faced, at the wrong moment, with a devastating muscle tear. The answer to this worrisome problem is not yet known, but perhaps a postulation is in order. It has been noted by the authors that hamstring tears tend to accompany a change in the position of the trunk of runners while they are in full stride. While trunk lean is associated with sprinting speed, it must be controlled or the athlete will fall. At periods of maximum velocity of running, no further acceleration is possible. Trunk lean must be lessened for control of the center of gravity. If the lessening takes place quickly (rather than gradually), the rectus femoris is stretched equally as rapidly and, in its attempt to respond to the stretch, contracts to cause sudden knee extension -- a condition that seems to be abhorrent to the hamstrings. Result -- a muscle tear. All of this is pure speculation. It is clear that more research must be done if we are to eliminate this insidious problem from the world of movement.

A quiz for this material can be found in the back of this book on page 295.

LABORATORY EXPERIENCES

1. Sit on a bench or table that is high enough to allow your feet to be off the floor and have a partner attach a 10-kilogram weight boot to your right foot. Gradually relax the muscles which cross the right knee as you palpate the space between the femur and tibia. You should notice a widening of the joint space and a feeling of tension in the collateral ligaments when the musculature has been completely relaxed. On the basis of what you have found, make a conclusion regarding the appropriate use of a weight boot in rehabilitation of the knee.

2. Sit in a chair which is low enough to allow you to flex the hip and knee joints to approximately 90 degrees when the foot is flat on the floor. Perform internal and external rotation of the knee joint as you palpate each set of agonists. The palpations may be enhanced if a partner applies resistance at the ankle joint.

3. Place electrodes on the three superficial muscles comprising the quadriceps and monitor their electrical activity as the knee joint is moved, against resistance, from 90 degrees of flexion to full extension. During what portion of the movement is each muscle active?

4. While continuing to monitor the electrical activity of the quadriceps, perform a knee bend to the point at which the back of the thigh and the calf touch, then return to standing position. Now perform a knee bend to the full squat position and, while in the position, allow the quadriceps to relax. Return to standing position. From a comparison of the two sets of electromyograms, determine (1) whether one knee bend elicits more activity than the other; (2) why the full squat is potentially dangerous to the knee joint.

5. Use an isokinetic measuring device to determine the maximum strength of a partner's knee extensors and knee flexors. Calculate the ratio of flexors to extensors. Does this ratio hold true for other members of the class?

6. Stand with the spine extended and heels on the floor. Slowly flex the knee joint while being careful to perpendicularly align the hip joint with the foot. How much flexion of the knee joint is allowed by surrounding musculature? Which muscle is acting as the major limiting factor to increased flexion?

THE ANKLE AND FOOT

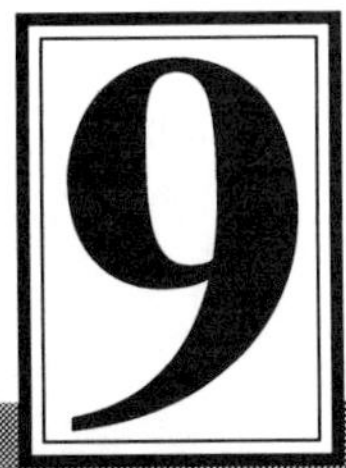

The ankle and foot have developed in man to provide for two functions -- static weight-bearing and propulsive weight-bearing. More than thirty joints between and among the twenty-six bones of the foot attest to the intricacy of the foot structure.

The ankle joint, or talocrural joint (Fig. 9.1), is formed through the articulation of the tibia and fibula with one of the tarsal bones, the talus. The talus articulates with a second bone, the calcaneus, to form the subtalar joint and with a third tarsal bone, the navicular, to

Bones of the Lower Leg and Foot

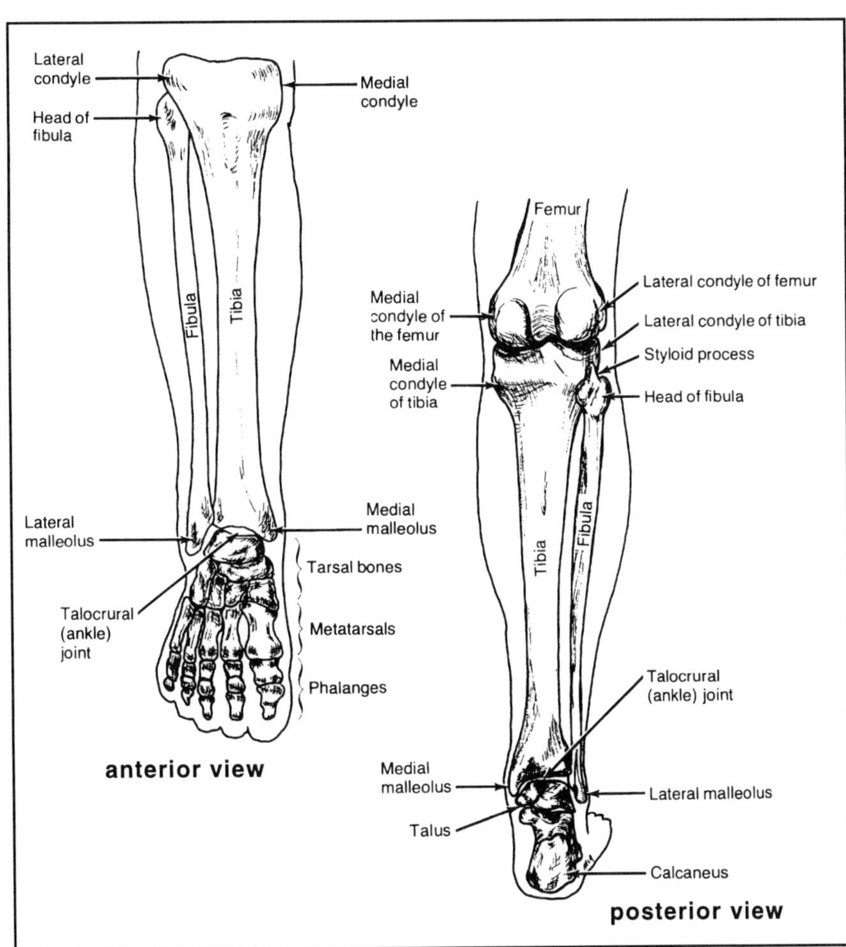

Fig. 9.1

comprise the talocalcaneonavicular joint. Through the calcaneocuboid articulation, the calcaneus communicates with a fourth tarsal, the cuboid. This joint, together with that between the talus and navicular form an S shaped articulation called the **midtarsal joint**. The navicular articulates with the remaining tarsals, the three cuneiforms, through the cuneonavicular joint, as well as the cuboid by the cuboideonavicular joint. Between the cuneiforms are the intercuneiform joints; the third cuneiform communicates with the cuboid through the cuneocuboid joint. All of the joints between the tarsals are referred to collectively as the **intertarsal joints** (Fig. 9.2).

The three cuneiforms and the cuboid articulate with the bases of the five metatarsals by the **tarsometatarsal** joints. The metatarsals articulate, in turn, with the phalanges by the **metatarsophalangeal** joints. Joints between the phalanges are referred to as the **interphalangeal joints** (Fig. 9.2). The metatarsals also articulate between themselves, at their bases, through joints called **intermetatarsal joints**.

Bones of the Foot

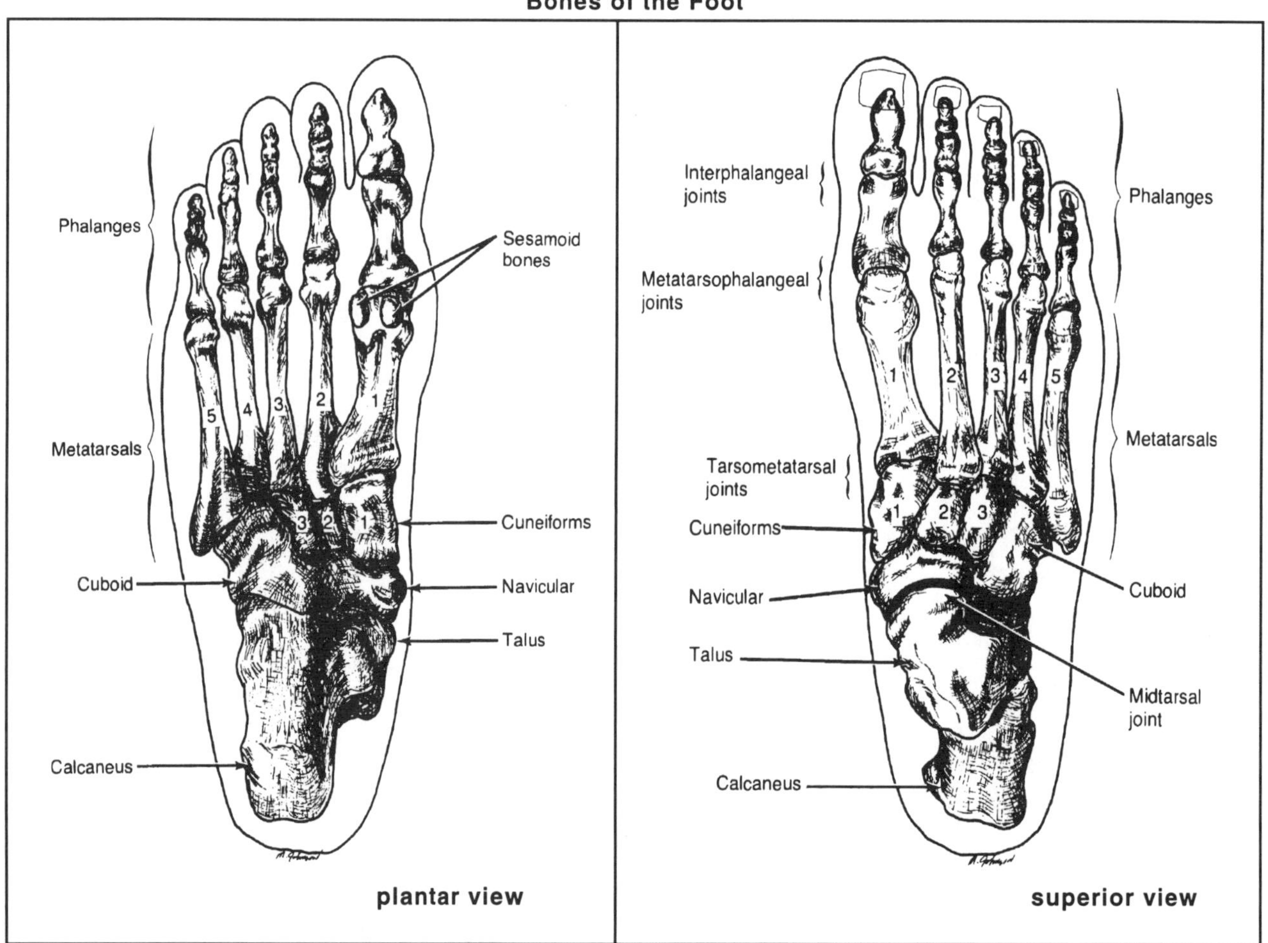

Fig. 9.2

BONE MARKINGS

Figures 9.1 and 9.2 present the bone markings referred to in the discussion of origins and insertions of the muscles. The illustrations should be used in conjunction with a skeleton.

JOINTS OF THE ANKLE AND FOOT

TALOCRURAL JOINT

The talocrural joint is formed by the tibia and its malleolus, the fibula and its malleous, and the inferior transverse ligament, which together present a receptacle for the talus. Unlike their proximal joint, the tibia and fibula are bound tightly together, and having no synovial capsule, form a cartilaginous joint. The talocrural joint, itself, is a hinge joint and is surrounding by a joint capsule which is thin and membranous. As a hinge joint, there is a single axis of rotation passing (approximately) through the two malleoli (Fig. 9.3). Movements of the joint are designated as **dorsiflexion** (raising the foot toward the anterior surface of the leg) and **plantar flexion** (lowering the foot as when "pointing the toes").

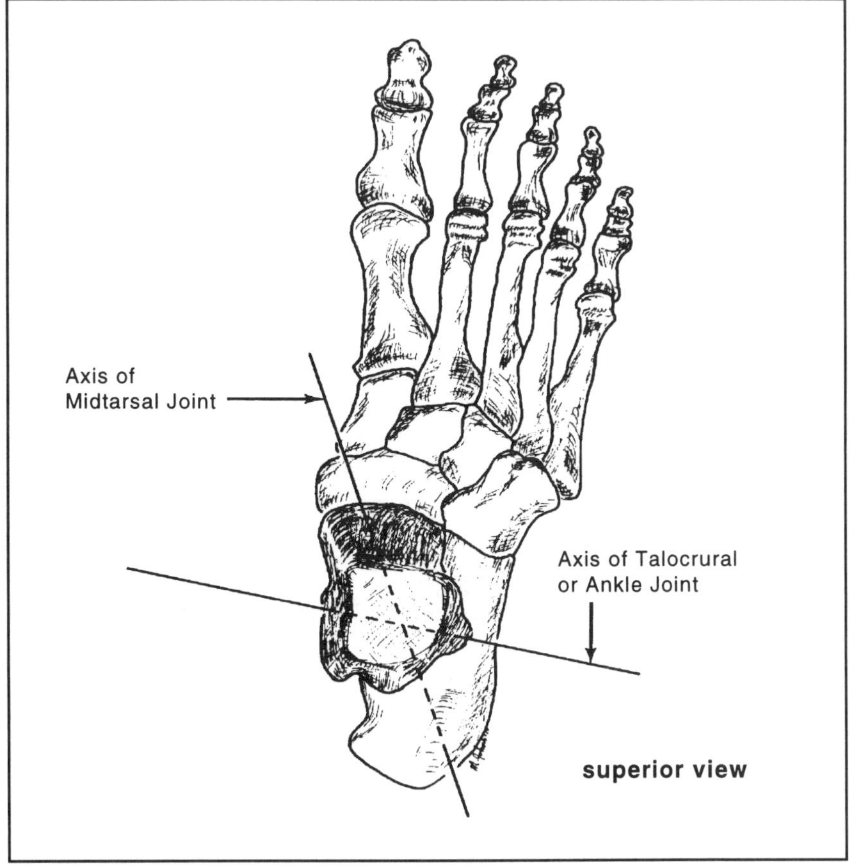

Axes of Rotation of Ankle and Foot

Fig. 9.3

Four ligaments connect the bones of the joint (Fig. 9.4). Three of these are located on the lateral aspect of the joint and are the anterior and posterior talofibular ligaments, and the calcaneofibular ligament. As their names imply, they course between the fibula and the talus, and fibula and calcaneus, respectively. The large, triangular deltoid ligament connects the tibial malleous with the talus, calcaneus, and navicular bones.

Ligaments of the Ankle and Foot

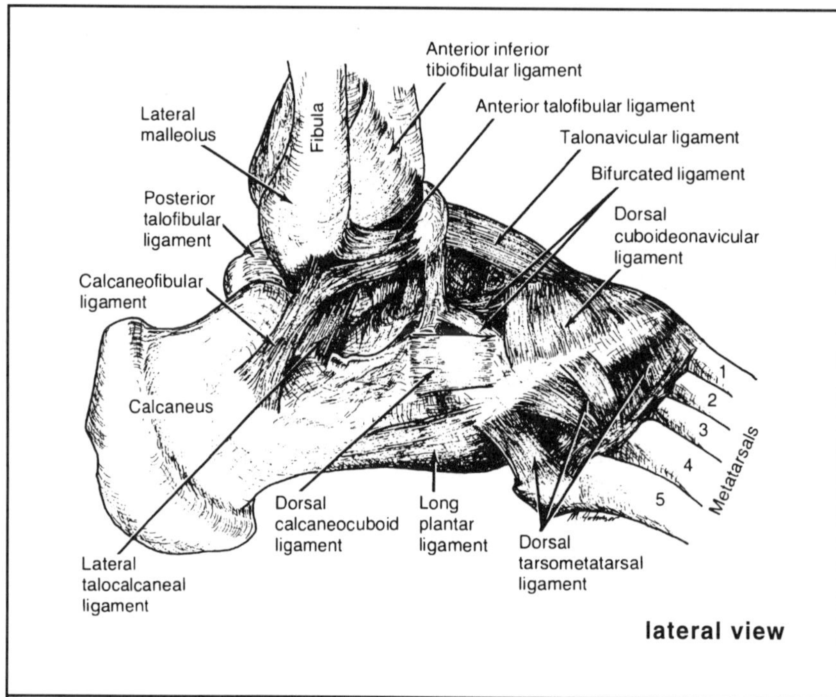

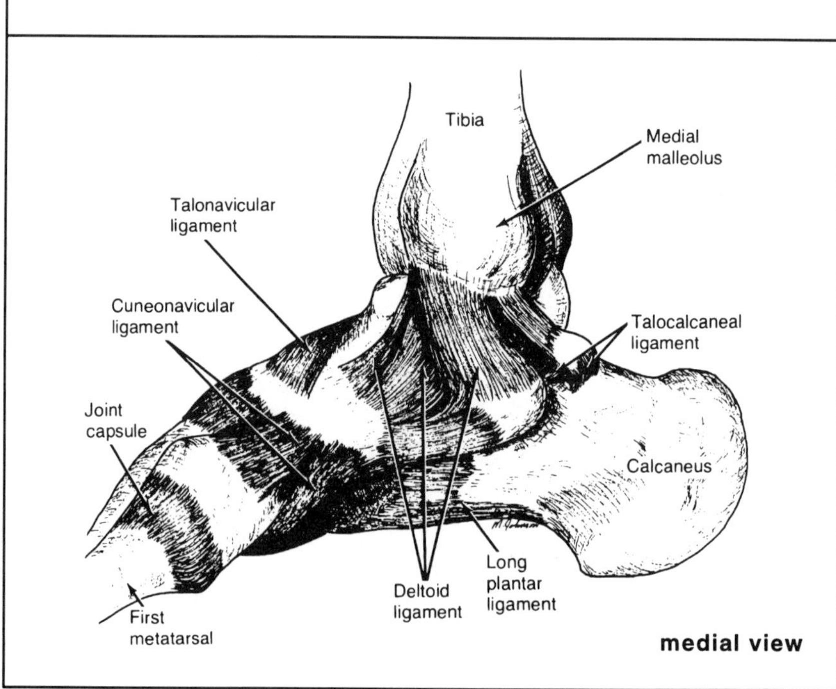

Fig. 9.4

INTERTARSAL JOINTS

The subtalar joint is the articulation between the talus, calcaneus, and navicular. It is synovial and nonaxial, and affords only gliding motion. Connecting the two bones are anterior, posterior, lateral, medial, and interosseus talocalcaneal ligaments, the dorsal talonavicular ligament, and the joint capsule.

The midtarsal joint, a double articulation including part of the subtalar joint, communicates the calcaneus with the cuboid, and the talus with the navicular. The joint permits a type of rotational movement by which the foot can be slightly dorsi- or plantar flexed while simultaneously being inverted (sole being turned inwardly) or everted (sole being turned outwardly). It is interesting to note that neither inversion nor eversion can be performed without an accompanying amount of adduction or abduction of the foot around the heel. Because of this, some kinesiologists use the terms **supination** and **pronation** to describe the combination movements of adduction/inversion and abduction/eversion, respectively. Those terms will not be employed in this text, however, since they are so frequently used to connote pathological conditions. Rather, inversion and eversion will be used with the understanding that adduction and abduction occur simultaneously. The axis of rotation (Fig. 9.3) takes an approximate direction from a lateral-posterior point on the heel to the articulation between the navicular and first cuneiform. This junction may be located easily by palpating the end of the medial malleolus, then moving the fingers about four centimeters toward the toes until a groove is felt between the prominent navicular bone and the cuneiform.

The ligaments of the midtarsal joint (Fig. 9.4 and Fig. 9.5) are the dorsal talonavicular and calcaneocuboid ligaments, part of the bifurcated ligament, and the long and short plantar ligaments. In addition, the plantar calcaneonavicular ligament, also called the **spring ligament**, spans the joint to support the head of the talus. This ligament is broad, thick, and considerably elastic to provide for shock absorption. Improper foot mechanics can cause a permanent stretch in the ligament resulting in the lowered arch associated with flat feet.

The remaining intertarsal articulations are the cuneonavicular, cuboideonavicular, intercuneiform, and cuneocuboid joints. They are all synovial gliding joints, and are reinforced by dorsal and plantar ligaments, and in the case of the latter three joints, by interosseus ligaments.

Ligaments of the Plantar Aspect of the Foot

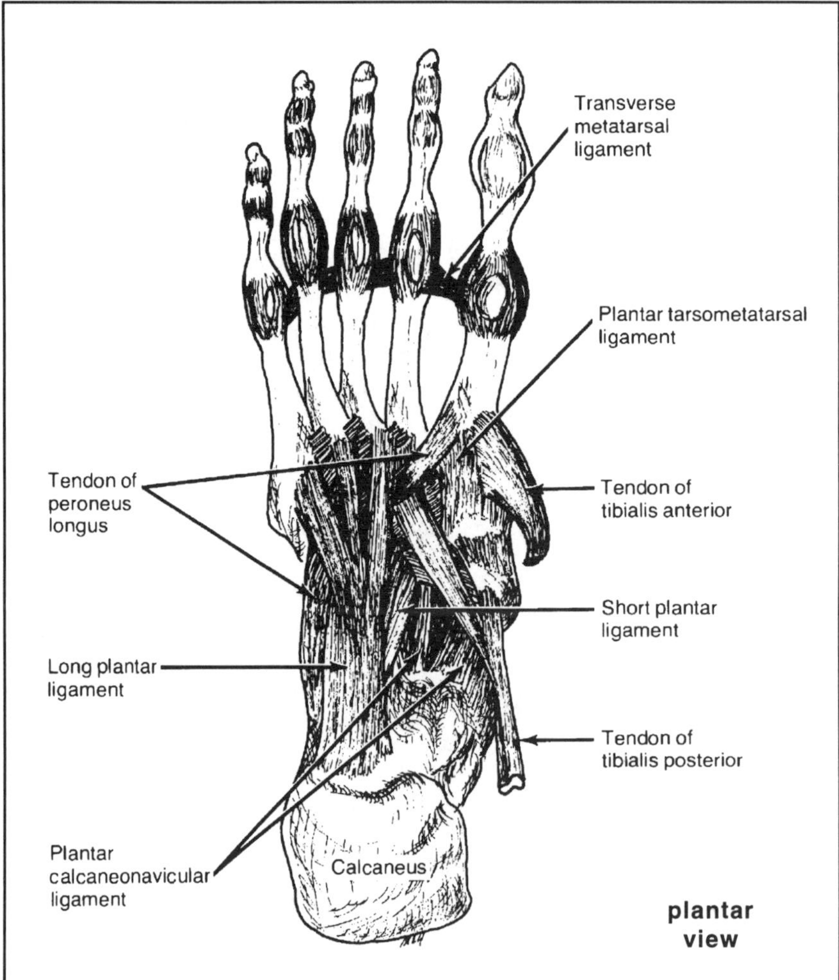

Fig. 9.5

TARSOMETATARSAL AND INTERMETATARSAL JOINTS

These are all nonaxial and synovial joints which permit only a slight gliding motion between the bones. Dorsal, plantar, and interosseus ligaments span the articulations.

The heads of the metatarsals are connected by the transverse metatarsal ligament. This ligament is a narrow band which holds the bones in some proximity when the foot bears weight.

INTERPHALANGEAL JOINTS

The interphalangeal joints are synovial hinge joints which permit only flexion and extension. Plantar and collateral ligaments connect the bones. The great toe has a single interphalangeal joint; the four lesser toes have two such joints.

MUSCULATURE

The muscles of the ankle and foot are divided into two groups, extrinsic and intrinsic. Extrinsic muscles originate in the lower leg or just above the knee and insert distal to the ankle. Intrinsic muscles originate and insert in the foot. In describing the actions of the muscles, the axis which passes through the two malleoli will be referred to as the **axis of the ankle**; the axis around which inversion and eversion are performed will be called the **midtarsal axis**.

EXTRINSIC MUSCLES

Tibialis Anterior (tibia'lis ante'rior)

The tibialis anterior (Fig. 9.6) is located on the anterior aspect of the lower leg. It can be palpated just lateral to the tibia and can be followed across the ankle almost to its insertion. Palpation is enhanced if the foot is dorsiflexed and inverted.

Tibialis Anterior

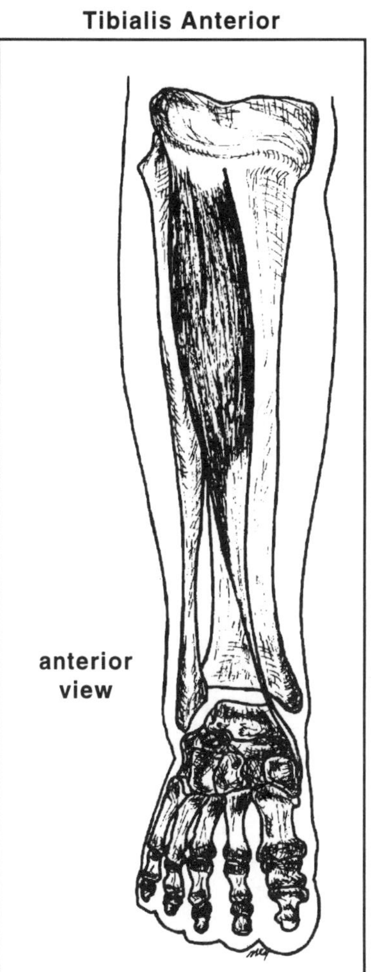

Fig. 9.6

Origin	Upper two-thirds of the lateral tibia and adjacent portion of the interosseus membrane which connects the tibia and fibula.
Insertion	Medial and plantar surface of first cuneiform and base of first metatarsal.
Innervation	Deep peroneal nerve.
Action	Dorsiflexion of the ankle joint; inversion of the midtarsal joint.

The tendon of tibialis anterior, which begins about two-thirds of the way down the leg, crosses the ankle joint anterior to the axis of the ankle and medial to the axis of the midtarsal joint. The muscle is, thus, an important one in both of its actions. The inversion action disappears, however, when the foot is held in plantar flexion. This is probably because forceful plantar flexion is accompanied by a certain amount of medial movement of the front of the foot -- just enough to place the insertion of the muscle in line with the axis of the midtarsal joint. This medial movement is termed, by dancers, sickling of the foot, and is deplored as being unattractive and undisciplined. Dismay is loudly voiced when it is realized after viewing slow motion film of leaps and other body elevations from the floor, that sickling is an unavoidable part of vertical projection of the body.

Extensor Digitorum Longus (exten'sor digito'rum lon'gus)

The extensor digitorum longus (Fig. 9.7) is located on the lateral and anterior aspect of the leg. It is best palpated where its tendon divides into four slips just distal to the ankle joint.

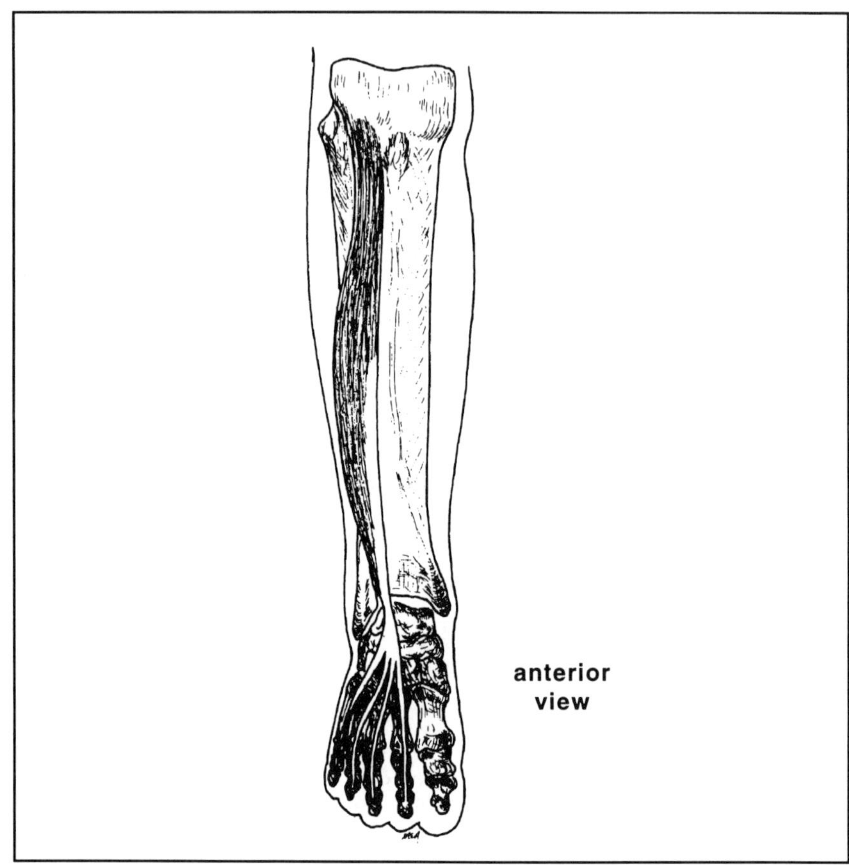

Fig. 9.7

Origin	Upper three-fourths of the anterior fibula; lateral condyle of the tibia; adjacent portions of the interosseus membrane between the tibia and fibula.
Insertion	Second and third phalanges of the four lesser toes.
Innervation	Deep peroneal nerve.
Action	Extension of the interphalangeal and metatarsophalangeal joints of the four toes; dorsiflexion of the ankle; eversion of the midtarsal joint.

The primary function of the muscle is extension of the interphalangeal joints; however, the muscle does cross the ankle and midtarsal joints, and must be examined for its contribution to their movements. These can best be explained by noting that the muscle crosses the ankle anterior to the axis of that joint and lateral to the axis of the midtarsal joint. The force arm is long to each axis indicating the importance of the muscle in both dorsiflexion and eversion.

Extensor Hallucis Longus (exten'sor hal'lucis lon'gus)

The extensor hallucis longus (Fig. 9.8) is located between the extensor digitorum longus and the tibialis anterior in the lower part of the leg. Its tendon can be palpated on the dorsum of the ankle as the great toe is raised and lowered.

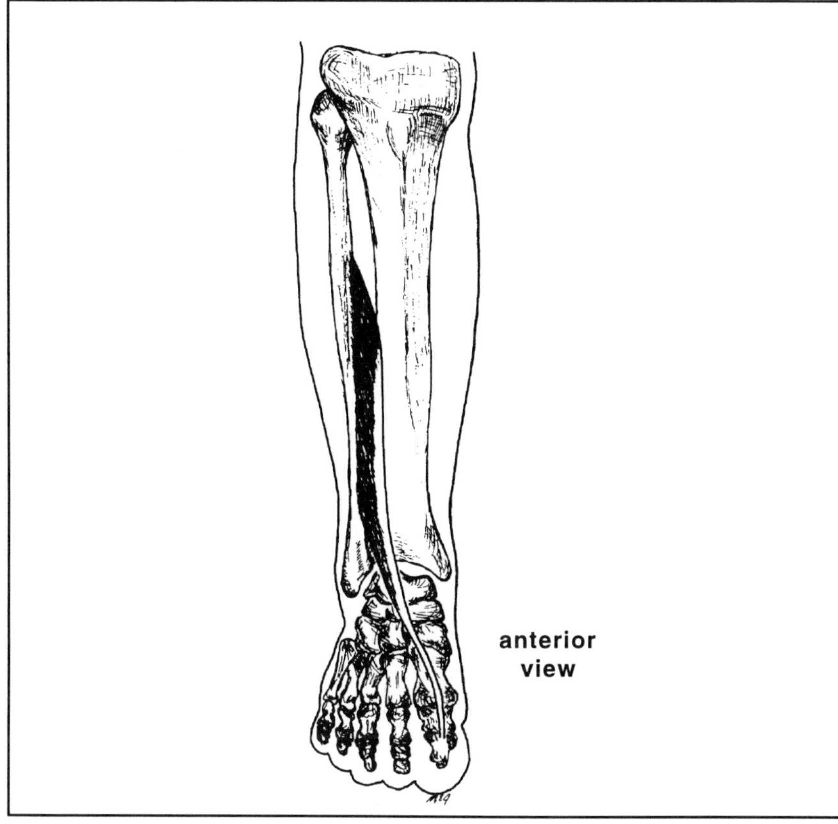

Extensor Hallucis Longus

Fig. 9.8

Origin —— Middle half of the anterior fibula and adjacent portions of the interosseus membrane between the tibia and fibula.
Insertion —— Base of the distal phalanx of the great toe.
Innervation — Deep peroneal nerve.
Action —— Extends the interphalangeal and metatarsophalangeal joints of the great toe; dorsiflexion of the ankle joint.

Movement of the great toe is the primary function of the extensor hallucis longus; however, since it is anterior to the axis of the ankle, it also functions as a dorsiflexor. The muscle has been variously reported as both an everter and an inverter of the midtarsal joint. Examination of its location indicates, however, that it lies on or very near the axis of the midtarsal joint and makes negligible contributions to either eversion or inversion.

Peroneus Tertius (perone'us ter'tius)

The peroneus tertius (Fig. 9.9) appears to be a part of the extensor digitorum longus and is often described as the fifth tendon of that muscle. It is difficult to distinguish from the extensor digitorum longus but may be palpated on the dorsum of the foot proximal to the prominent base of the fifth metatarsal.

Peroneus Tertius

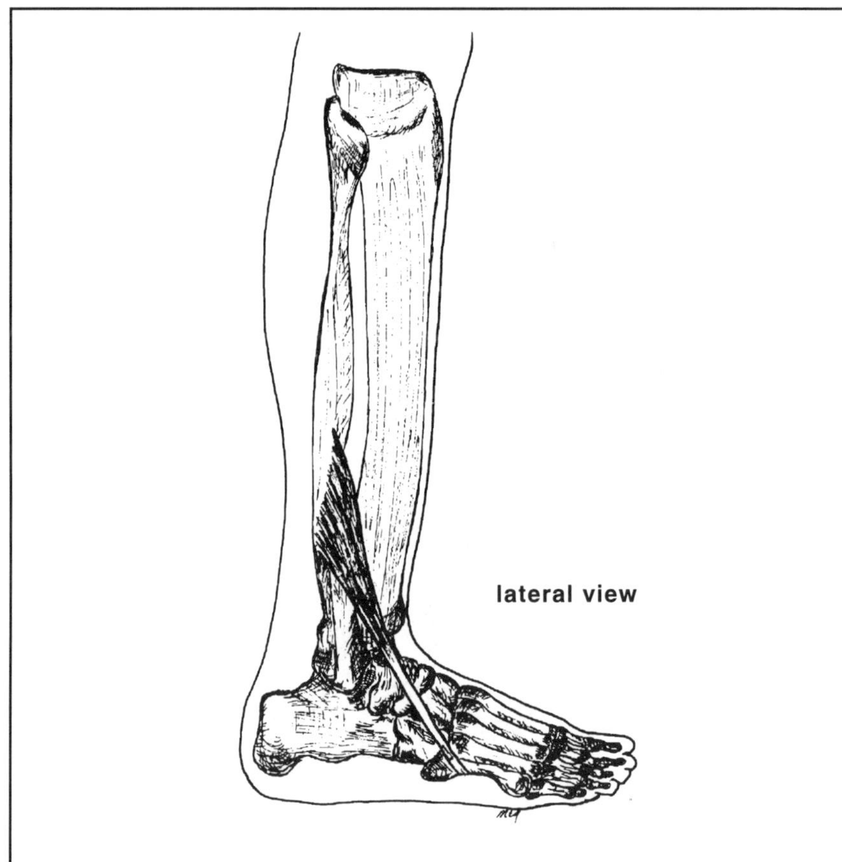

Fig. 9.9

Origin —	Distal third of the anterior fibula and adjacent portions of the interosseus membrane between the tibia and fibula.
Insertion —	Dorsal surface of the base of the fifth metatarsal.
Innervation —	Deep peroneal nerve.
Action —	Dorsiflexion of the ankle joint; eversion of the midtarsal joint.

The line of pull of the peroneus tertius is similar to that of the extensor digitorum longus as the latter muscle crosses the ankle and midtarsal joints. It can be credited therefore, with the same actions. The muscle is often missing.

Peroneus Longus (perone'us lon'gus)

The peroneus longus (Fig. 9.10) is located on the lateral aspect of the lower leg. Its tendon is easily palpated above and slightly behind the lateral malleolus as the foot is held in eversion.

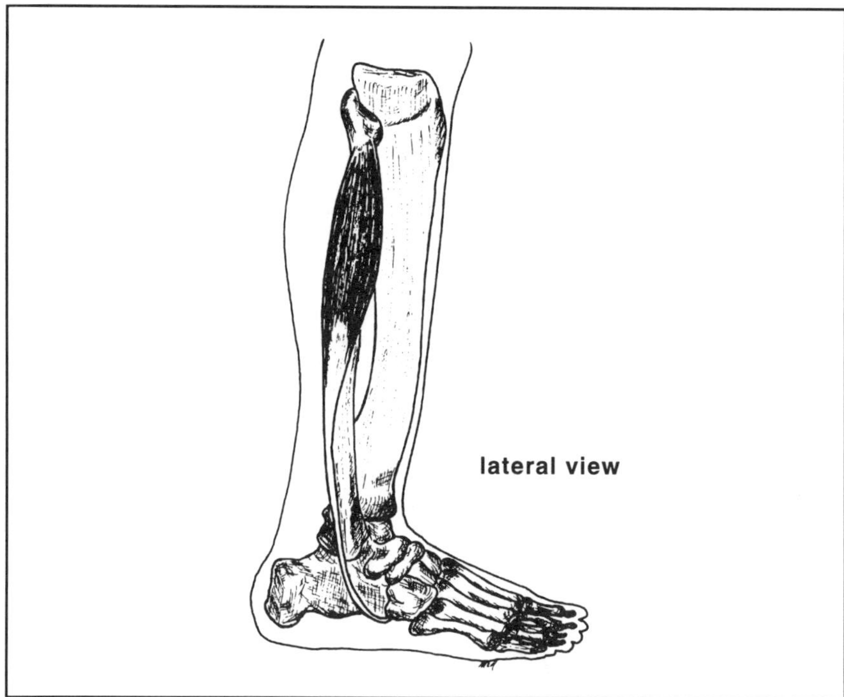

Peroneus Longus

Fig. 9.10

Origin — Head and upper two-thirds of fibula; occasionally from the lateral condyle of the tibia.
Insertion — Lateral surface of the first cuneiform and adjacent portion of the first metatarsal.
Innervation — Superficial peroneal nerve.
Action — Eversion of the midtarsal joint; aids in plantar flexion of the ankle joint.

The tendon of the peroneus longus changes direction twice before its insertion. From its downward run on the outside of the leg, it passes behind the lateral malleolus, using that bony prominence as a pulley around which the tendon passes to direct itself toward the toes. It maintains this direction until it reaches the cuboid where it finds a groove that turns it at an approximate right angle to pass diagonally across the sole of the foot to attach near the tibialis anterior. Through its progress, the muscle passes the midtarsal joint lateral to the axis with a long force arm. It passes close but posterior to the axis of the ankle and hence can contribute only assistively to plantar flexion.

Peroneus Brevis (perone'us bre'vis)

The peroneus brevis (Fig. 9.11) is shorter and smaller than the peroneus longus. It lies beneath the latter muscle and cannot be palpated except where its tendon approaches the prominent base of the fifth metatarsal.

Peroneus Brevis

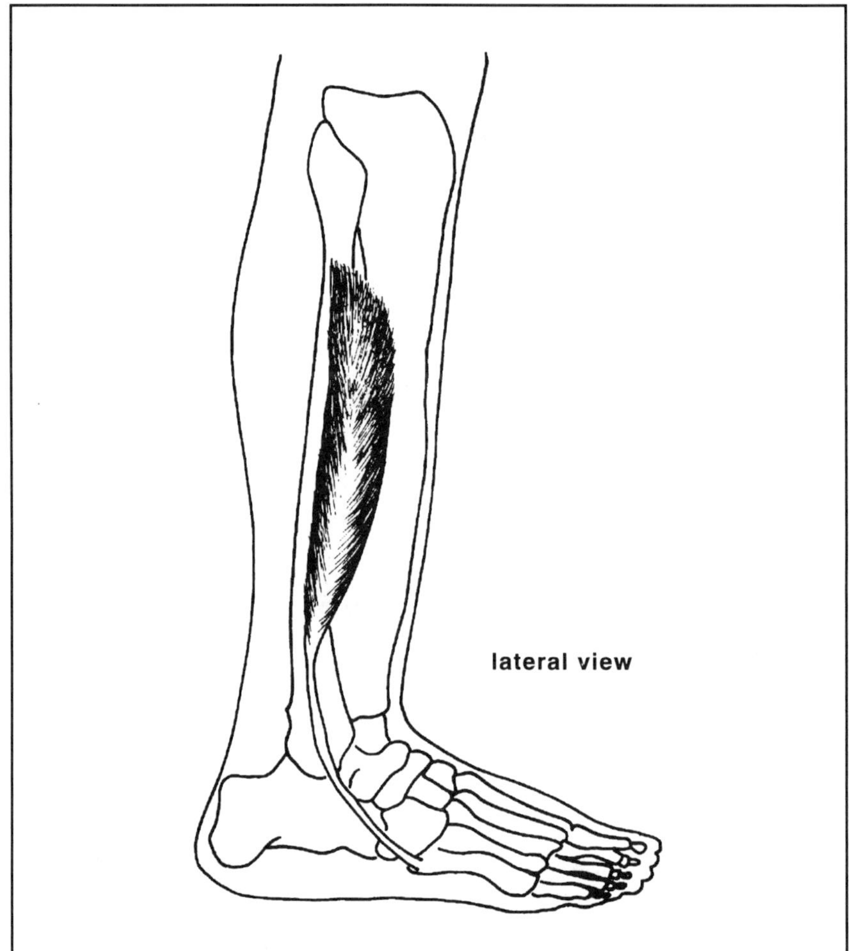

Fig. 9.11

Origin —	Distal two-thirds of the fibula.
Insertion —	Lateral side of the base of the fifth metatarsal.
Innervation —	Superficial peroneal nerve.
Action —	Eversion of the midtarsal joint; aids in plantar flexion of the ankle joint.

The line of pull is similar to that of the peroneus longus, and the resulting actions are essentially the same as those of that muscle.

Gastrocnemius (gastrocne'mius)

The gastrocnemius (Fig. 9.12) is the large superficial muscle on the posterior portion of the lower leg. It is often referred to as the **calf muscle**, and is easily palpated between the knee and heel.

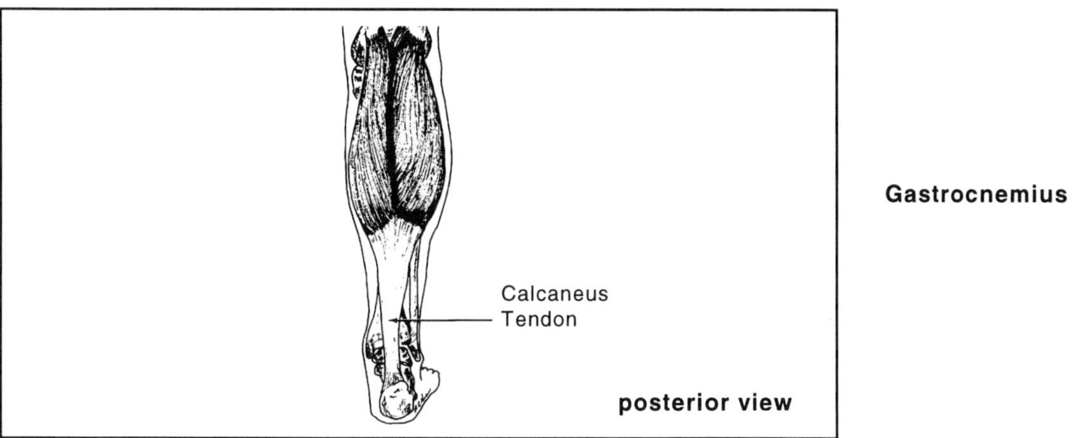

Gastrocnemius

Fig. 9.12

Origin	By two heads, from the posterior surface of the condyles of the femur.
Insertion	Posterior surface of the calcaneus by the calcaneal (Achilles) tendon.
Innervation	Tibial nerve.
Action	Plantar flexion of the ankle joint; weak inversion of the midtarsal joint.

The calcaneus, by virtue of its posterior projection, offers optimum insertion for the gastrocnemius by way of the calcaneal tendon. The force arm of this muscle is the longest it can be from the axis of the ankle and this, paired with the muscle's large size, allows for forceful plantar flexion. The gastrocnemius is not recruited, however, during standing at ease but only when ankle motion is required. The gastrocnemius aids weakly in inversion of the midtarsal joint since the calcaneal tendon attaches to the calcaneus just medial to the axis of that joint. The force arm is extremely short, however, and any contribution to inversion is so overshadowed by the ability of the gastrocnemius to plantar flex that it is usually considered negligible. Its action as an inverter can be seen well, however, through slow-motion photography. Films exposed in a camera situated to record the front view of runners will show that the foot inverts immediately after it leaves the ground. The gastrocnemius accompanied by the soleus are the major muscles involved in providing thrust to the ground for each running step. Their attachment to the lateral side of the inversion axis is responsible for the brief pigeon-toed look of the foot. This same phenomenon can be seen, also, during the vertical jump. The strong contraction of the gastrocnemius and soleus manifests itself first in forceful plantar flexion to elevate the body and then in inversion (or in the dancers' terminology, "sickling") when ground contact is lost.

Soleus (so'leus)

The soleus (Fig. 9.13) is located beneath the gastrocnemius except along its lower and lateral aspect where a portion protrudes and may be palpated.

Soleus

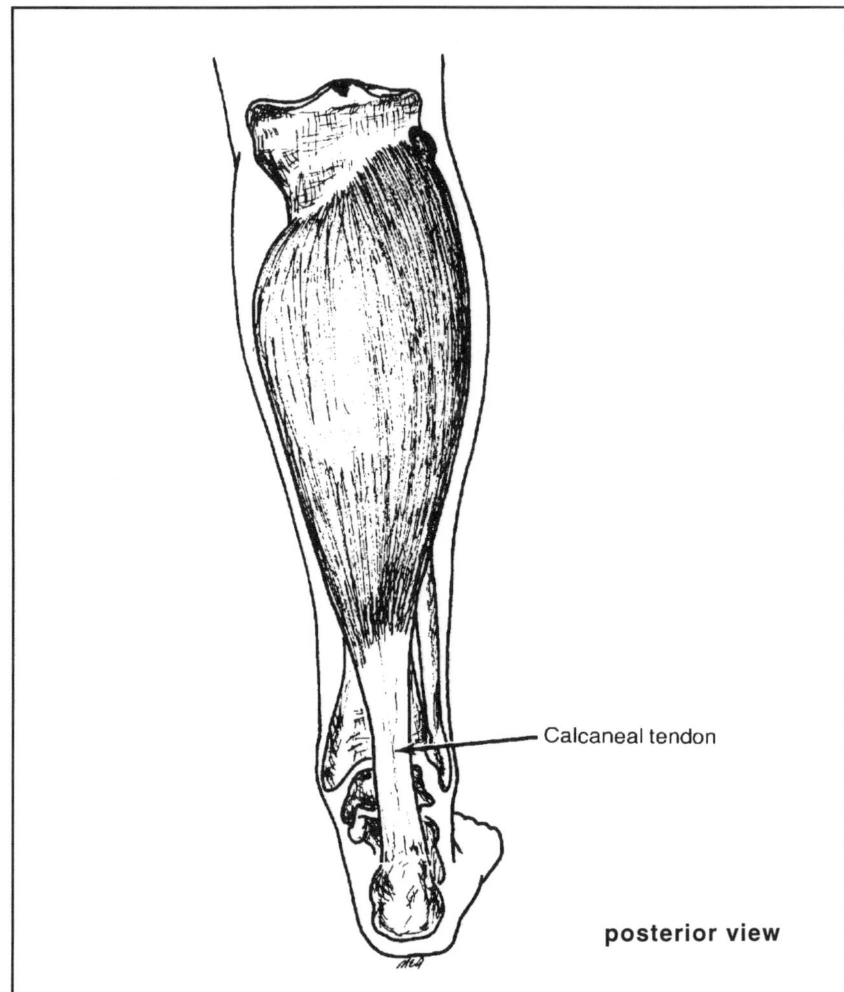

Fig. 9.13

Origin ——— Upper posterior surface of the fibula, tibia, and interosseus membrane.
Insertion —— Posterior surface of the calcaneus by means of the calcaneal (Achilles) tendon.
Innervation— Tibial nerve.
Action ——— Plantar flexion of the ankle joint; weak inversion of the midtarsal joint.

The soleus is an associate of the gastrocnemius and with that muscle forms the muscular unit called the triceps surae. The muscular activity of the soleus differs from the gastrocnemius only in that the soleus is involved more constantly in static standing.

Plantaris (planta'ris)

The plantaris (Fig. 9.14) is a small muscle located deep in the back of the knee. Its tendon runs between the gastrocnemius and soleus; it cannot be palpated.

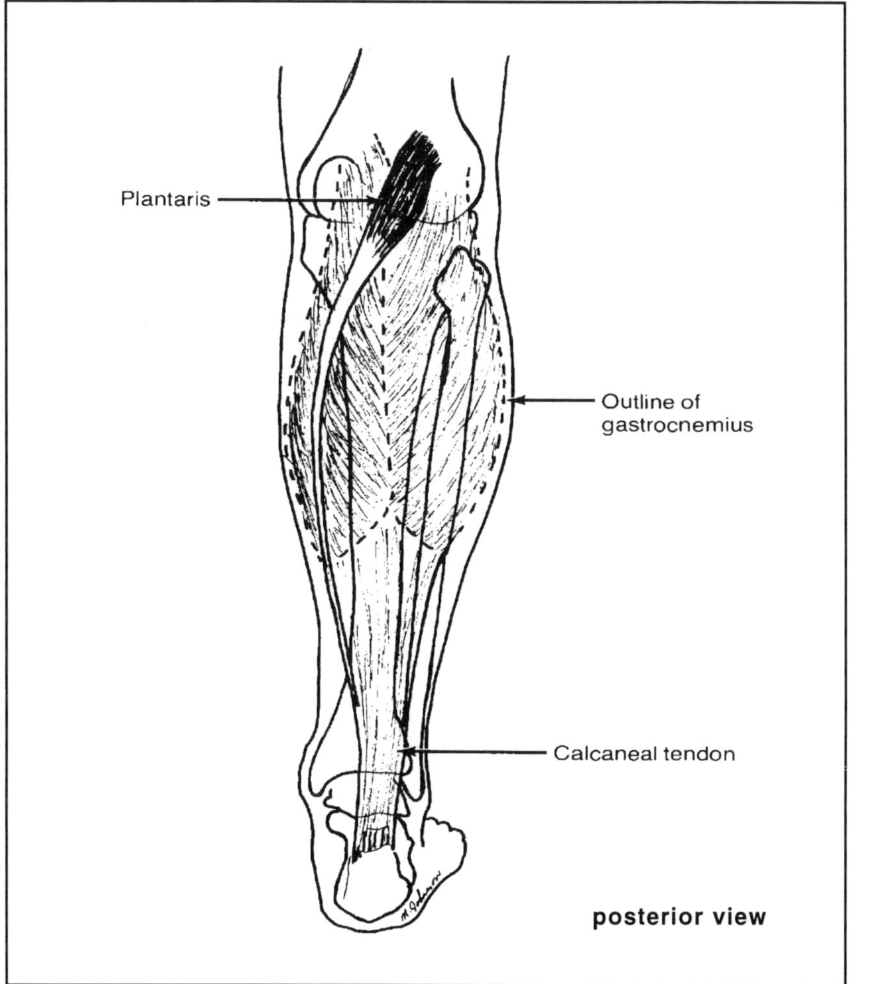

Fig. 9.14

Plantaris

Origin —— Distal portion of the linea aspera and oblique popliteal ligament.
Insertion —— Calcaneus just medial to the calcaneal (Achilles) tendon.
Innervation — Tibial nerve.
Action —— Aids in plantar flexion of the ankle joint.

The plantaris has the same force arm to the axis of the ankle that the soleus and gastrocnemius do, since their tendons insert side by side; however, the small size of the plantaris enables it to contribute only weak assistance of plantar flexion.

Flexor Digitorum Longus (flex'or digito'rum lon'gus)

The flexor digitorum longus (Fig. 9.15) is located deep on the back of the lower leg. It cannot be palpated.

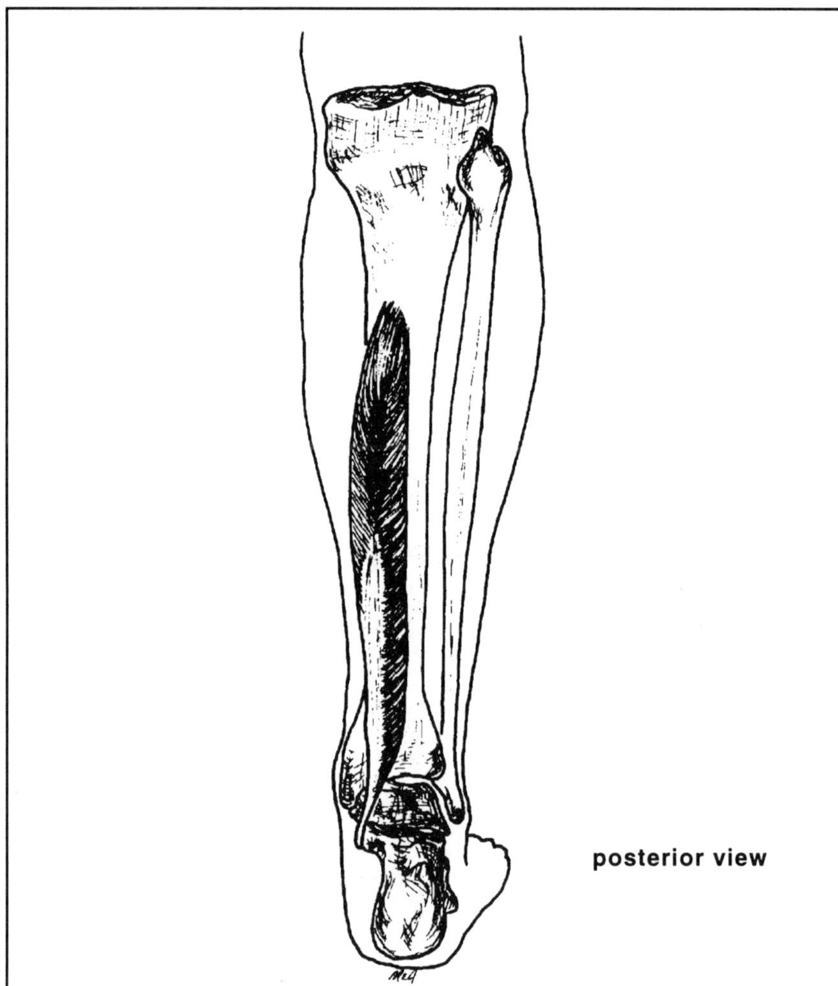

Fig. 9.15

Origin —— Posterior surface of the tibia from just below the popliteal line.
Insertion —— Base of distal phalanges of four lesser toes.
Innervation — Tibial nerve.
Action —— Flexion of the interphalangeal and metatarsophalangeal joints of the four lesser toes; plantar flexion of the ankle joint; inversion of the midtarsal joint.

The responsibility of the flexor digitorum longus is primarily that of moving the toes; however, it contributes also to the movement of the other joints it crosses. The muscle runs posterior to the axis of the ankle and medial to the midtarsal axis to be a plantar flexor and inverter, respectively.

Flexor Hallucis Longus (flex'or hal'lucis lon'gus)

The flexor hallucis longus (Fig. 9.16) is located to the lateral side of the flexor digitorum longus deep in the back of the leg. It cannot be palpated.

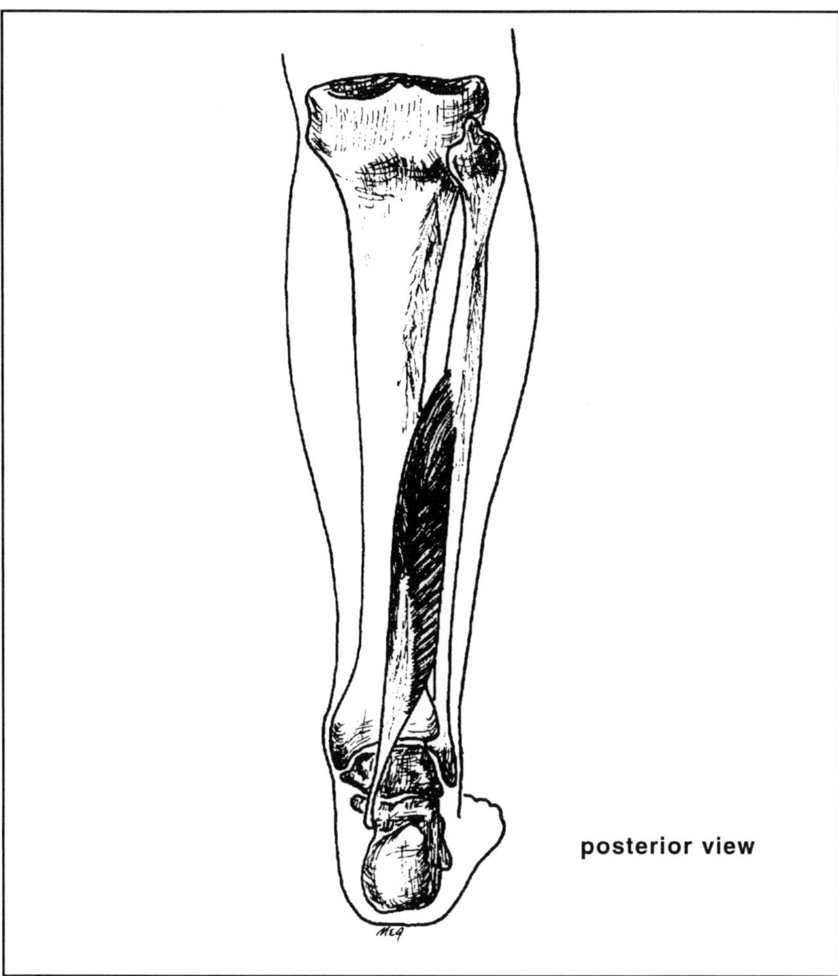

Flexor Hallucis Longus

Fig. 9.16

Origin	Lower two-thirds of the posterior surface of the fibula and the distal portion of the interosseus membrane between the tibia and fibula.
Insertion	Base of the distal phalanx of the great toe.
Innervation	Tibial nerve.
Action	Flexion of the interphalangeal and metatarsophalangeal joints of the great toe; plantar flexion of the ankle joint; inversion of the midtarsal joint.

The tendon of the flexor hallucis longus crosses the axis of the ankle and midtarsal joints just to the posterior side of the tendon of the flexor digitorum longus; hence, the two muscles function similarly on those joints. The major responsibility of the muscle is, however, movement of the great toe.

Tibialis Posterior (tibia'lis poste'rior)

The tibialis posterior (Fig. 9.17) lies beneath the triceps surae on the back of the lower leg. It cannot be palpated.

Tibialis Posterior

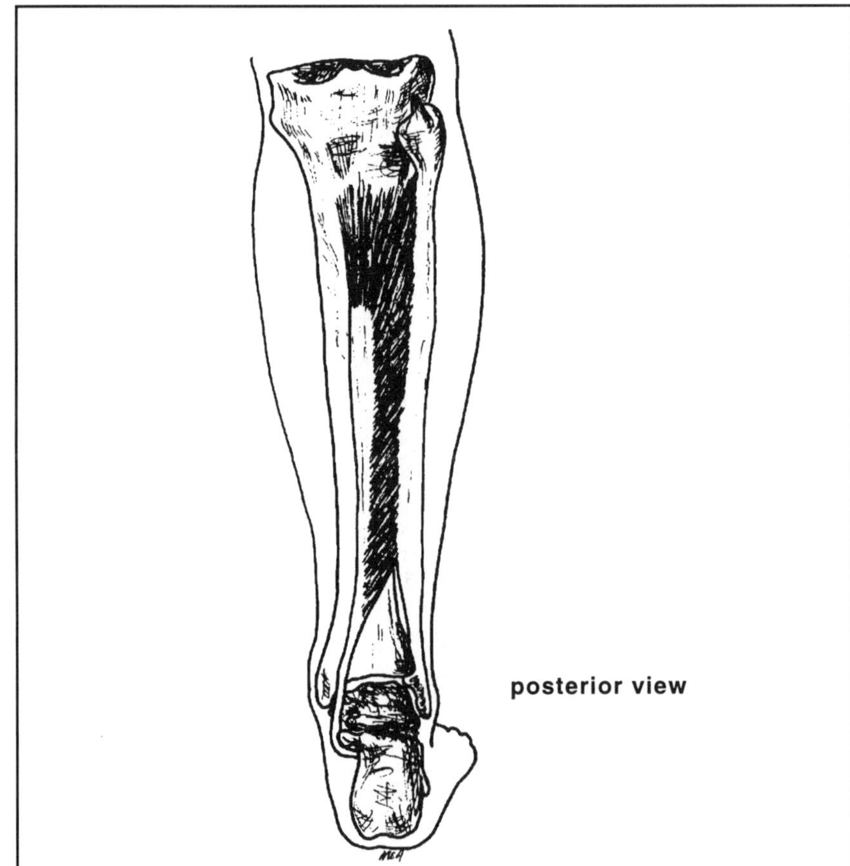

Fig. 9.17

Origin — Posterior surface of upper two-thirds of the tibia, medial surface of upper two-thirds of the fibula, and adjacent portion of interosseus membrane between the tibia and fibula.
Insertion — Tuberosity of the navicular with fibrous slips to the calcaneus, cuboid, the three cuneiforms, and the bases of the second through fourth metatarsals.
Innervation — Tibial nerve.
Action — Plantar flexion of the ankle joint; inversion of the midtarsal joint.

The tendon of the tibialis posterior crosses the ankle and midtarsal joints, with the tendons of the flexor digitorum longus and the flexor hallucis longus, and functions with them at these joints. These three muscles are often referred to as the **Tom, Dick, and Harry** muscles: **Tom** for tibialis posterior, **Dick** for flexor digitorum longus, and **Harry** for flexor hallucis longus.

INTRINSIC MUSCLES

The instrinsics of the foot lie in one dorsal layer and four plantar layers. The muscles of the plantar aspect are covered by a strong layer of fibrous tissue called the plantar fascia or plantar aponeurosis. It attaches to the medial tubercle of the calcaneus and spreads toward the heads of the metatarsals where it divides into five slips and attaches to the skin and the tendons of the flexor muscles. It supports the foot during all forms of weight-bearing and, with the ligaments of the foot, is a primary contributor to its arched contour.

The First Plantar Layer

Flexor Digitorum Brevis (flex'or digito'rum bre'vis)

The flexor digitorum brevis (Fig. 9.18) lies immediately beneath the central portion of the plantar aponeurosis. It cannot be palpated.

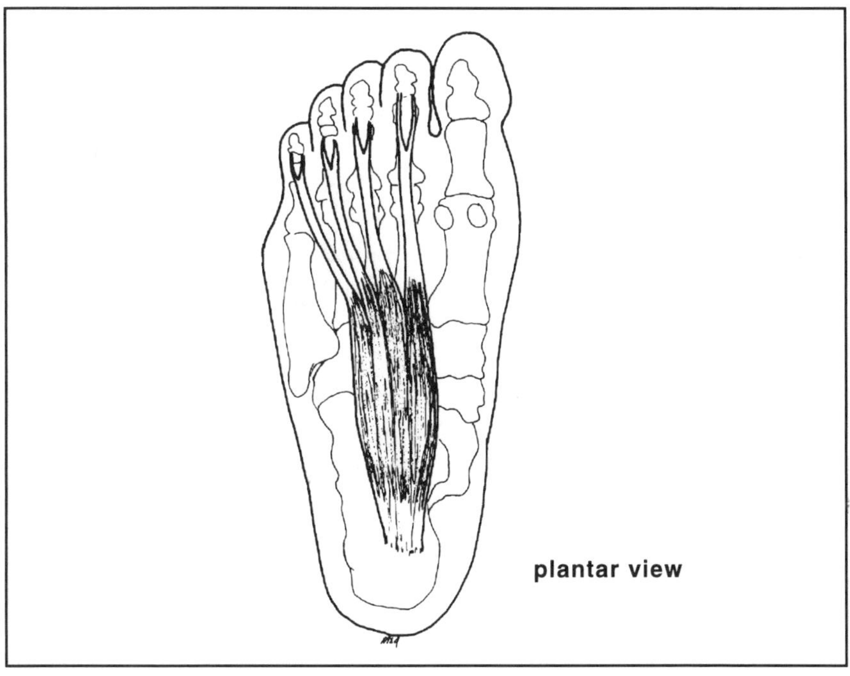

Flexor Digitorum Brevis

Fig. 9.18

Origin — Tuberosity of the calcaneus and the central part of the plantar aponeurosis.
Insertion — By four tendons which divide distally to insert on the sides of the middle phalanges of the four lesser toes.
Innervation — Medial plantar nerve.
Action — Flexion of the proximal interphalangeal joints and metatarsophalangeal joints of four lesser toes.

Abductor Hallucis (abduc'tor hal'lucis)

The muscle is located to the medial side of the flexor digitorum brevis (Fig. 9.19). It cannot be palpated.

Abductor Hallucis

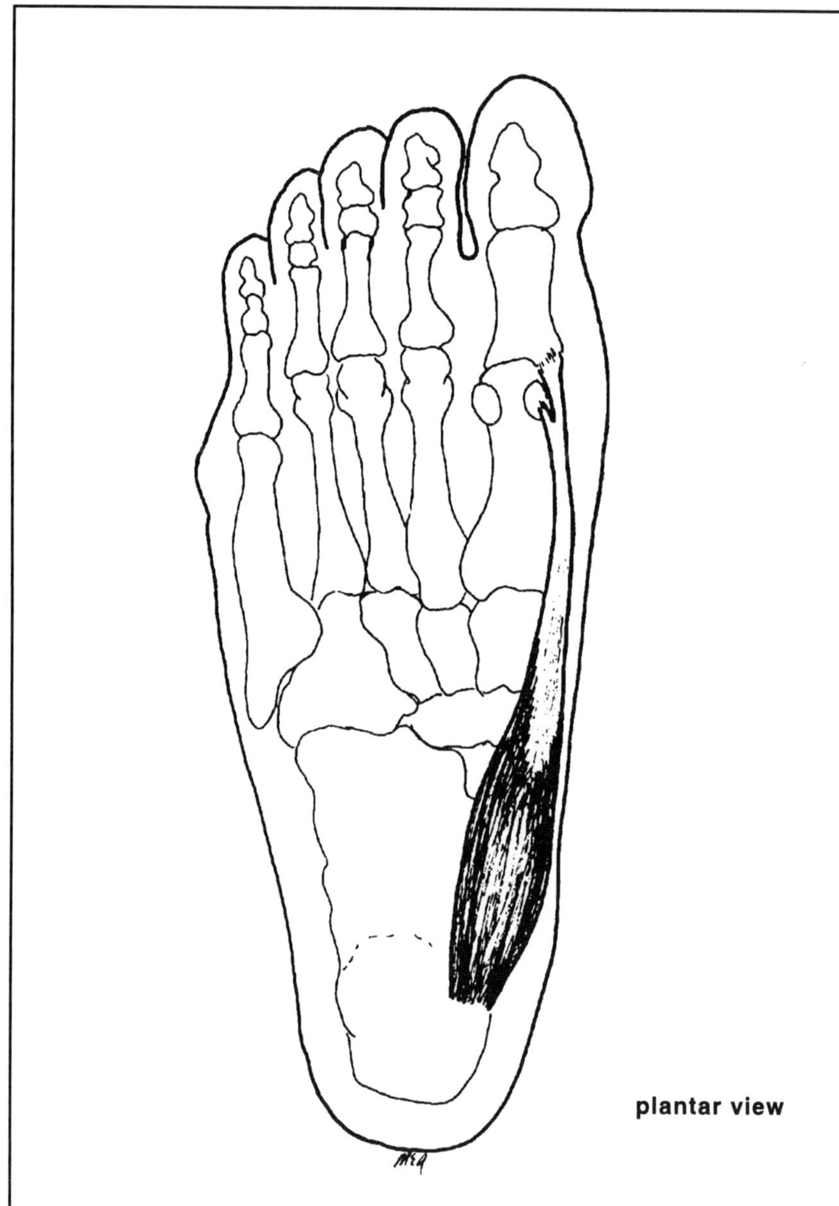

Fig. 9.19

Origin	Tuberosity of the calcaneus, the flexor retinaculum, and the plantar aponeurosis.
Insertion	Tibial side of the base of the proximal phalanx of the great toe.
Innervation	Medial plantar nerve.
Action	Abduction of the metatarsophalangeal joint of the great toe.

Abductor Digiti Minimi (abduc'tor dig'iti min'imi)

The abductor digiti minimi (Fig. 9.20) is located along the lateral side of the foot beneath the plantar aponeurosis. It cannot be palpated.

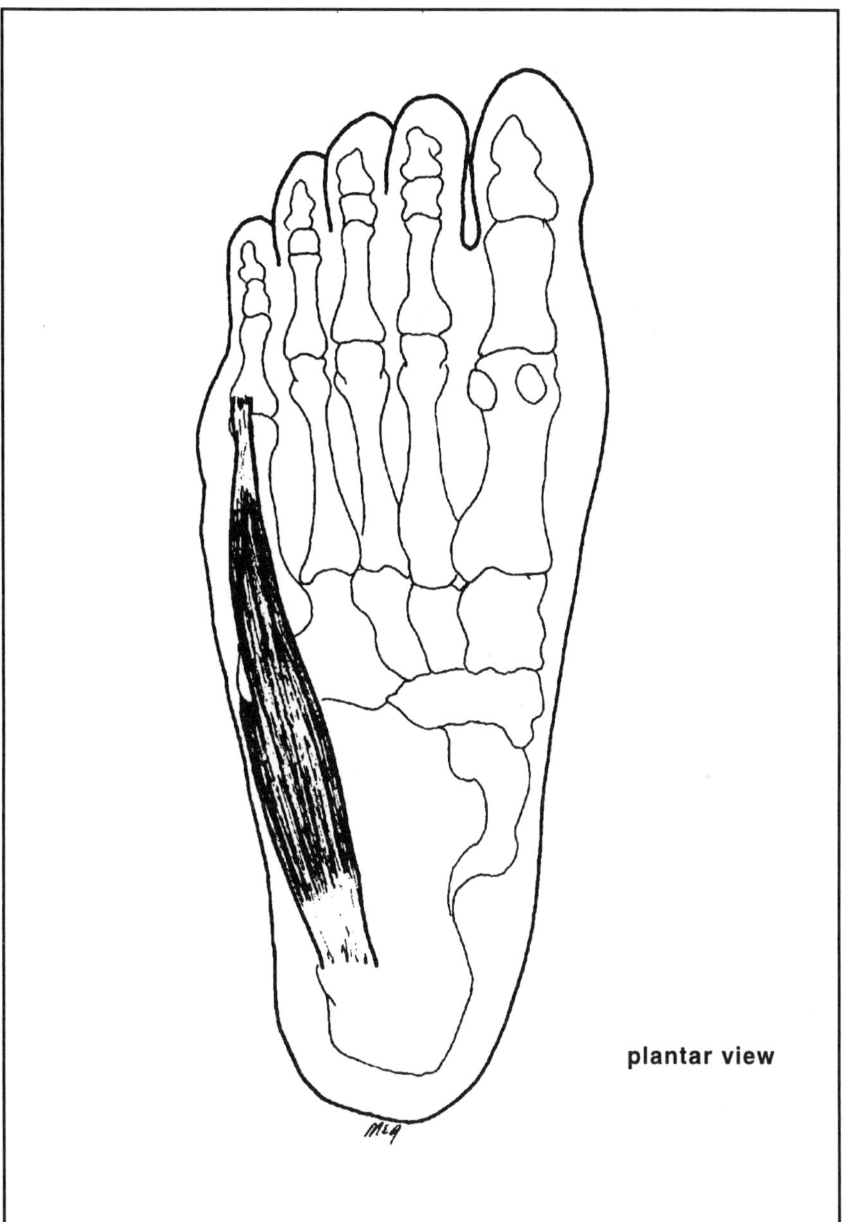

Abductor Digiti Minimi

Fig. 9.20

Origin —— Tuberosity and plantar surface of the calcaneus and plantar aponeurosis.
Insertion —— Fibular side of the base of the first phalanx of the little toe.
Innervation — Lateral plantar nerve.
Action —— Abduction of the metatarsophalangeal joint of the little toe.

The Second Plantar Layer

Quadratus Plantae (quadra'tus plan'tae)

The quadratus plantae (Fig. 9.21) is beneath the muscles of the first layer but is separated from them by a plantar nerve and blood vessels.

Quadratus Plantae

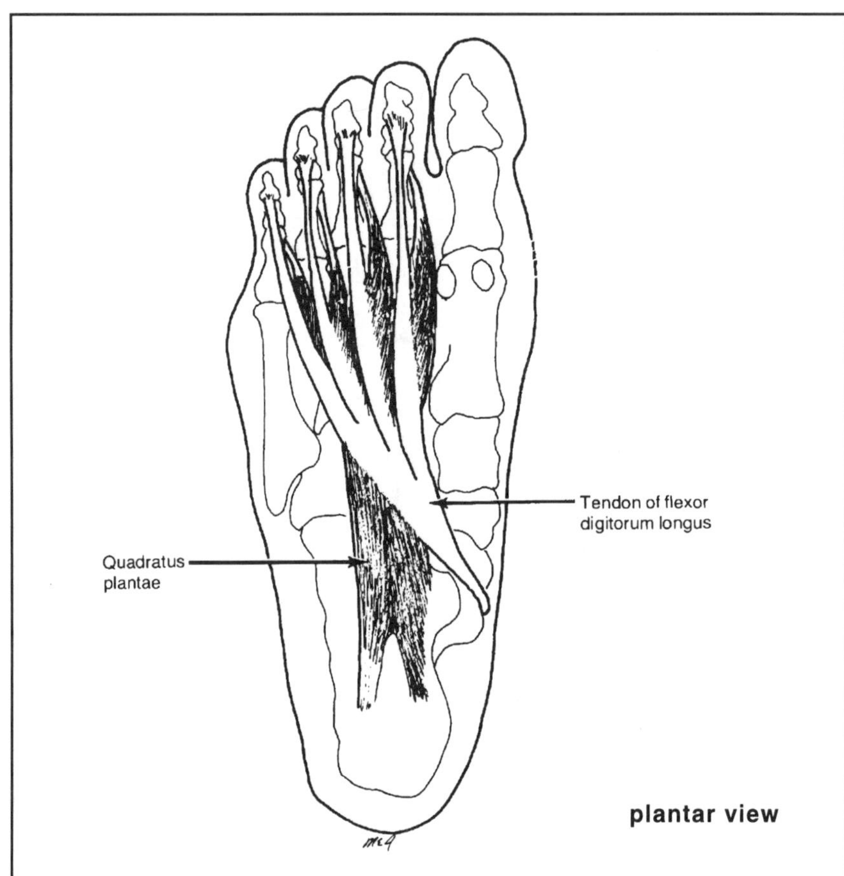

Fig. 9.21

Origin	By two heads, from the tibial and fibular surfaces of the calcaneus.
Insertion	Tendon of the flexor digitorum longus just before it divides.
Innervation	Lateral plantar nerve.
Action	Through the tendon of the flexor digitorum longus, flexion of the distal interphalangeal joints of the four lesser toes.

Lumbricales (lumbrica'les)

The lumbricales (Fig. 9.22) are four small muscles located in conjunction with the tendons of the flexor digitorum longus. They are numbered from the tibial side of the foot.

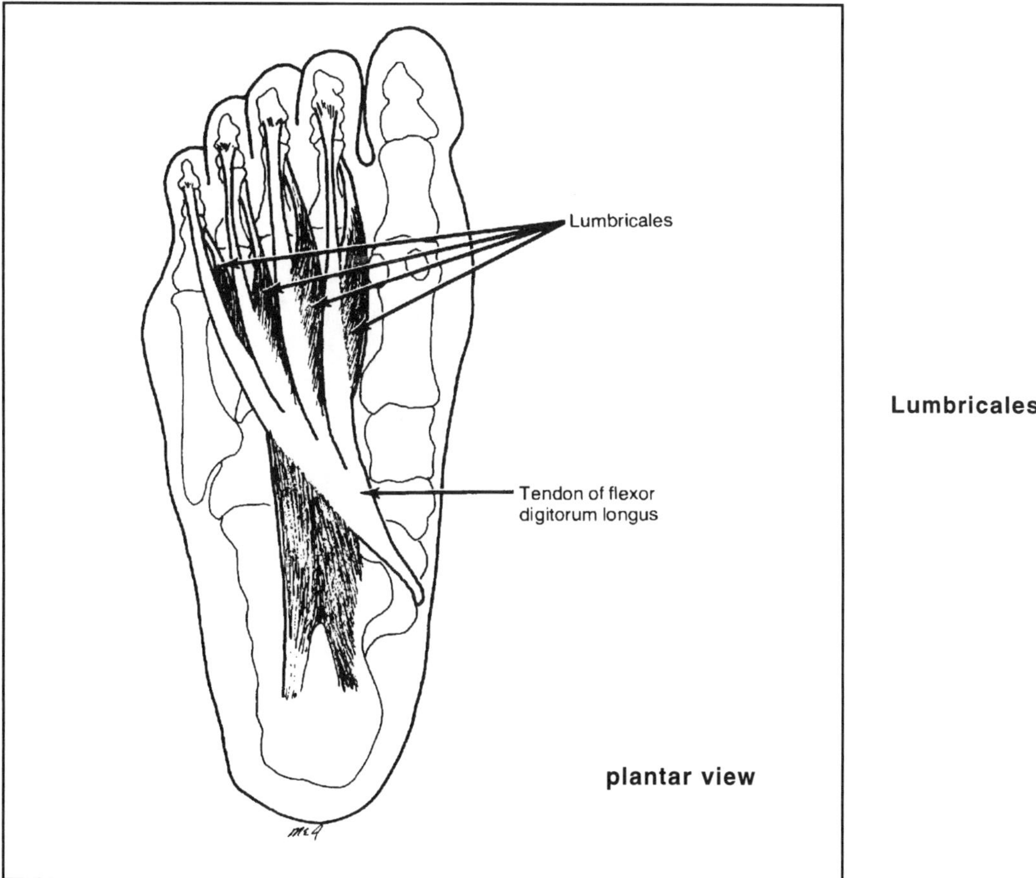

Fig. 9.22

Lumbricales

Origin —	Tendons of the flexor digitorum longus.
Insertion —	After passing to the tibial side of the four lesser toes, the muscles insert on the tendons of the extensor digitorum longus.
Innervation —	Medial and lateral plantar nerves.
Action —	Through the tendons on which the muscles originate and insert, they flex the metatarsophalangeal joints of the four lesser toes and extend the interphalangeal joints of these toes.

The Third Plantar Layer

Flexor Hallucis Brevis (flex'or hal'lucis bre'vis)

The flexor hallucis brevis (Fig. 9.23) is sometimes described as the first plantar interosseus. It is analogous to the flexor pollicis brevis in that respect.

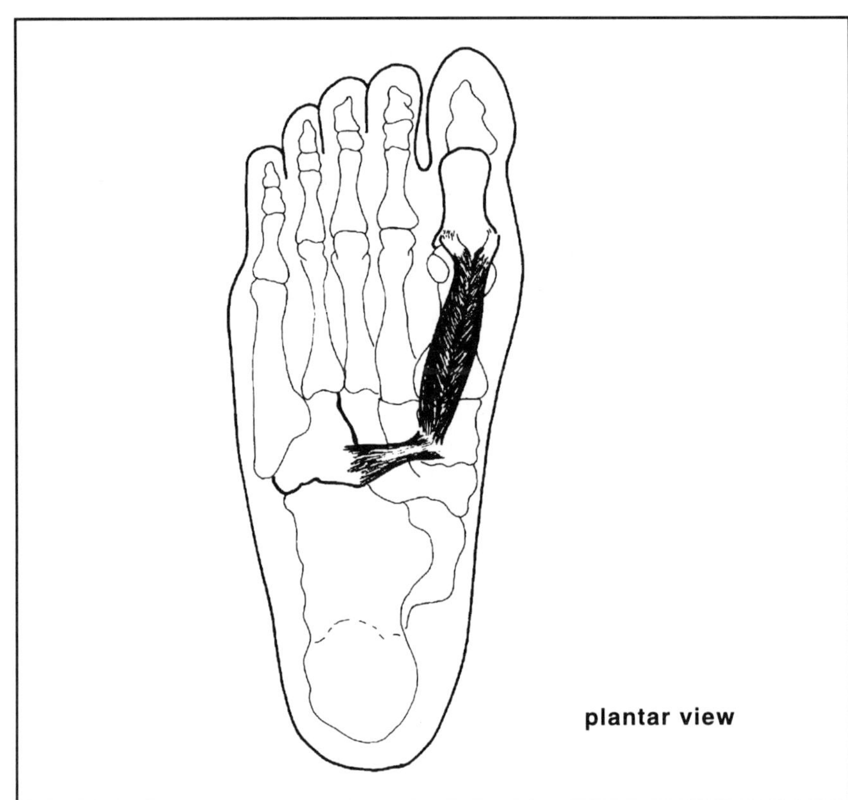

Fig. 9.23

Origin —— Cuboid and third cuneiform bones.
Insertion —— By two heads, to the sides of the base of the proximal phalanx of the great toe.
Innervation — Medial plantar nerve.
Action —— Flexion of the metatarsophalangeal joint of the great toe.

Adductor Hallucis (adduc'tor hal'lucis)

The adductor hallucis (Fig. 9.24) is characterized by two widely separated heads. Except for its common tendon of attachment, it would appear to be two muscles.

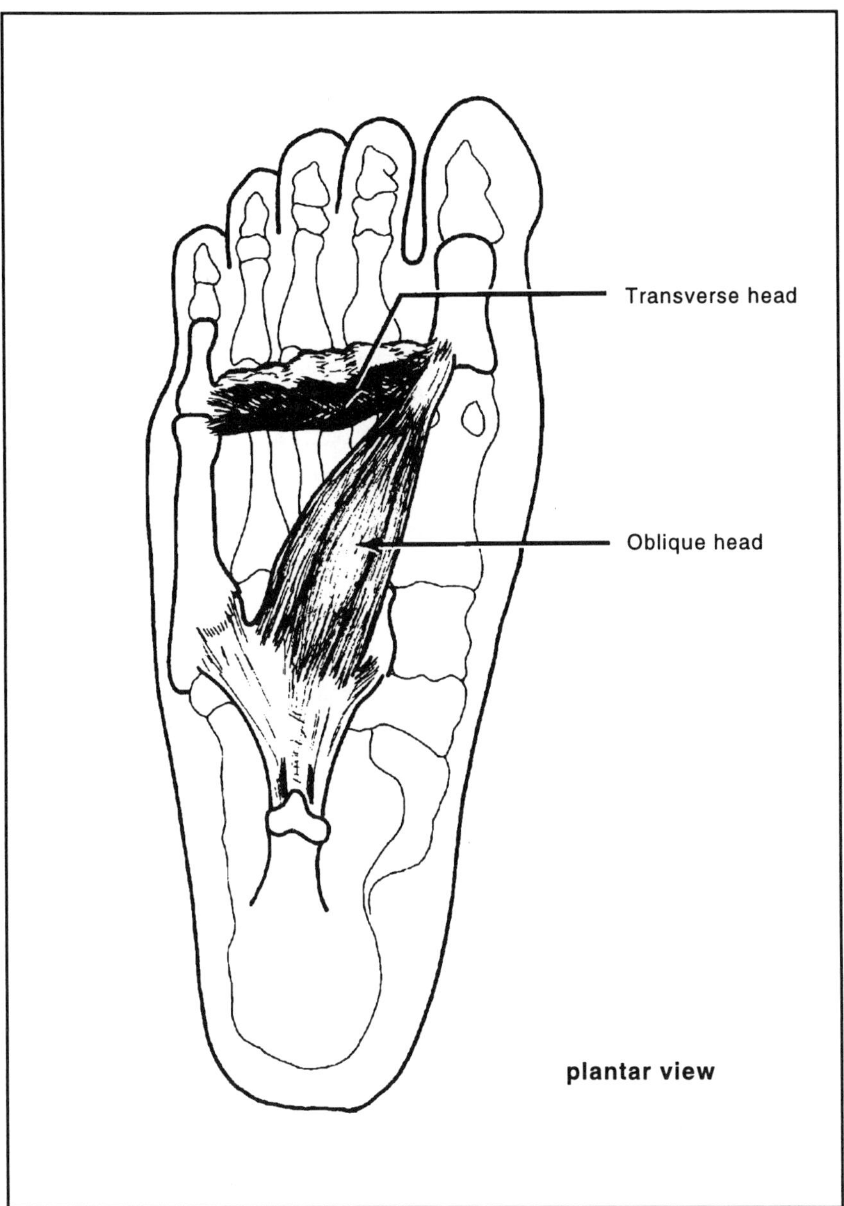

Fig. 9.24

Adductor Hallucis

Origin —— Oblique head: Base of second through fourth metatarsals. Transverse head: Metatarsophalangeal ligaments of the third through fifth toes.
Insertion —— Fibular side of the base of the proximal phalanx of the great toe.
Innervation – Lateral plantar nerve.
Action —— Adduction of the metatarsophalangeal joint of the great toe.

Flexor Digiti Minimi Brevis (flex'or dig'iti min'imi bre'vis)

The flexor digiti minimi brevis (Fig. 9.25) lies along the metatarsal of the little toe. It resembles an interosseus muscle.

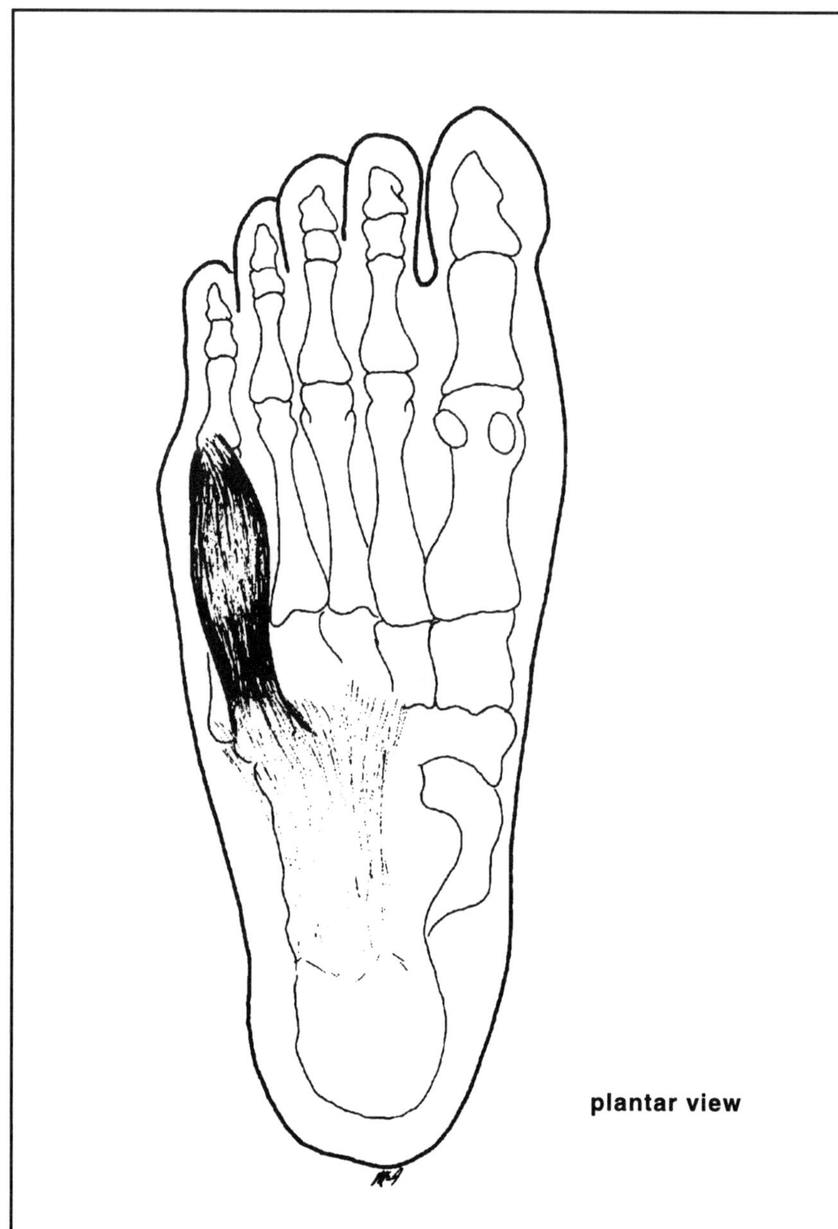

Fig. 9.25

Origin —— Base of the fifth metatarsal.
Insertion —— Lateral side of the base of the first phalanx of the little toe.
Innervation – Lateral plantar nerve.
Action —— Flexion of the metatarsophalangeal joint of the little toe.

The Fourth Plantar Layer

The Dorsal Interossei (dor'sal interos'sei)

The dorsal interossei (Fig. 9.26) are four small muscles occupying the spaces between the metatarsals. They are numbered from the tibial side of the foot.

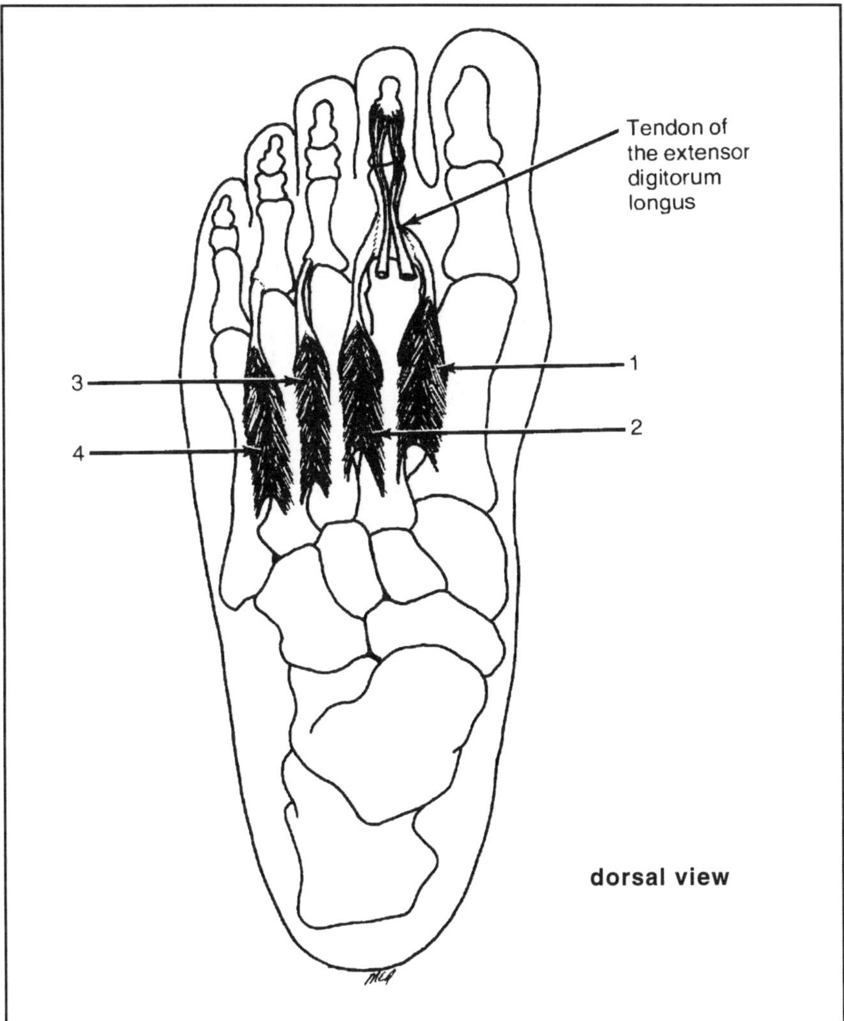

Fig. 9.26

Dorsal Interossei

Origin — Each muscle originates by two heads from the sides of adjacent metatarsals.

Insertion — Bases of proximal phalanges of the four lesser toes, and the tendons of the extensor digitorum longus as shown in Fig. 9.26.

Innervation — Lateral plantar nerve.

Action — Abduction of third and fourth metatarsophalangeal joints, and tibial and fibular deviation of that joint of the second toe; flexion of the metatarsophalangeal joints and extension of the interphalangeal joints of the second, third, and fourth toes.

Plantar Interossei (plan'tar interos'sei)

The plantar interossei (Fig. 9.27) are three small muscles which lie beneath the third, fourth, and fifth metatarsals. They are numbered from the tibial side of the foot.

Plantar Interossei

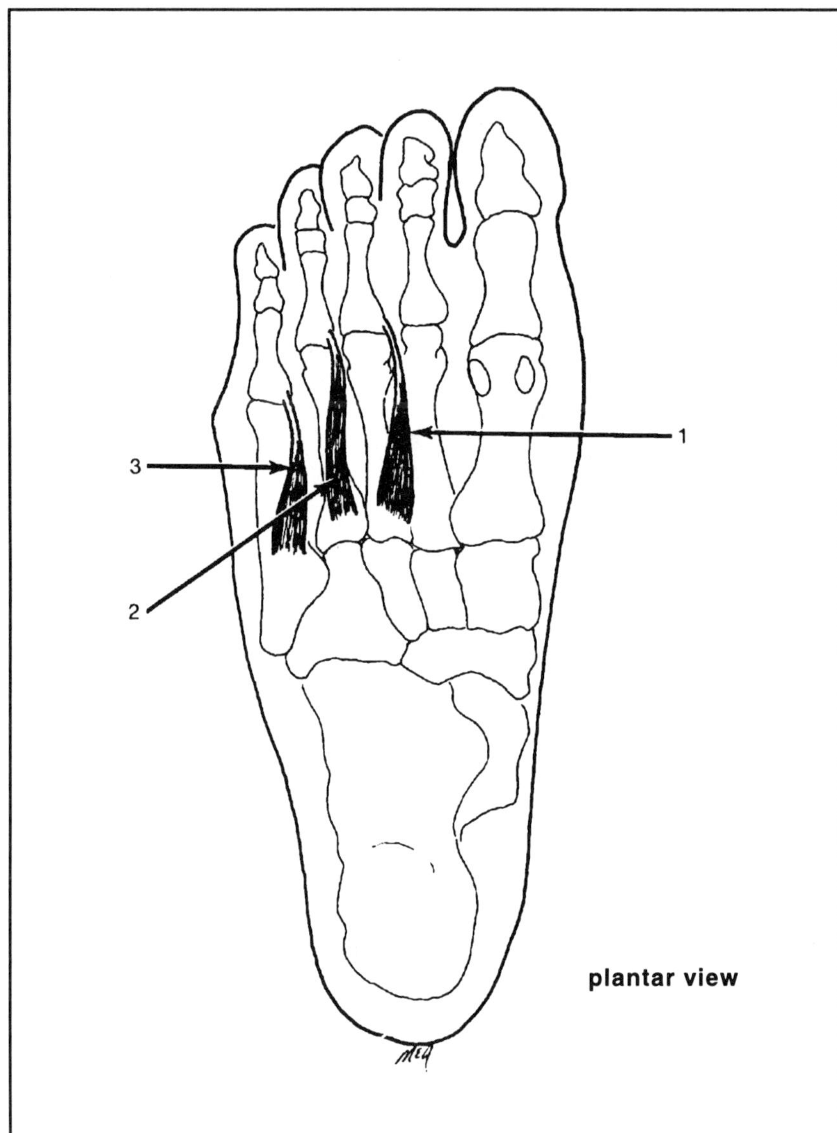

Fig. 9.27

Origin ——	Tibial side of the third through fifth metatarsals.
Insertion ——	Tibial sides of the bases of the first phalanges of the third through fifth toes.
Innervation —	Lateral plantar nerve.
Action ——	Adduction of the metatarsophalangeal joints of the third, fourth, and fifth toes; flexion of the metatarsophalangeal joints and extension of the interphalangeal joints of those toes.

The Dorsal Layer

Extensor Digitorum Brevis (exten'sor digito'rum bre'vis)

The extensor digitorum brevis (Fig. 9.28) is the only intrinsic muscle on the dorsum of the foot. It is superficial in some of its parts but is difficult to palpate because it is easily confused with the long extensor.

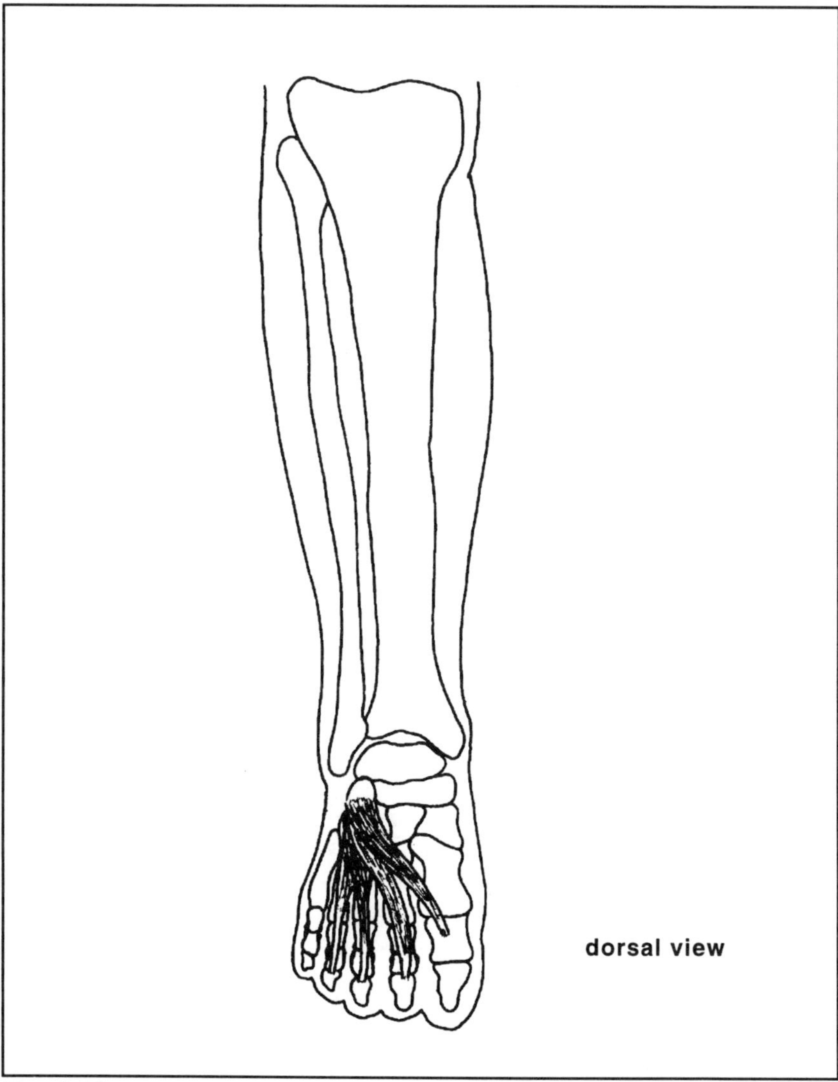

Fig. 9.28

Extensor Digitorum Brevis

Origin — Lateral surface of the distal portion of the calcaneus.
Insertion — By four tendons, to the base of the proximal phalanx of the great toe, and the tendons of the extensor digitorum longus of the second, third, and fourth toes.
Innervation — Deep peroneal nerve.
Action — Extension of the metatarsophalangeal joints of the first through the fourth toes.

COMMENTS

So little research has been completed which relates to the ankle and foot that it is difficult, or impossible, to state any generalizations; however, a few isolated examples may suffice as "takeoff" points on which relevant movement concepts can be built. One such example concerns the frequent alternation between footwear with low heels (or no footwear at all) and footwear comprising the popular two- or three-inch heel. While wearing the low-heel shoes, or no shoes, the foot enjoys maximum contact with the floor, and the weight of the body is spread over its total surface. Shoes with higher heels cause the body weight to be localized over the metatarsophalangeal joints, and especially over the second of these joints since the second metatarsal is the longest of the five. There is frequent soreness in the ball of the foot below the head of that metatarsal because of underlying bruised tissue.

A difficulty of the same origin often befalls those individuals who habitually wear shoes with high heels, and suddenly note, with alarm, that they cannot place their heels on the floor. The triceps surae and other plantar flexors have shortened in response to the carriage demanded by the shoes.

Sprains of the ankle joint are quite common and usually occur from forceful inversions of the ankle. Study of the ligamentous structure will indicate, however, that the ankle is better protected from this type of sprain than from eversion sprains because there are more lateral than medial ligaments. It must follow that the foot is more prone to accidental inversion than eversion -- a conclusion that will be verified when the weight-bearing surface of the foot is examined. Since the weight of the body is spread along the lateral margin of the foot, only a slight miscue in stepping can result in weight placement to the outside of the foot -- the inversion sprain. A gross misplacement is required, however, for the weight line to exceed the foot's medial margin and cause an eversion sprain. Unfortunately, the added ligamentous protection against inversion sprains can be somewhat obscured by inappropriate choice of shoes. A generalization is offered -- if one looks down upon the top of the shoe while the foot is bearing weight, the sole should be seen projecting along the entire circumference of the forepart of the shoe. Otherwise, the foot can too easily roll laterally over the sole and sprain may result.

A quiz for this material can be found in the back of this book on page 297.

LABORATORY EXPERIENCES

1. Examine the ankle mechanism on a human skeleton and note that one of the malleoli is longer than the other. Keeping this in mind, visualize the ankle joint in an inversion sprain and in an eversion sprain. In which of the two sprains will the tarsal bones of the foot be made to contact a malleolus? Which of the two sprains is seen more commonly? Do you agree that most inversion accidents result in sprains while most eversion accidents result in fractures to the fibula?

2. Draw an outline of your foot on a piece of paper. Make a mark on the outline directly below each malleolus, and below the joint space between the navicular and first cuneiform bones. Finally, make a mark slightly lateral to the line of insertion of the gastrocnemius. Join the two malleoli marks with a straight line, and then join the remaining two marks with a straight line. The result should be a large *X* on the diagram which represents the two axes of the ankle joint. Label each quadrant-like area according to the movement of the ankle which will occur if a muscle in that quadrant contracts. For example, the medial-anterior quadrant should be labeled dorsiflexion and inversion.

3. Palpate the tendons of the extrinsic muscles of the foot as they cross the ankle joint and locate them as precisely as possible on the diagram completed in Experience #2. Does your drawing show agreement with the actions stated in this chapter for the muscles concerned? Can you determine, from your drawing, whether the muscles will be relatively weak or strong movers according to their relationships to the two axes?

4. Examine the metatarsals of a human skeleton. Which metatarsal is longest? Now, rise on your toes and note that the area of the ball of the foot which supports the greatest weight is under the first and second metatarsals. Further examination of the skeleton will indicate that the first metatarsal is considerably larger than the second; the force of the body weight transmitted through the first metatarsal is thus spread over a larger area than is the case with the second metatarsal. Can you now determine why the ball of the foot under the second metatarsal often becomes sore and tender after wearing shoes with elevated heels? or after running or dancing with bare feet?

MUSCLES OF RESPIRATION

10

The thorax as a unit, comprises the sternum, the costal cartilages, the ribs, and the thoracic vertebrae (Fig. 10.1). The sternum consists of three portions -- manubrium, body, and xiphoid process -- which are joined by fibrocartilage and fibrous tissue. The manubrium supports the two clavicles through synovial joints of a modified ball-and-socket nature (see Chapter 2) and articulates with the first rib by means of an immovable cartilaginous joint. The body of the sternum articulates with the costal cartilages of the second through the seventh ribs; these joints are synovial and nonaxial. The xiphoid process is the smallest of the three portions and is a thin, long cartilage which gradually ossifies with age.

The Thorax

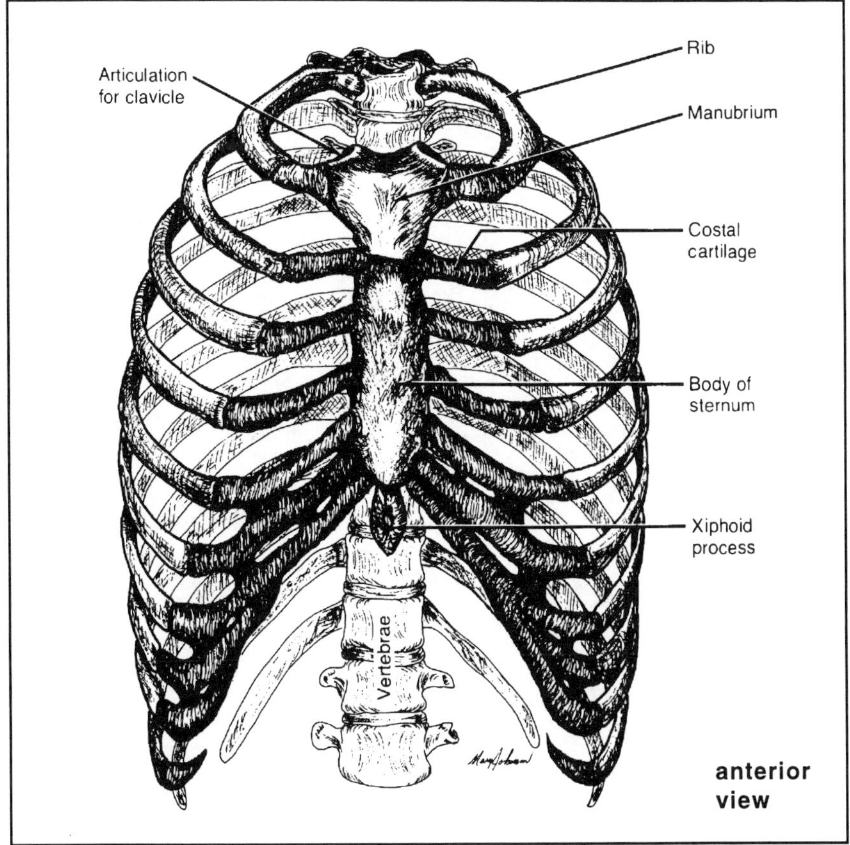

Fig. 10.1

The ribs are pliable bony arches which form the major part of the thorax. The first seven are designated **true ribs** because they articulate, through their costal cartilages, with the sternum. The lower five ribs are called **false ribs** and of these, the last two, being free at their anterior ends, are termed the **floating ribs**. The ribs have in common the characteristics of vertebral and sternal extremities, and a body. The vertebral extremity presents a tubercle which articulates with the transverse process of its thoracic vertebra, a head which articulates with the bodies of two adjacent vertebrae, and a flattened portion lateral to the head called **the neck**. Both articulations of the vertebral extremity are synovial and of the gliding type. The sternal extremity presents a shallow concavity into which the costal cartilage is inserted. The body of the rib is the bony expanse between the two extremities and is characterized by the internal and external surfaces, superior and inferior borders, and a point of sharpest curvature called the angle.

Movements of the thorax are mainly those of the ribs and are described as **elevation** and **depression**. These movements occur in conjunction with the breathing movements of inspiration and expiration. During inspiration, the ribs are elevated to enlarge the size of the thorax. During expiration, if breathing is at resting levels, the muscles relax and gravity depresses the ribs. No muscular contraction is required unless the expiration is forced. In this event, activity of the abdominals and rib depressors is required.

MUSCLES OF THE THORAX

The muscles acting on the thorax during resting respiration are:

Diaphragm	External intercostals	Internal intercostals

Additional recruitment of the following muscles is necessary during forced inspiration:

Sternocleidomastoid	Pectoralis minor	Levators costarum
Trapezius Part 1	Scaleni	Levator scapulae
Serratus posterior superior	Rhomboids	

These muscles combine actions to elevate the clavicle, scapula, and ribs in order to further increase the size of the thorax beyond that required by resting respiration. All of these muscles, with the exception of the serratus posterior superior, are discussed fully in chapters devoted to the shoulder joint or the spine and will not be duplicated in this chapter.

Muscles recruited to action during forced expiration are:

Internal intercostals	Serratus posterior inferior	Transversus abdominis
Transversus thoracis	Rectus abdominis	External oblique
Internal oblique	Quadratus lumborum	

These muscles join in depressing the rib cage beyond that which is possible because of the passive depression accomplished by gravity, and the elasticity of the relaxed muscles of inspiration. Only the internal intercostals, serratus posterior inferior, transverus abdominis, and transversus thoracis will be discussed in this section since the others have been covered fully under muscles of the spine.

The Diaphragm (di'aphragm)

The diaphragm (Fig. 10.2) is the dividing muscle between the thoracic and abdominal cavities. It is tendinous along its dome and muscular along its sides. It cannot be palpated.

Diaphragm

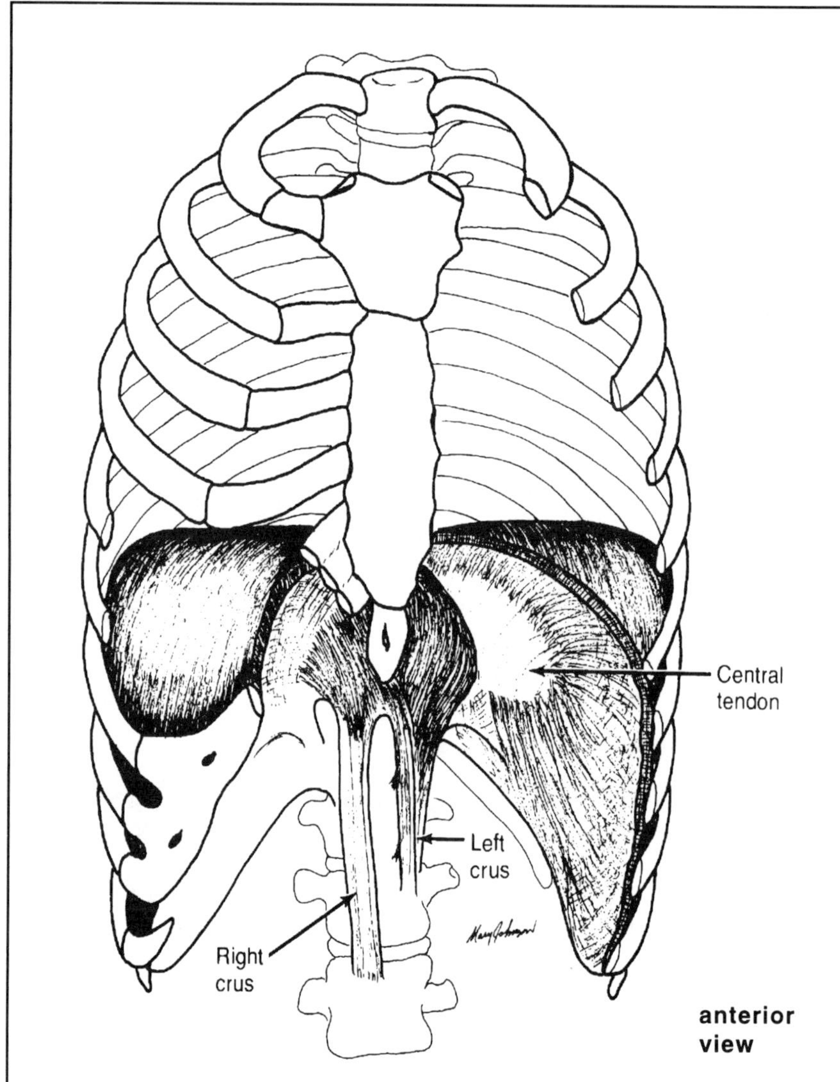

Fig. 10.2

Origin — Like a circular rim, from the upper two lumbar vertebrae, the lumbar fascia, the inner portions of the last six ribs around to the inner surface of the xiphoid process of the sternum.

Insertion — The central tendon which forms the dome of the muscle.

Innervation — Phrenic nerve.

Action — Depression of the central tendon which in turn increases the diameter of the thorax.

External Intercostals (exter'nal intercos'tals)

The external intercostals are eleven thin sheets of fibers located between the ribs (Fig. 10.3). They can be palpated on lean individuals anterior to the serratus anterior.

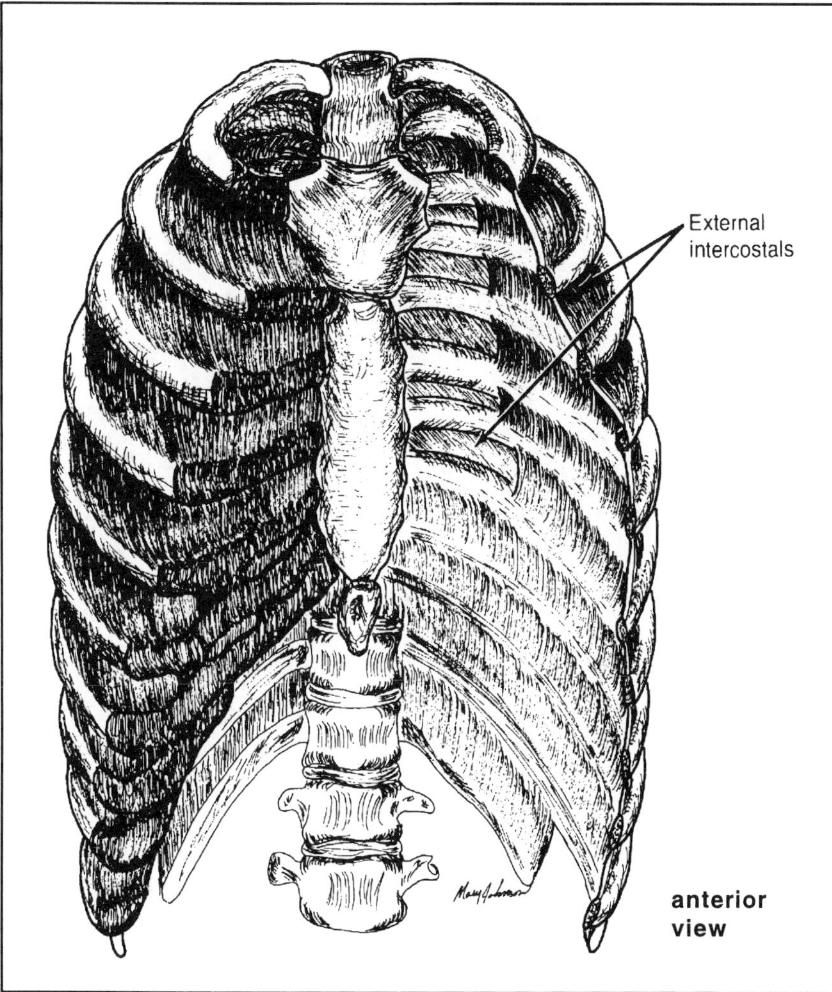

External Intercostals

Fig. 10.3

Origin —— Inferior border of the ribs.
Insertion —— Superior border of the rib below that of the rib of origin.
Innervation — Intercostal nerves.
Action —— Elevation of the ribs thereby increasing the size of the thorax.

Internal Intercostals (inter'nal intercos'tals)

The internal intercostals (Fig. 10.4) are eleven sheets of muscular fibers located just beneath the external intercostals. The direction of their fibers is at right angles to that of their external counterparts. They cannot be palpated.

Internal Intercostals

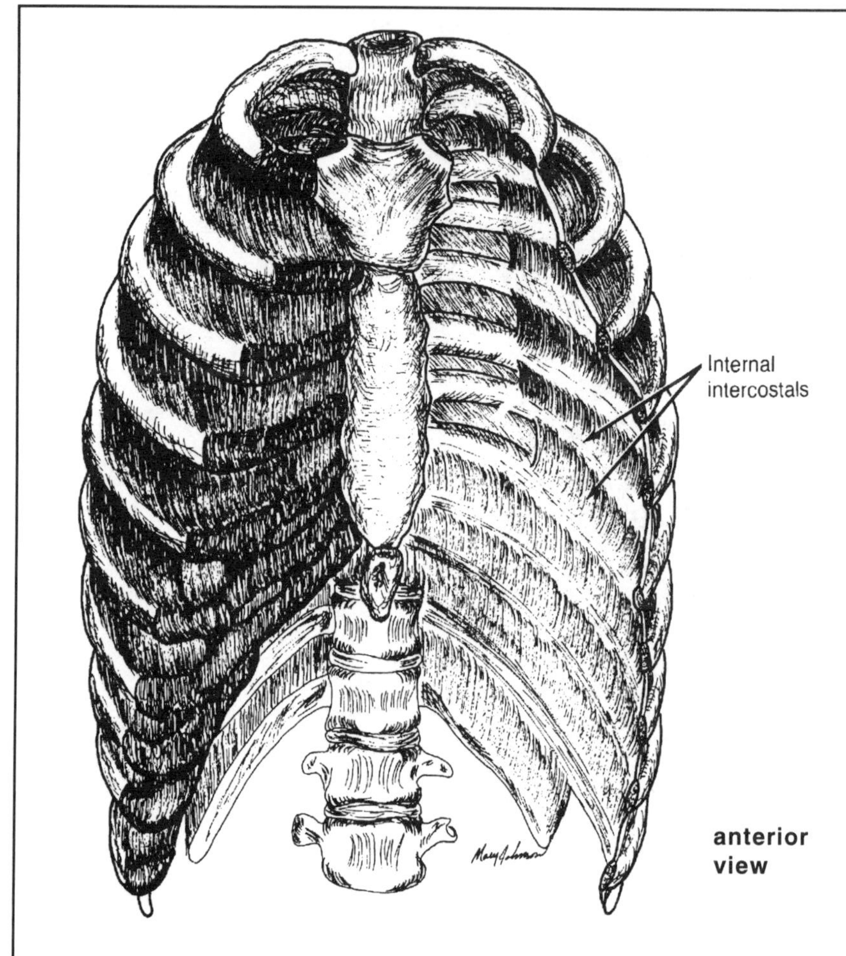

Fig. 10.4

Origin —	Inner surface of a rib or its costal cartilage.
Insertion —	Superior surface of the rib below that of the origin.
Innervation —	Intercostal nerves.
Action —	Slight contraction during resting respiration; depression of the ribs during forced expiration in order to decrease the size of the thorax.

Serratus Posterior Superior (serra'tus poste'rior supe'rior)

This muscle is comprised of a flat sheet of muscle fiber located beneath the scapula (Fig. 10.5). It cannot be palpated.

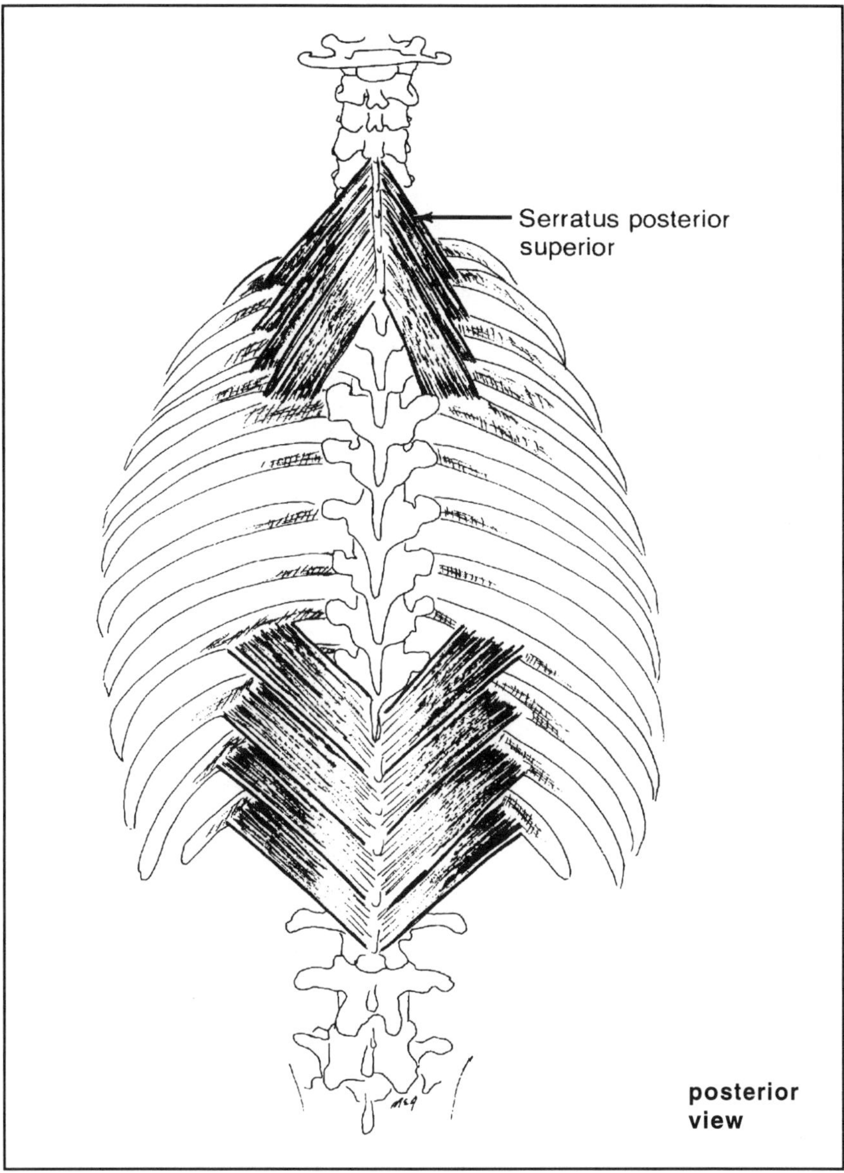

Fig. 10.5

The Serratus Posterior Superior

Origin	Posterior portion of the ligamentum nuchae; spinous processes of the last cervical and first two or three thoracic vertebrae.
Insertion	Superior borders of the second through the fifth ribs in the vicinity of their angles.
Innervation	First four thoracic nerves.
Action	Elevation of the ribs on which the muscle is inserted, increasing the size of the thorax.

Serratus Posterior Inferior (serra'tus poste'rior infe'rior)

The serratus posterior inferior (Fig. 10.6) is located in the middle of the back. It is a second-layer muscle, lying beneath the trapezius and latissimus dorsi, and cannot be palpated.

The Serratus Posterior Inferior

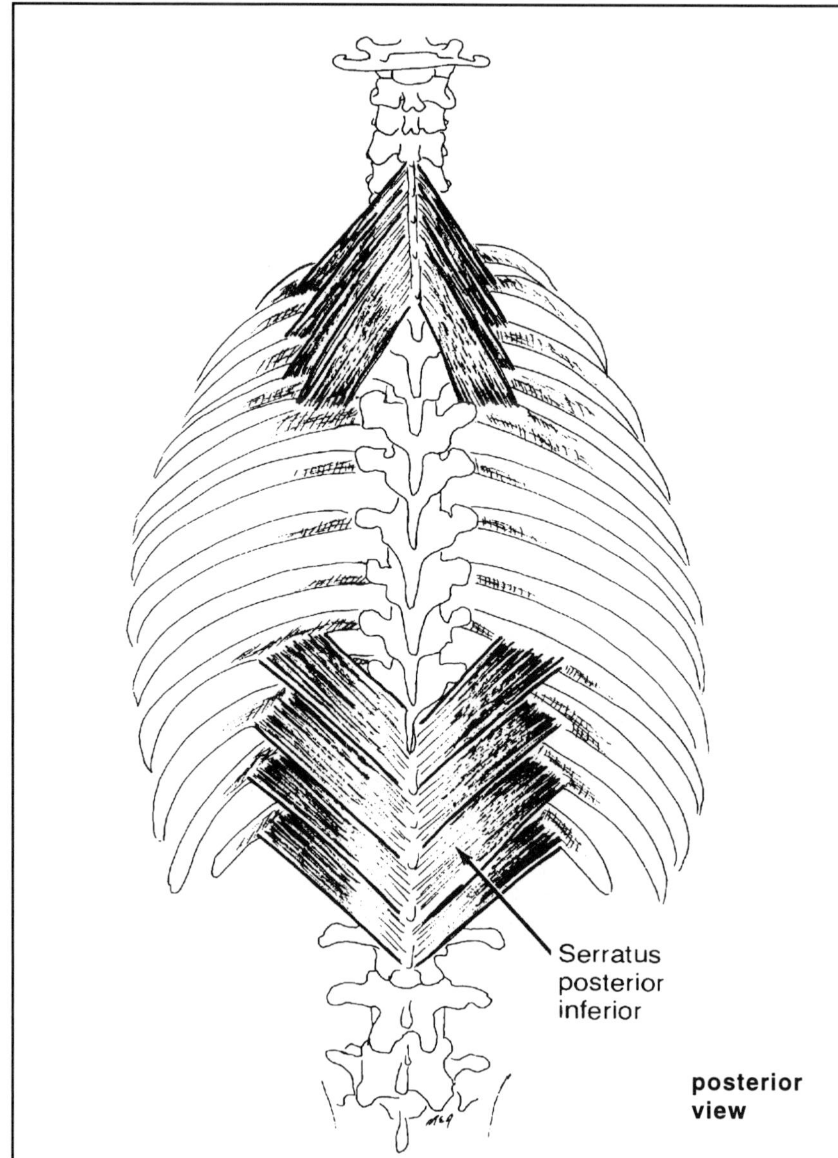

Fig. 10.6

Origin	Spinous processes of last two thoracic and first two or three lumbar vertebrae.
Insertion	Inferior borders of lower four ribs in the vicinity of their angles.
Innervation	Ninth to twelfth thoracic nerves.
Action	Depression of the ribs on which the muscle inserts, acting mainly to neutralize the inward pull of the diaphragm.

Transversus Abdominis (transver'sus abdom'inis)

The transversus abdominis (Fig. 10.7) is the deepest of the abdominal muscles. It cannot be palpated.

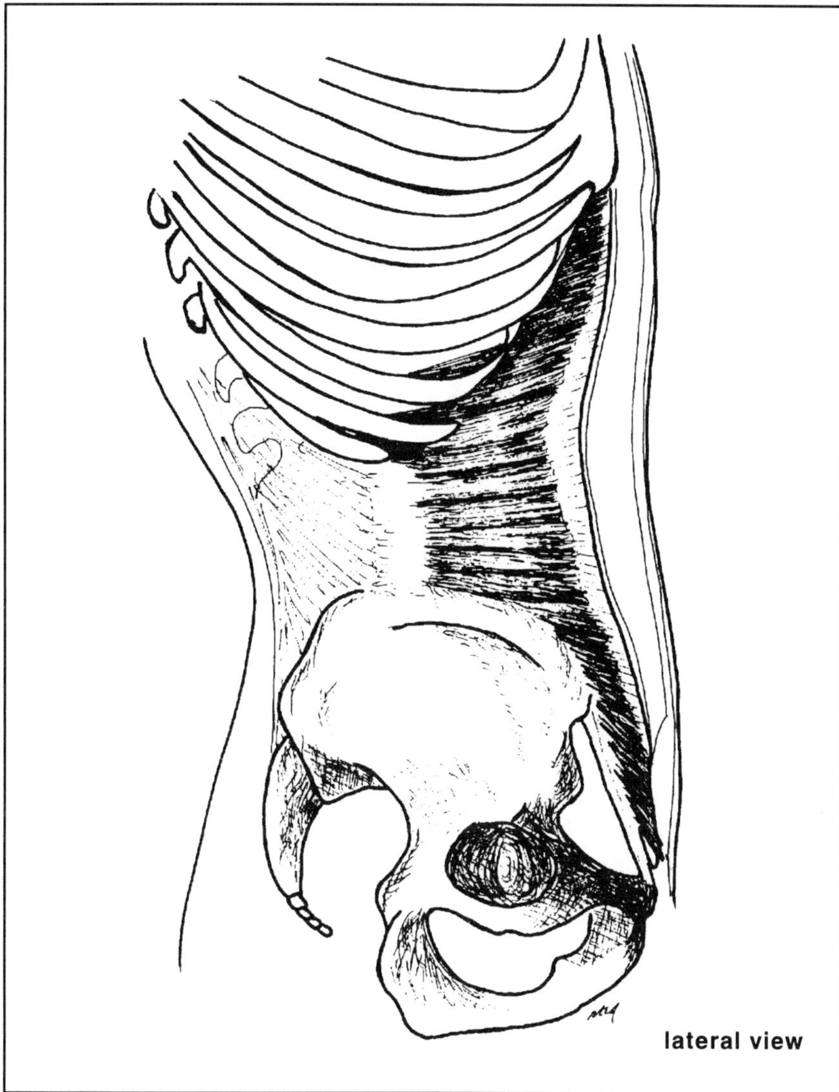

Transversus Abdominis

Fig. 10.7

Origin —	Lateral portion of the inguinal ligament; inner portion of the iliac crest; thoracolumbar fascia; inner surfaces of last six ribs.
Insertion —	Linea alba.
Innervation —	Seventh to twelfth intercostal nerves; iliohypogastric and ilioinguinal nerves.
Action —	Compresses the abdomen during forced expiration.

Transversus Thoracis (transver'sus thora'cis)

The transversus thoracis is a thin sheet of muscle and tendon located on the inner surface of the anterior wall of the thorax. It cannot be palpated.

Origin —— Posterior third of inner surface of the sternal body and xiphoid process; costal cartilages of last three or four true ribs.
Insertion —— Costal cartilages of second through sixth ribs.
Innervation – Intercostal nerve.
Action —— Depresses the anterior portions of the ribs on which the muscle inserts, decreasing the size of the thorax.

COMMENTS

Respiration, when the body is at rest, involves low muscular activity. During exercise, however, the rib cage must be expanded to greater dimensions, and activity of the involved musculature increases surprisingly. The individual exercising, requires increased circumference of the thorax to accommodate the air-filled lungs, exhibits activity in the muscles which are associated with forced inspiration. The expiration phase of thorax movement is, largely, a passive one, therefore the muscles of forced expiration are not recruited. Any muscle which is continuously active tends to hypertrophy. So it is with the muscles of inspiration, and since these muscles are located primarily in the region of the neck, they give rise to the thickness so frequently noted there.

A quiz for this material can be found in the back of this book on page 299.

LABORATORY EXPERIENCES

1. Palpate the sternocleidomastoid during forced inspiration. What degree of involvement in respiration do they have?

2. Determine, through palpation or electromyography the involvement of the superficial abdominal muscles during resting and forced expiration. What sports might entail the recruitment of the superficial abdominals to affect efficient respiration?

BIBLIOGRAPHY

A

Adrian, M. J., and Cooper, J. M. *The Biomechanics of Human Movement.* Indianapolis: Benchmark Press, Inc., 1989.

Adrian, M. J., Cooper, J. M., and Glassow, R. B. *Kinesiology.* 5th ed. St. Louis: C. V. Mosby Company, 1982.

American Academy of Orthopaedic Surgeons. *Athletic Training and Sports Medicine.* 2nd ed. Park Ridge, IL: American Academy of Orthopaedic Surgeons, 1991.

American Physical Therapy Association. "Focus on the lower back." *Physical Therapy* 59 (1979):965-1076.

American Society for Surgery of the Hand. *The Hand: Examination and Diagnosis.* 3rd ed. New York: Churchill Livingstone, 1990.

American Society for Surgery of the Hand. *The Hand: Primary Care of Common Problems.* 2nd ed. New York: Churchill Livingstone, 1990.

Arnheim, D. D., and Schlaich, J. *Dance Injuries: Their Prevention and Care.* 3rd ed. Princeton, NJ: Princeton Book Co., 1991.

Ariyan, S. *The Hand Book,* 2nd ed. Baltimore: The Williams & Wilkins Company, 1983.

Asmussen, E. "Movement and man and study of man in motion: A scanning review of the development of biomechanics." In *Biomechanics V-A,* ed. P.V. Komi. Baltimore: University Park Press, 1976.

B

Barham, J. N. *Mechanical Kinesiology.* St. Louis: C. V. Mosby Company, 1978.

Barham, J. N., and Wooten, E. P. *Structural Kinesiology.* New York: Macmillan Company, 1973.

Basmajian, J. V. *Muscles Alive.* 5th ed. Baltimore: The Williams & Wilkins Company, 1985.

Basmajian, J. V., and S. L. Wolf, eds. *Therapeutic Exercise.* 5th ed. Baltimore: The Williams & Wilkins Company, 1990.

Bareman, J. E., and Trott, A. W. *The Foot and Ankle.* New York: Thieme-Stratton, Inc., 1980.

Bechtol, C. O. "Biomechanics of the shoulder." *Clinical Orthopaedics,* 146:37-41.

Borenstein, D. G., and Wiesel, S. W. *Low Back Pain.* Philadelphia: W. B. Saunders Co., 1989.

Bowling, R. W., Rochar Jr., P. A., and Erhard, R. "Examination of the shoulder complex." *Physical Therapy* 66 (1986):1866-1877.

Brand, P. W., and Hollister, A. *Clinical Mechanics and the Hand*. 2nd ed. St. Louis: C. V. Mosby Company, 1993.

Brantigan, O. C. *Clinical Anatomy*. New York: McGraw-Hill Book Company, 1963.

Broer, M. R., and Zernicke, R. F. *Efficiency of Human Movement*. 4th ed. Philadelphia: W. B. Saunders Company, 1979.

C

Chaffin, D. B., and Andersson, G. B. *Occupational Biomechanics*. 2nd ed. New York: John Wiley & Sons, Inc., 1991.

Chase, R. Anatomy and Kinesiology of the Hand. In Hunter, J. M., Schneider, L. H., Mackin, E. J., and Callahan, A. D. (eds.) *Rehabilitation of the Hand: Surgery and Therapy*. 3rd ed. St. Louis: C. V. Mosby, 1990.

Clayson, S. J., Newman, I. M., Debevec, D. F., Anger, R. W., Skowland, H. V., and Kottke, F. J. "Evaluation of mobility of hip and lumbar vertebrae of normal young women." *Archives of Physical Medicine and Rehabilitation* 43(1962):1-8.

Close, J. R. *Motor Function in the Lower Extremity*. Springfield, IL: Charles C. Thomas Publisher, 1964.

Conolly, W. B. *Color Atlas of Hand Conditions*. Chicago: Yearbook Medical Publishers, 1980.

Crowe, P., O'Connell, A. L., and Gardner, E. B. "An electromyographic study of the role of the abdominal muscles and certain hip flexors during sit-ups." Report presented at the National Convention of the American Association for Health, Physical Education, and Recreation, Minneapolis, MN, 1963.

D

deVries, H. A. "Muscle tonus in postural muscles." *American Journal of Physical Medicine* 44 (1965):275-291.

DeSousa, O. M., DeMoraes, J. L., and Vieria, F. L. deM. "Electromyographic study of the brachioradialis muscle." *Anatomical Record* 139 (1961):125-131.

Dorland, W. A. N. *Dorland's Illustrated Medical Dictionary*. 27th ed. Philadelphia: W. B. Saunders Company, 1988.

Duvall, E. M. *Kinesiology: The Anatomy of Motion*. Englewood Cliffs, NJ: Prentice-Hall, 1959.

E

Eaton, R. G. *Joint Injuries of the Hand*. Springfield, IL: Charles C. Thomas Publisher, 1971.

Edington, D. W., and Edgerton, V. R. *The Biology of Physical Activity*. Boston: Houghton Mifflin Company, 1976.

Edelson, J. G., Taitz, C., and Grishkan, A. "The coracohumeral ligament: Anatomy of a substantial but neglected structure." *Journal of Bone and Joint Surgery* 73B(1991): 150-153.

Evans, F. G. *Biomechanical Studies of the Musculo-Skeletal System.* Springfield, IL: Charles C. Thomas Publisher, 1961.

F

Featherstone, D. F. *Dancing Without Danger.* Cranbury, NJ: A. S. Barnes & Company, 1970.

Ferrari, D. A. "Capsular ligaments of the shoulder: Anatomical and functional study of the anterior superior capsule. *American Journal of Sports Medicine* 18(1990):20-24.

Ficat, R. P., and Hungerford, D. S. *Disorders of the Patello-Femoral Joint.* Baltimore: The Williams & Wilkins Company, 1979.

Fischer, F. J., and Houtz, S. J. "Evaluation of the function of the gluteus maximus muscle." *American Journal of Physical Medicine* 47 (1968):182-191.

Flint, M. M. "An electromyographic comparison of the function of the iliacus and the rectus abdominis muscles." *Journal of American Physical Therapy Association* 45 (1965):248-252.

Floyd, W. F., and Silver, P. H. S. "Electromyographic study of patterns of activity of the anterior abdominal wall muscles in man." *Journal of Anatomy* 84(1950):132-145.

Freedman, L., and Munro, R. R. "Abduction of the arm in the scapular plane; scapular and glenohumeral movements." *Journal of Bone and Joint Surgery* 48A (1966):1503-1510.

G

Giannestras, N. J. *Foot Disorders Medical and Surgical Management.* 2nd ed. Philadelphia: Lea & Febiger, 1973.

H

Harris, M. L. "Flexibility," (Review of Literature). *Journal of American Physical Therapy Association* 49 (1969):491-601.

Hay, J. G. *Anatomical and Mechanical Bases of Human Motion,* Englewood Cliffs, NJ: Prentice Hall, 1982.

Hay, J. G., and Reid, J. G. Anatomy, Mechanics, and Human Motion. 2nd ed. Englewood Cliffs, NJ: Prentice Hall, 1988.

Herman, R., and Bragin, S. J. "Function of the gastrocnemius and soleus muscles." *Journal of American Physical Therapy Association* 47 (1967):105-113.

Hertling, D., and Kessler, R. M. *Management of Common Musculoskeletal Disorders.* 2nd ed. Philadelphia: Lippincott, 1990.

Hlavac, H. F. *The Foot Book.* Mountain View, CA: World Publications, 1977.

Holland, G. J. The physiology of flexibility; a review of the literature. In *Kinesiology Review.* Washington, DC: American Association of Health, Physical Education, and Recreation, 1968.

Hollinshead, W. H. "Anatomy of the spine." *Journal of Bone and Joint Surgery* 47A (1965):209-215.

Hoppenfield, S. *Physical Examination of the Spine and Extremities.* New York: Appleton-Century-Crofts, 1976.

Hopper, B. J. *The Mechanics of Human Movement.* New York: American Elsevier Publishing Company, 1973.

House, E. L., and Pansky, B. A. *A Functional Approach to Neuroanatomy.* 3rd ed. New York: McGraw-Hill Book Company, 1979.

I

Inman, V. T. "The shoulder as a functional unit." *Journal of Bone and Joint Surgery* 44A (1962):977-978.

Inman, V. T., Saunders, J. B. deC. M., and Abbott, L. C. "Observations on the function of the shoulder joint." *Journal of Bone and Joint Surgery* 26(1944):1-30.

J

Jenkins, D. B. *Hollinshead's Functional Anatomy of the Limbs and Back.* 6th ed. Philadelphia: W. B. Saunders, 1991.

Jensen, C. R., Schultz, G. W., and Bangerter, B. L. *Applied Kinesiology and Biomechanics.* New York: McGraw-Hill Book Company, 1983.

Jenson, D. B. *Hollinshead's Functional Anatomy of the Limbs and Back.* 6th ed. Philadelphia: W. B. Saunders Company, 1991.

K

Kendall, F. P., McCreary, E. K., and Provance, P.G. *Muscles: Testing and Function with Posture and Pain.* 4th ed. Baltimore: The Williams & Wilkins Company, 1993.

Kent, B. "Functional anatomy of the shoulder complex," *Journal of American Physical Therapy Association* 51(1971):867-888.

Kessler, R. M., and Hertling, D. *Management of Common Musculoskeletal Disorders: Physical Therapy, Principles and Methods.* Philadelphia: Harper & Row, 1990.

Klein, K. K. "The knee and the ligaments." *Journal of Bone and Joint Surgery* 44A (1962):1191-1192.

Klein, K. K., and Allman, F. L. *The Knee in Sports.* Del Mar, CA: Academic Publishers, 1985.

Krause, J. V., and Barham, J. N. *The Mechanical Foundations of Human Motion.* St. Louis: C. V. Mosby Company, 1975.

L

LaBan, M. M., Raptou, A. D, and Johnson, E. W. "Electromyographic study of function of iliopsoas muscles." *Archives of Physical Medicine and Rehabilitation* 46 (1965):676-679.

Larson, R. F. "Forearm positioning on maximal elbow-flexor force." *Journal of American Physical Therapy Association* 49 (1969):748-756.

Lehmkuhl, L. D., and Smith, L. K. *Brunnstrom's Clinical Kinesiology.* 4th ed. Philadelphia: F. A. Davis Company, 1984.

LeVeau, B. *Williams and Lessner: Biomechanics of Human Motion.* Philadelphia: W. B. Saunders Company, 1977.

Lewis, R. W. *The Joints of the Extremities.* Springfield, IL: Charles C. Thomas Publisher, 1955.

Lucas, G. L. *Examination of the Hand.* Springfield, IL: Charles C. Thomas Publisher, 1972.

M

MacConail, M. A., and Basmajian, J. V. *Muscles and Movements: A Basis for Human Kinesiology.* Huntington, NY: R. E. Krieger Publishing Company, 1977.

Magee, D. J. *Orthopedic Physical Assessment.* Philadelphia: W. B. Saunders Company, 1992.

Malcolm, P. "Functional Anatomy of the Shoulder Complex". *Physical Therapy* 66 (1986):1855-1865.

Malick, M., & Cash, M. *Manual on Management of Specific Hand Problems.* Pittsburgh: American Rehabilitation Network Publications, 1984.

Margaria, R. *Biomechanics and Energetics of Muscular Exercise.* Oxford: Clarendon Press, 1976.

McCraw, L. W. "Effects of variations of forearm position in elbow flexion." *Research Quarterly* 35(1964):504-510.

McMinn, R. M. H., Hutchings, R. T., Pegington, J., and Abrahams, P. *Color Atlas of Human Anatomy.* 3rd Ed. St. Louis: Mosby Year Book, Inc., 1993.

Merrifield, H. H. "An electromyographic study of the gluteus maximus, the vastus lateralis and the tensor fasciae latae." *Dissertation Abstracts* 21 (1961):1833.

Michele, A. A. *Iliopsoas Development of Anomalies in Man.* Springfield, IL: Charles C. Thomas Publisher, 1962.

Milford, L. *The Hand.* 3rd ed. St. Louis: C. V. Mosby Company, 1988.

Morris, C. B. "The measurement of the strength of muscle relative to the cross section." *Research Quarterly* 19 (1948):295-303.

N

Northrip, J. W., Logan, G. A., and McKinney, W. C. *Introduction to Biomechanic Analysis of Sport.* Dubuque, IA: Wm. C. Brown Company Publishers, 1974.

O

O'Donoghue, D. H. *Treatment of Injuries to Athletes.* Philadelphia: W. B. Saunders Company, 1984.

P

Partridge, M. J., and Walters, C. E. "Participation of the abdominal muscles in various movements of the trunk in man." *Physical Therapy Review* 39(1959):791-800.

Pauly, J. E. "An electromyographic analysis of certain movements and exercises. I. Some deep muscles of the back." *Anatomical Record* 155 (1966):223-234.

Pauly, J. E., Rushing, J. L., and Scheving, L. E. "An electromyographic study of some muscles crossing the elbow joint." *Anatomical Record* 159 (1967):47-53.

Peat, M. "Functional anatomy of the shoulder complex." *Physical Therapy*, 60:1855-1865.

Pecina, M. *Overuse Injuries of the Musculoskeletal System.* Boca Raton, FL: CRC Press, 1993.

Perrott, J. W. *Structural and Functional Anatomy.* 3rd ed. Great Britain: Edward Arnold, Ltd., 1977.

Pink, M., and Jobe, F. W. "Shoulder injuries in athletes." *Orthopedics* 11(6) (1991):39-47.

Plagenhoef, S. *Patterns of Human Motion: A Cinematographic Analysis.* Englewood Cliffs, NJ: Prentice-Hall, 1971.

Pocock, G. S. "Electromyographic study of the quadriceps during resistive exercise." *Journal of American Physical Therapy Association* 43 (1963):426-434.

Poppen, N.K., and Walker, P.S. "Normal and abnormal motion of the shoulder." *Journal of Bone and Joint Surgery*, 58 (1976):195-201.

Poppen, N.K., and Walker, P.S. "Forces at the glenohumeral joint in abduction." *Clinical Orthopaedics*, 135 (1978):165-170.

Pratt, N. E. "Neurovascular entrapment in the regions of the shoulder and posterior triangle of the neck." *Physical Therapy* 66 (1986):1894-1899.

Q

Quiring, D. P., and Warfel, J. H. *The Head, Neck, and Trunk.* 3rd ed. Philadelphia: Lea & Febiger, 1967.

Quiring, D. P., and Warfel, J. H. *The Extremities.* 3rd ed. Philadelphia: Lea & Febiger, 1967.

R

Rasch, P. J. *Kinesiology and Applied Anatomy.* 7th ed. Philadelphia: Lea & Febiger, 1989.

Rettig, & Strickland, R. *Hand Injuries in Athletes.* Philadelphia: W. B. Saunders Company, 1992.

Rockwood, C. A., and Matsen, F. A. *The Shoulder,* Vol. 1. Philadelphia: W. B. Saunders Company, 1990.

Root, M. L., Orien, W. P., and Weed, J. H. *Normal and Abnormal Function of the Foot,* Vol. 2. Los Angeles: Clinical Biomechanics Corporation, 1977.

Root, M. L., Orien, W. P., Weed, J. H., and Hughes, R. J. *Biomechanical Examination of the Foot,* Vol 1. Los Angeles: Clinical Biomechanics Corporation, 1971.

S

Shevlin, M. G., Lehmann, J. F., and Lucci, J. A. "Electromyographic study of the function of some muscles crossing the glenohumeral joint." *Archives of Physical Medicine and Rehabilitation* 50 (1969):264-270.

Singleton, M. C. "Functional anatomy of the shoulder." *Journal of American Physical Therapy Association* 46 (1966):1043-1051.

Singleton, M. C., and LeVeau, B. F. "The hip joint: structure, stability, and stress." *Journal of American Physical Therapy Association* 55 (1975):957-973.

Soderberg, G. L. *Kinesiology: Application to Pathological Motion.* Baltimore: TheWilliams & Wilkins Company, 1986.

Spinner, M. *Kaplan's Functional and Surgical Anatomy of the Hand.* 3rd ed. Philadelphia: J. B. Lippincott, 1984.

Steindler, A. *Kinesiology of the Human Body Under Normal and Pathological Conditions.* Springfield, IL: Charles C. Thomas Publisher, 1955.

Subotnick, S. I. *Podiatric Sports Medicine.* Mount Kisco, NY: Futura Publishing Company, Inc., 1975.

Subotnick, S. I. *Sports Medicine of the Lower Extremity.* New York: Churchill Livingstone, 1989.

Subotnick, S. I. *The Running Foot Doctor.* Mountain View, CA: World Publications, 1977.

Sweigard, L. E. *Human Movement Potential: Its Ideokinetic Facilitation.* New York: Dodd, Mead & Company, 1974.

T

Torg, J. S., Vegso, J. J., and Torg, E. *Rehabilitation of Athletic Injuries.* Chicago: Year Book Medical Publishers, Inc., 1987.H)279

Tubiana, R., ed. *The Hand.* Philadelphia: W. B. Saunders Company, 1981.

Tubiana, R., Thomine, J. M., and Mackin, E. *Examination of the Hand and Upper Limb.* Philadelphia: W. B. Saunders, 1984.

W

Walters, C. E., and Partridge, M. J. "Electromyographic study of the differential action of the abdominal muscles during exercise." *American Journal of Physical Medicine* 36 (1957):259-268.

Weineck, J. *Functional Anatomy in Sports.* 2nd ed. Chicago: Year Book Medical Publishers, Inc., 1990.

Wheatley, M. S., and Jahnke, W. D. "Electromyographic study of the superficial thigh and hip muscles in normal individuals." *Archives of Physical Therapy* 31 (1951): 508-522.

Williams, P. L., ed. *Gray's Anatomy of the Human Body.* 37th ed. Philadelphia: Lea & Febiger, 1989.

QUIZZES

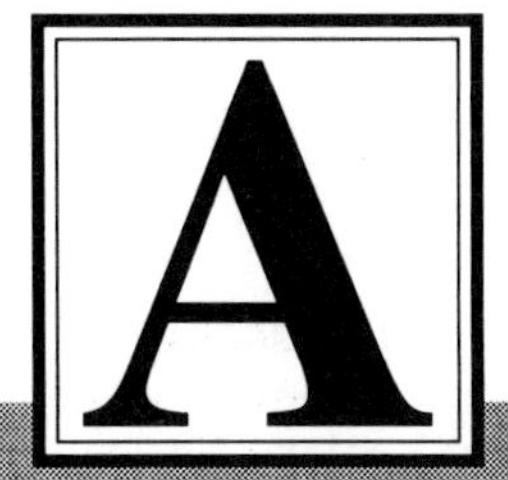

(Quizzes Answer Key for chapters 2 - 10 is found on page 329.)

CHAPTER 2 - QUIZ

	True	False
1. The sagittal plane passes through the body from side to side.	☐	☐
2. The axis around which frontal plane actions occur is known as the sagittal axis.	☐	☐
3. A triaxial joint allows for movement in two planes only.	☐	☐
4. A person should hold a heavy weight close to the body to prevent a drastic shift of the center of gravity.	☐	☐
5. The higher the center of gravity the more stable the object.	☐	☐
6. Only a first class lever can have a mechanical advantage of one.	☐	☐
7. A wheelbarrow acts as a second class lever.	☐	☐
8. A third class lever has the resistance located between the force and the axis.	☐	☐
9. Force is a vector quantity as it has both magnitude and direction.	☐	☐
10. The strongest muscle fiber type is longitudinal.	☐	☐

Answer

11. Who is most stable while standing upright?
    a. child
    b. man
    c. woman

12. As a backpack is put on, the center of gravity moves
    a. up and forward
    b. up and backward
    c. down and forward
    d. down and backward

13. To apply force in the sagittal plane, widen the base of support by taking a
    a. side-to-side stance
    b. front-to-back stance
    c. feet together stance

14. A lever is comprised of
    a. a force and a resistance
    b. a force, resistance, and axis
    c. a force, resistance, and rigid bar
    d. a force, resistance, axis, and rigid bar

15. Which lever is known as the strong lever?
    a. first class
    b. second class
    c. third class

16. If a lever has a mechanical advantage of .5, how much resistance can it balance with 20 units of force?
    a. 10 units of resistance
    b. 40 units of resistance
    c. it depends on the length of the force arm
    d. insufficient information is given

17. A muscle which is directly involved in causing a movement is referred to as a(n)
    a. agonist
    b. antagonist
    c. neutralizer
    d. stabilizer

18. To achieve mobility rather than stability
    a. widen the base of support
    b. shorten the base of support
    c. lower the center of gravity
    d. raise the center of gravity
    e. b and d above

19. The perpendicular line that passes through the center of gravity is the
    a. midpoint of gravity
    b. pull of gravity
    c. line of gravity
    d. none of the above

20. Which muscle fiber type would be easiest to stretch?
    a. multipenniform
    b. triangular
    c. fusiform
    d. penniform

CHAPTER 3 - QUIZ

SCAPULA

True False

1. Of the two articulations of the clavicle, the sternoclavicular articulation is stronger.

2. All movements of the scapula occur in the frontal plane.

3. The levator scapula elevates and abducts the scapula.

4. Part 2 of the trapezius is an upward rotator of the scapula.

5. Parts 1 and 3 of the trapezius are agonists during elevation of the scapula.

6. The serratus anterior inserts on the upper 9 ribs.

7. The subclavius is located just below the scapular spine.

8. The pectoralis minor is a depressor of the scapula.

9. Dislocations of the acromioclavicular joint are called "shoulder separations."

Answer

10. Which of the following muscles does not attach to the scapula?
    a. rhomboids
    b. pectoralis minor
    c. serratus anterior
    d. subclavius
    e. part 2, trapezius

11. The action common to the rhomboids and part 3 of the trapezius is
    a. adduction of the scapula
    b. elevation of the scapula
    c. depression of the scapula
    d. upward rotation of the scapula
    e. downward rotation of the scapula

12. The origin of part 1 of the trapezius is
    a. clavicle
    b. acromion process
    c. scapular spine
    d. axillary border of scapula
    e. occipital bone

13. Resolution of the line of pull of the rhomboids yields
    a. an adducting vector only
    b. an elevating vector only
    c. an adducting and an elevating vector
    d. an abducting and an elevating vector
    e. an abducting and a depressing vector

Answer ☐

14. The two portions of the trapezius that are agonists during upward rotation of the scapula are
    a. portions 1 and 3
    b. portions 2 and 4
    c. portions 2 and 3
    d. portions 3 and 4
    e. portions 1 and 4

☐

15. Which of the following muscles act together to hold the scapula next to the ribs?
    a. part 1 of the trapezius and levator scapulae
    b. pectoralis minor and subclavius
    c. rhomboids and serratus anterior
    d. part 4 of the trapezius and serratus anterior

☐

16. Which of the following muscles acts as an antagonist during downward rotation of the scapula?
    a. part 2 of the trapezius
    b. rhomboids
    c. pectoralis minor
    d. subclavius
    e. levator scapulae

☐

	True	False
17. The levator scapulae is innervated by the dorsal scapular nerve and cervical nerves 5 and 6.	☐	☐
18. The serratus anterior is innervated by the long thoracic nerve.	☐	☐
19. Pectoralis minor is innervated by the lateral anterior thoracic nerve.	☐	☐
20. The subclavius is innervated by the 5 and 6 cervical nerves.	☐	☐

SHOULDER

	True	False
1. The shoulder joint is known as the glenohumeral joint.		
2. Flexion and extension of the shoulder joint are performed around the frontal axis.		
3. The movements of the humerus occur in the frontal, sagittal, and transverse planes.		
4. As a whole, the deltoid adducts the humerus.		
5. The latissimus dorsi is an external rotator of the glenohumeral joint.		
6. The anterior deltoid and posterior deltoid are antagonists during internal and external rotation of the glenohumeral joint.		
7. The pectoralis major inserts on the humerus just below the humeral head.		
8. The teres minor is known as the latissimus dorsi's "little helper."		
9. The coracobrachialis is a large and powerful mover of the humerus.		
10. Both heads of the biceps brachii cross the glenohumeral joint.		

Answer

11. Which muscle does not belong to the rotator cuff?
    a. subscapularis
    b. supraspinatus
    c. infraspinatus
    d. teres minor
    e. teres major

12. A glenohumeral joint action common to the latissimus dorsi and the sternal portion of pectoralis major is
    a. adduction
    b. external rotation
    c. horizontal adduction
    d. abduction
    e. hyperextension

13. The origin of teres minor is
    a. clavicle
    b. acromion process of the scapula
    c. scapular spine
    d. axillary border of the scapula
    e. vertebral border of the scapula

14. The actions of the biceps brachii at the glenohumeral joint can be enhanced by
   a. flexing the glenohumeral joint
   b. internally rotating the glenohumeral joint
   c. flexing the elbow joint
   d. extending the elbow joint
   e. adducting the glenohumeral joint

Answer

15. If the suprascapular nerve were blocked, which of the following glenohumeral actions would be impeded?
   a. internal rotation
   b. adduction
   c. horizontal adduction
   d. external rotation
   e. none of the above

16. Which of the following muscles act to form a force couple during abduction of the glenohumeral joint?
   a. pectoralis major and deltoid
   b. pectoralis major and latissimus dorsi
   c. deltoid and rotator cuff muscles
   d. coracobrachialis and biceps brachii

17. Which of the following muscles acts as an antagonist during flexion of the glenohumeral joint?
   a. latissimus dorsi
   b. anterior deltoid
   c. clavicular portion of the pectoralis major
   d. subscapularis
   e. biceps brachii

18. The coracobrachialis is innervated by the _____ nerve.
   a. suprascapular
   b. thoracodorsal
   c. musculocutaneous
   d. axillary
   e. subscapular

19. The latissimus dorsi is innervated by the ______ nerve.
   a. suprascapular
   b. thoracodorsal
   c. medial anterior thoracic
   d. medial lateral thoracic
   e. axillary

20. The long head of the triceps brachii is innervated by the _____ nerve.
   a. axillary
   b. subscapular
   c. radial
   d. musculocutaneous
   e. thoracodorsal

CHAPTER 4 - QUIZ

		True	False
1.	The elbow joint is the articulation between the humerus and the ulna.	☐	☐
2.	Pronation and supination are performed around the long axis.	☐	☐
3.	The elbow and radioulnar joints each has two degrees of freedom.	☐	☐
4.	The biceps brachii and the supinator are antagonists.	☐	☐
5.	The triceps brachii has three heads, only one of which crosses the glenohumeral joint.	☐	☐
6.	Of the two pronator muscles, the pronator quadratus is the larger.	☐	☐
7.	The anconeus is a large and powerful extensor of the elbow joint.	☐	☐
8.	The flexion action of the biceps brachii is enhanced when the hand is in a supinated position.	☐	☐
9.	Palpate the brachioradialis between the lateral epicondyle and mid-radius.	☐	☐
10.	The triceps brachii and the anconeus are innervated by the same nerve.	☐	☐

Answer

11. Which nerve supplies the brachioradialis? ☐
    - a. median
    - b. musculocutaneous
    - c. radial

12. The muscle known as the "workhorse of the elbow joint" is the ☐
    - a. biceps brachii
    - b. brachialis
    - c. brachioradialis
    - d. triceps brachii

13. The origin of the pronator teres is ☐
    - a. radius
    - b. lateral epicondyle of the humerus
    - c. radius and ulna
    - d. ulna and medial epicondyle of the humerus

Answer

14. Which of the following actions would be effected if the median nerve were blocked?
    a. extension of the elbow joint
    b. pronation of the radioulnar joint
    c. supination of the radioulnar joint

15. What is the nerve supply to the supinator?
    a. median
    b. musculocutaneous
    c. radial

16. Which of the following muscles is not innervated by the musculocutaneous nerve?
    a. biceps brachii
    b. brachioradialis
    c. brachialis

17. Which of the following muscles would still function as an elbow flexor if the radial and musculocutaneous nerves were blocked?
    a. biceps brachii
    b. brachioradialis
    c. brachialis
    d. pronator quadratus
    e. pronator teres

CHAPTER 5 - QUIZ

		True	False
1.	The wrist joint is formed by the articulation of the ulna with the carpal bones.	☐	☐
2.	Flexion and extension of the wrist joint are performed around the frontal axis.	☐	☐
3.	There are eight carpal bones in the hand.	☐	☐
4.	There are three muscles on the palmar surface of the forearm that deviate the wrist.	☐	☐
5.	The extensor digitorum extends the DIP joints.	☐	☐
6.	The extensor carpi radialis longus inserts on the second metacarpal.	☐	☐
7.	The palmaris longus originates on the ulna.	☐	☐
8.	All muscles that originate proximal to the wrist that have "extensor" in their name are innervated by the radial nerve.	☐	☐
9.	The extensor pollicis brevis performs ulnar deviation.	☐	☐
10.	The intrinsic muscles of the hand are innervated by the median and radial nerves.	☐	☐

Answer

11. The nerve supply to the flexor pollicis brevis is ☐
    a. median
    b. radial
    c. ulnar
    d. median and ulnar

12. The insertion of the opponens pollicis is ☐
    a. 1st metacarpal
    b. proximal phalanx of the thumb
    c. distal phalanx of the thumb

13. The flexor retinaculum is comprised of the ☐
    a. palmar aponeurosis
    b. palmar carpal ligament
    c. transverse carpal ligament
    d. both a and b
    e. both b and c

Answer

14. The muscle that extends the IP joint of the thumb is the
    a. extensor pollicis longus
    b. 1st dorsal interosseus muscle
    c. extensor pollicis brevis
    d. abductor pollicis longus
    e. adductor pollicis

15. Which of the following muscles acts as an *agonist,* during radial deviation of the wrist joint?
    a. extensor digitorum
    b. flexor digitorum superficialis
    c. abductor pollicis longus
    d. flexor carpi ulnaris
    e. none of the above

16. Which of the following muscles acts as an antagonist during extension of the MCP joints?
    a. extensor digitorum
    b. flexor carpi ulnaris
    c. opponens digiti minimi
    d. extensor carpi radialis longus
    e. interosseus muscles

17. The opponens digiti minimi is innervated by the _____ nerve.
    a. median
    b. ulnar
    c. radial

18. The extensor carpi ulnaris is innervated by the _____ nerve.
    a. median
    b. ulnar
    c. radial

19. The extensor indicis is innervated by the _____ nerve.
    a. median
    b. ulnar
    c. radial

20. The opponens pollicis is innervated by the _____ nerve.
    a. median
    b. ulnar
    c. radial

CHAPTER 6 - QUIZ

True False

1. The primary curves of the spine are thoracic and sacral.
2. Flexion and extension of the spine are performed around the frontal axis.
3. The movements of the spine can occur in the frontal, sagittal, and transverse planes.
4. Lordosis is more commonly thought of as a condition of the cervical rather than the lumbar spine.
5. The straight leg lift from supine position is the best exercise for strengthening the abdominals.
6. The scaleni and the semispinalis muscles are agonists during lateral flexion of the spine.
7. The rectus abdominis inserts on ribs 5, 6, and 7.
8. Strong hip flexors and weak abdominals often lead to lower back pain.
9. The erector spinae is active through the complete range of spinal flexion.
10. To prevent back injury, take care to bend the knees and keep the head above the hips during lifting tasks.

Answer

11. Which muscle rotates the spine to the same side?
    a. sternocleidomastoid
    b. erector spinae
    c. rectus abdominis
12. An action common to the external oblique and the semispinalis muscles is
    a. flexion of the spine
    b. extension of the spine
    c. rotation of the spine to the same side
    d. rotation of the spine to the opposite side
13. The insertion of the sternocleidomastoid is the
    a. clavicle
    b. sternum
    c. mastoid
    d. a and b above
    e. a and c above

Answer

14. The actions of the levator scapulae on the spine are
    a. flexion
    b. extension
    c. lateral flexion
    d. stabilization
    e. c and d above

15. The internal oblique, suboccipitals, and splenius muscle are agonists during
    a. internal rotation of the spine
    b. external rotation of the spine
    c. rotation of the spine to the same side
    d. rotation of the spine to the opposite side
    e. none of the above

16. The origin of the internal oblique is on the
    a. iliac crest
    b. pubis via the linea alba
    c. lower 4 ribs
    d. ribs 5, 6, and 7

17. Which of the following muscles act as antagonists during extension of the spine?
    a. levator scapulae and part 1 of the trapezius
    b. prevertebrals and suboccipitals
    c. scaleni and rectus abdominis
    d. splenius muscles and quadratus lumborum

CHAPTER 7 - QUIZ

True False

1. The hip joint has three degrees of freedom.
2. Flexion and extension of the hip joint are performed around the frontal axis.
3. The movements of the femur can occur in the frontal, sagittal, transverse planes.
4. The rectus femoris and iliospoas muscles are antagonists during hip flexion.
5. The gluteus maximus is an external rotator of the hip joint.
6. The gluteus medius and gluteus minimus are antagonists during abduction of the hip.
7. The sartorius inserts on the upper medial fibula.
8. The pectineus is an adductor and a flexor of the hip joint.
9. All of the hamstrings originate on the ischial tuberosity.
10. Both heads of the adductor magnus originate on the pubis.

Answer

11. Which muscle is not one of the hamstrings?
    a. gracilis
    b. semitendinosus
    c. semimembranosus
    d. biceps femoris
12. An action common to the hamstrings and the adductor magnus is
    a. abduction of the hip joint
    b. outward rotation of the hip joint
    c. extension of the hip joint
    d. flexion of the hip joint
13. The origin of the sartorius is
    a. upper medial tibia
    b. upper tibia and fibula
    c. linea aspera of the femur
    d. anterior superior iliac spine
    e. anterior inferior iliac spine

Answer

14. An action of the pectineus at the hip joint is
    a. flexion
    b. internal rotation
    c. extension
    d. external rotation
    e. none of the above

15. If the obturator nerve were blocked, which of the following hip actions would be impeded?
    a. external rotation
    b. abduction
    c. extension
    d. internal rotation
    e. none of the above

16. Which of the following muscles is an antagonist during internal rotation of the hip joint?
    a. pectineus
    b. gluteus maximus
    c. rectus femoris
    d. semitendinosus

17. Which of the following muscles acts as an agonist during flexion of the hip joint?
    a. biceps femoris
    b. gluteus maximus
    c. rectus femoris
    d. semimembranosus

18. The adductor longus is innervated by the _____ nerve.
    a. femoral
    b. gluteal
    c. obturator
    d. sciatic

19. The biceps femoris is innervated by the _____ nerve.
    a. femoral
    b. gluteal
    c. obturator
    d. sciatic

20. The tensor fasciae latae is innervated by the _____ nerve.
    a. femoral
    b. gluteal
    c. obturator
    d. sciatic

CHAPTER 8 - QUIZ

True False

1. The knee joint is formed by the articulation of the fibula and the femur.
2. Flexion and extension of the knee are performed around the frontal axis.
3. The meniscus of the knee is referred to as cartilage.
4. The rectus femoris extends and internally rotates the knee.
5. The sartorius is a flexor and internal rotator of the knee.
6. The biceps femoris crosses the knee joint posterior to the frontal axis.
7. The gracilis inserts on the fibula and tibia.
8. All of the quadricep muscles are innervated by the same nerve.
9. The plantaris is a powerful extensor of the knee.
10. All of the hamstring muscles are rotators of the knee joint.

Answer

11. All of the hamstring muscles originate on the
    a. pubis
    b. iliac crest
    c. ischial tuberosity
    d. femoral tuberosity
    e. sacrum
12. The action common to all of the hamstring muscles is
    a. extension of the knee joint
    b. flexion of the knee joint
    c. internal rotation of the knee joint
    d. external rotation of the knee joint
    e. all of the above
13. The origin of the rectus femoris is
    a. anterior superior iliac spine
    b. anterior inferior iliac spine
    c. patella
    d. pubis
    e. iliac crest

14. The line of pull of the vastus lateralis on the patella is **Answer**
   a. upward and inward
   b. downward and inward
   c. downward and outward
   d. upward and outward

15. The two quadricep muscles which exert the same line of pull on the patella are the
   a. rectus femoris and vastus intermedius
   b. vastus intermedius and vastus lateralis
   c. vastus lateralis and vastus medialis
   d. rectus femoris and vastus medialis
   e. vastus intermedius and vastus medialis

16. Which of the following muscles acts as an agonist during flexion of the knee joint?
   a. rectus femoris
   b. vastus lateralis
   c. sartorius
   d. vastus lateralis
   e. none of the above

17. Which of the following muscles acts as an antagonist during internal rotation of the knee joint?
   a. semitendinosus
   b. semimembranosus
   c. vastus medialis
   d. rectus femoris
   e. biceps femoris

18. The gracilis is innervated by the _____ nerve.
   a. femoral
   b. obturator
   c. sciatic
   d. tibial

19. The popliteus is innervated by the _____ nerve.
   a. femoral
   b. obturator
   c. sciatic
   d. tibial

20. The semimembranosus is innervated by the _____ nerve.
   a. femoral
   b. obturator
   c. sciatic
   d. tibial

Chapter 9 - Quiz

	True	False
1. The talocrural joint is formed by the articulation of the tibia and the talus.	☐	☐
2. Plantar flexion and dorsiflexion of the talocrural joint are performed around the frontal axis.	☐	☐
3. The lateral malleolus is the distal end of the tibia.	☐	☐
4. The gastrocnemius dorsiflexes the talocrural joint.	☐	☐
5. The peroneus tertius everts and dorsiflexes.	☐	☐
6. The tibialis anterior crosses the midtarsal joint medial to the midtarsal axis.	☐	☐
7. The calcaneal tendon inserts on the talus and calcaneus.	☐	☐
8. The triceps surae muscles are innervated by the same nerve.	☐	☐
9. The plantaris is a powerful plantar flexor.	☐	☐
10. All of the peroneus muscle are everters of the midtarsal joint.	☐	☐

Answer

11. The 'shin splint' muscle is the ☐
    a. soleus
    b. gastrocnemius
    c. tibialis anterior
    d. tibialis posterior
    e. plantaris

12. The action(s) common to the triceps surae muscles are ☐
    a. dosiflexion
    b. plantar flexion
    c. dorsiflexion and inversion
    d. plantar flexion and inversion
    e. none of the above

13. The insertion of the extensor hallucis longus is the ☐
    a. dorsum of the foot
    b. plantar surface of the foot
    c. anterior surface of the tibia
    d. posterior surface of the tibia
    e. lateral malleolus

Answer

14. The tendon of the peroneus longus passes posterior to the lateral malleolus to act as a(n)
    a. inverter
    b. dorsiflexor
    c. plantar flexor

15. The 'Tom, Dick, and Harry' muscles are the tibialis posterior, the flexor hallucis longus, and the
    a. flexor digitorum longus
    b. extensor hallucis longus
    c. tibialis anterior
    d. extensor digitorum longus
    e. none of the above

16. Which of the following muscles acts as an agonist during inversion of the talocrural joint?
    a. extensor hallucis longus
    b. peroneus tertius
    c. tibialis anterior
    d. tibialis posterior
    e. c and d above

17. Which of the following muscles are involved during sagittal plane movement of the ankle?
    a. gastrocnemius
    b. soleus
    c. peroneus brevis
    d. flexor hallucis longus
    e. all of the above

18. The soleus is innervated by the _____ nerve.
    a. peroneal
    b. tibial

19. The peroneus tertius is innervated by the _____ nerve.
    a. peroneal
    b. tibial

20. The tibialis anterior is innervated by the _____ nerve.
    a. peroneal
    b. tibia

CHAPTER 10 - QUIZ

True False

1. The thorax is comprised of the sternum, the costal cartilages, the ribs, and the cervical vertebrae.

2. The muscles acting on the thorax during resting respiration are the diaphragm, external intercostals, and internal intercostals.

3. The diaphragm is the dividing muscle between the thoracic and abdominal cavities.

4. The rectus abdominis is a muscle of respiration.

5. During expiration, the ribs are elevated to enlarge the size of the thorax.

6. If expiration is not forced, no muscular contraction is required.

7. Movements of the thorax are described as elevation and depression.

Answer

8. The diaphragm is innervated by the _____ nerve(s).
   a. phrenic
   b. intercostal
   c. thoracic
   d. iliohypogastric
   e. ilioinguinal

9. The transversus thoracis is innervated by the _____ nerve.
   a. phrenic
   b. intercostal
   c. thoracic
   d. iliohypogastric
   e. ilioinguinal

10. The serratus posterior superior is innervated by the _____ nerve.
   a. phrenic
   b. intercostal
   c. thoracic
   d. iliohypogastric
   e. ilioinguinal

CERVICAL PLEXUS

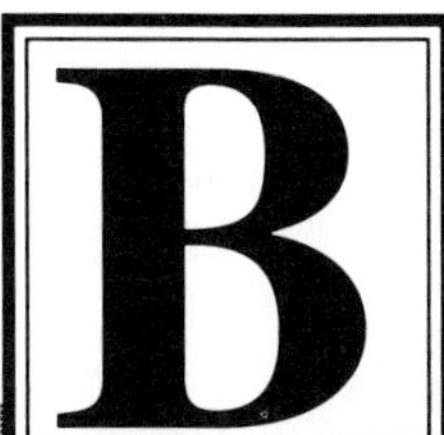

The cervial plexus is formed by the ventral primary rami of spinal nerves C1 through C4 with a small contribution from C5. Peripheral nerves arising from it innervate most of the anterior and lateral muscles of the neck, and supply sensory fibers to part of the head and much of the neck.

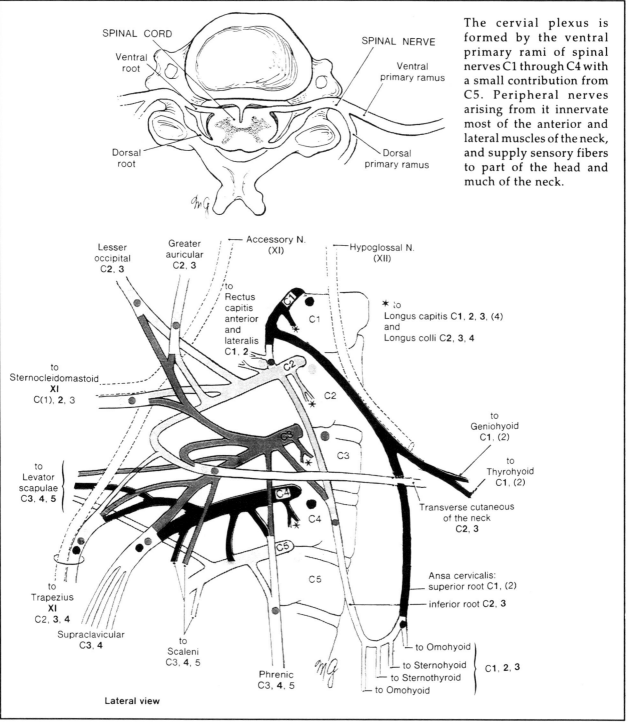

SPINAL CORD
Ventral root
Dorsal root
SPINAL NERVE
Ventral primary ramus
Dorsal primary ramus

Lesser occipital C2, 3
Greater auricular C2, 3
Accessory N. (XI)
Hypoglossal N. (XII)
to Rectus capitis anterior and lateralis C1, 2
* to Longus capitis C1, 2, 3, (4) and Longus colli C2, 3, 4
to Sternocleidomastoid XI C(1), 2, 3
to Geniohyoid C1, (2)
to Thyrohyoid C1, (2)
to Levator scapulae C3, 4, 5
Transverse cutaneous of the neck C2, 3
Ansa cervicalis: superior root C1, (2)
inferior root C2, 3
to Trapezius XI C2, 3, 4
Supraclavicular C3, 4
to Scaleni C3, 4, 5
Phrenic C3, 4, 5
to Omohyoid
to Sternohyoid
to Sternothyroid
to Omohyoid
C1, 2, 3
C1
C2
C3
C4
C5

Lateral view

Reproduced with permission from Kendall, F., McCreary, E., and Provance, P. Muscles, Testing and Function, 4th ed. Baltimore: Williams and Wilkins.

BRACHIAL PLEXUS

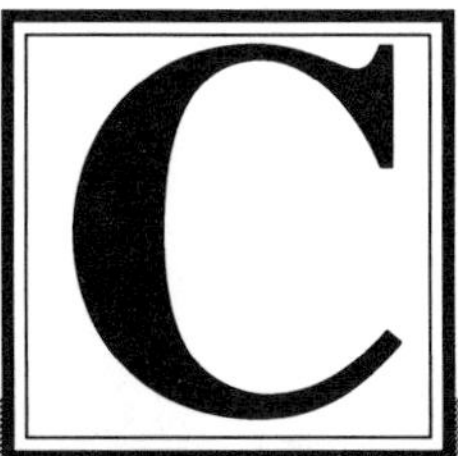

Nerves are susceptible to the same types of trauma that affect other soft tissue: contusion, compression, crush, stretch, avulsion, and laceration. Particular kinds of trauma are more likely to occur at certain sites along the nerve.

These sites will be pointed out as the nerve pathways of the upper extremity are traced from origin in the spinal cord to termination in the digits. Much of the anatomical description is taken from the work of Haymaker and Woodhall.

Roots

The roots of the brachial plexus, C5, C6, C7, C8 and T1 anterior primary rami, exit the spinal column at the intervertebral foramina (Fig. 1). They then pass between the anterior and medial scalenes in the posterior triangle of the neck which is formed by the sternocleidomastoid, the trapezius, and the middle third of the clavicle. The scalenes comprise the lower part of the floor of the triangle and are the primary lateral flexors of the neck. Spasm, hypertrophy, and variations in scalene attachment to the clavicle are included among the causes of thoracic outlet syndrome, the symptoms of which are related to compression of the C8 and T1 fibers of the plexus.

The nerve roots give rise to two nerves.

- The long thoracic comes off C5, C6, and C7 and innervates the serratus anterior. It travels in a straight line behind the cords of the plexus, through the medial aspect of the axilla and down the lateral wall of the thorax. Because it is anchored by the scalenes and by the muscle slips of the serratus anterior, it has been noted to be subject to stretch injuries in, for example, furniture movers.
- The second nerve derived from the roots is the dorsal scapular, comprised mainly of fibers from C5. It provides partial innervation for the levator scapulae and full innervation for the rhomboids.

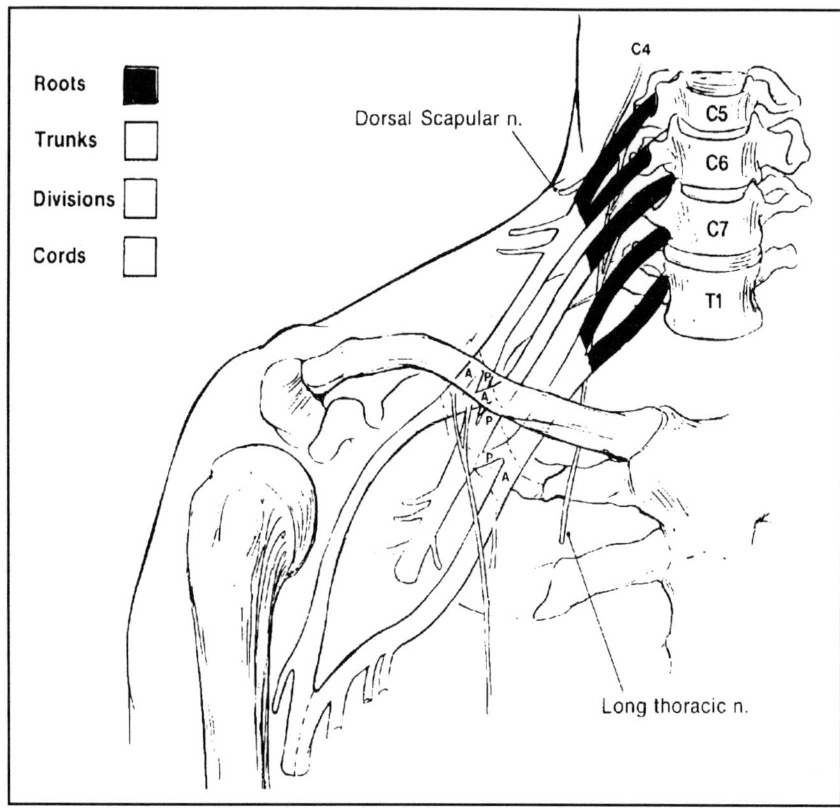

Fig. 1

Reproduced with permission from Malick, M., and Cash, M., ed. *Manual on Management of Specific Hand Problems.* Pittsburgh: American Rehabilitation Network.

Trunks

The roots combine to form upper, middle, and lower trunks at the level of the scalenes. (Fig. 2) Fibers from C4, C5, C6 combine to form the upper trunk. The middle trunk is a continuation of C7 fibers. C8 and T1 fibers combine to form the lower trunk. These trunks are located mainly in the supraclavicular fossa.

Two nerves come off the upper trunk.

- The subclavian nerve innervates the subclavian muscle (this acts as a depressor of the lateral head of the clavicle).
- The suprascapular nerve passes superficial to the cords of the brachial plexus, then passes through the suprascapular notch to reach the dorsal surface of the scapula where it innervates supraspinatus and infraspinatus.

Interruption of the upper trunk results in motor and sensory deficits in the C5-C6 distribution, known as "Erb's palsy." Injury to the middle trunk affects the C7 (radial nerve) distribution. Injury to the lower trunk affects the C8-T1 motor and sensory distribution in a pattern known as "Klumpke's paralysis."

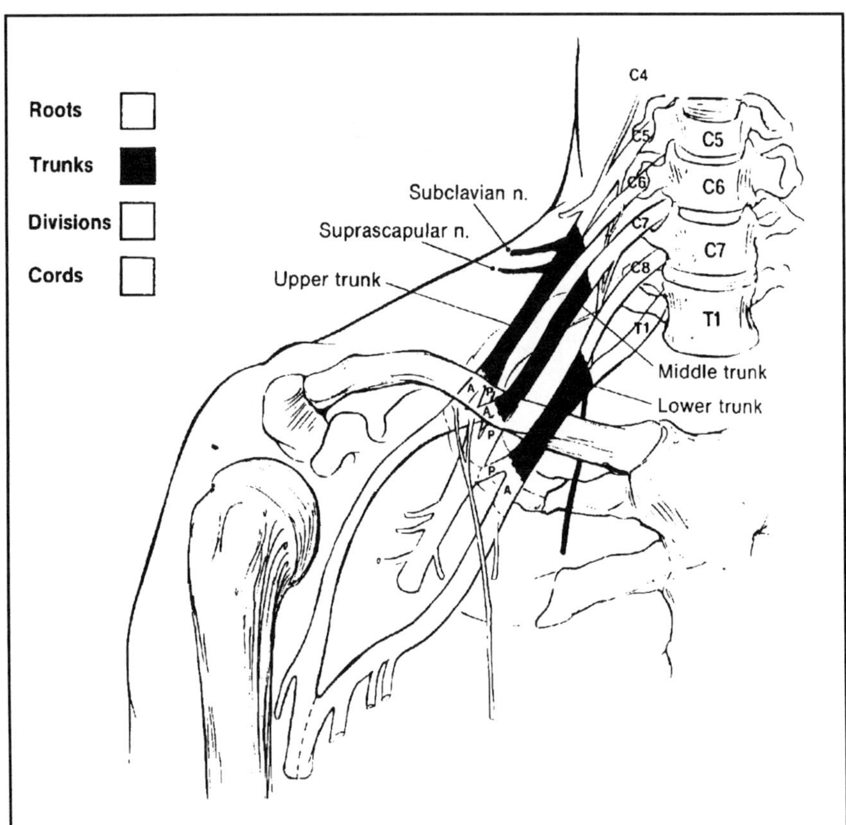

Fig. 2

Reproduced with permission from Malick, M., and Cash, M., ed. *Manual on Management of Specific Hand Problems.* Pittsburgh: American Rehabilitation Network.

Divisions

Each of the three trunks divides into an anterior and posterior division. (Fig. 3) Fibers in the anterior divisions eventually innervate the anterior (volar) aspect of the upper extremity; those in the posterior divisions eventually innervate the posterior (dorsal) aspect of the extremity. The divisions are located deep to the middle third of the clavicle and extend distally to the lateral border of the first rib.

One nerve comes off the combined anterior divisions of the upper and middle trunks: the lateral anterior thoracic. It innervates the upper portion of pectorals major.

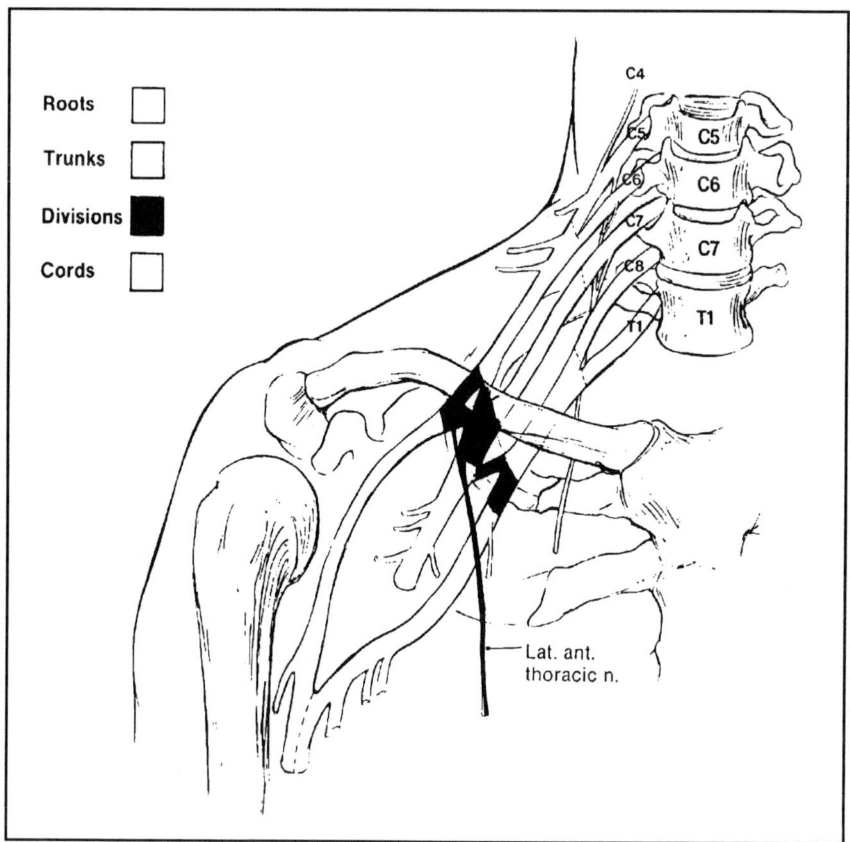

Fig. 3

Reproduced with permission from Malick, M., and Cash, M., ed. *Manual on Management of Specific Hand Problems.* Pittsburgh: American Rehabilitation Network.

Cords

The divisions unite to form the lateral, posterior, and medial cords, so named because of their position relative to the axillary artery. (Fig. 4) The cords are situated below the clavicle in the axilla behind the pectoralis minor tendon. The anterior divisions of the upper and middle trunks form the lateral cord; the anterior division of the lower trunk forms the medial cord (frequently with a contribution from the middle trunk). The posterior divisions from all three trunks form the posterior cord.

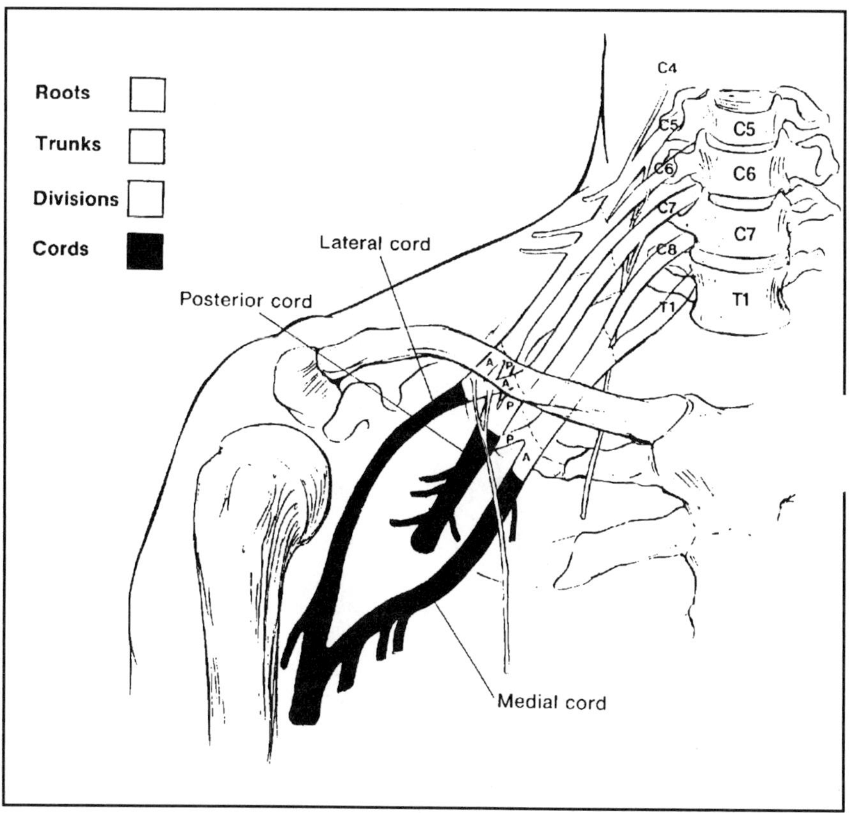

Fig. 4

Reproduced with permission from Malick, M., and Cash, M., ed. *Manual on Management of Specific Hand Problems.* Pittsburgh: American Rehabilitation Network.

The Lateral Cord (Fig. 5) gives rise to two nerves:

- musculocutaneous nerve (motor to coracobrachialis, biceps, and brachialis; sensory to lateral aspect of forearm on both the dorsal and volar surfaces. (This is the lateral cutaneous nerve of the forearm.) Fig. 6
- lateral head of the median nerve (motor to all median nerve muscles except for the intrinsic muscles in the hand.)

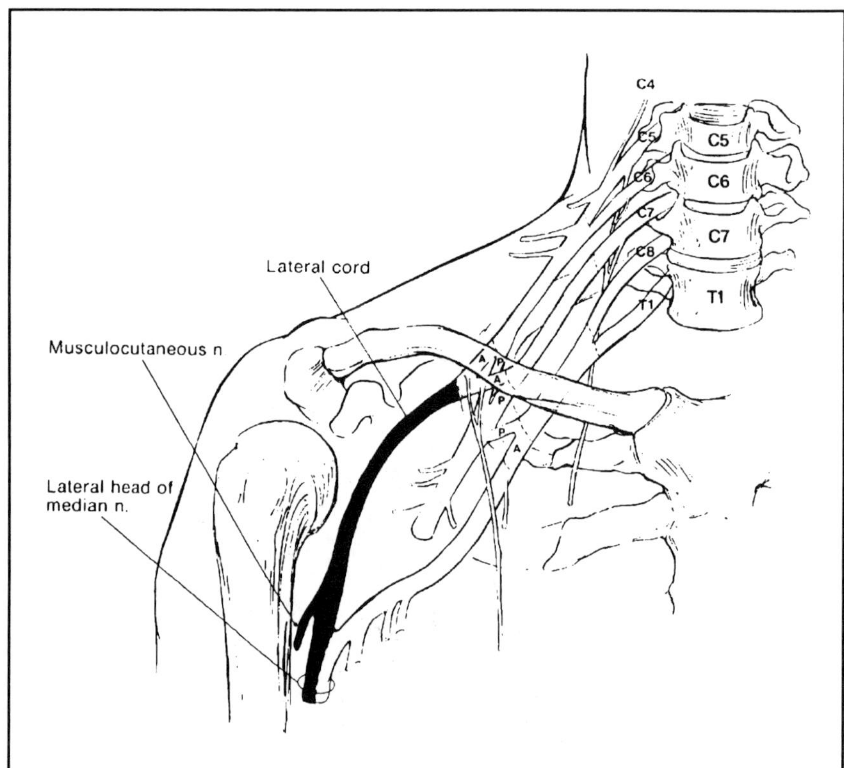

Fig. 5

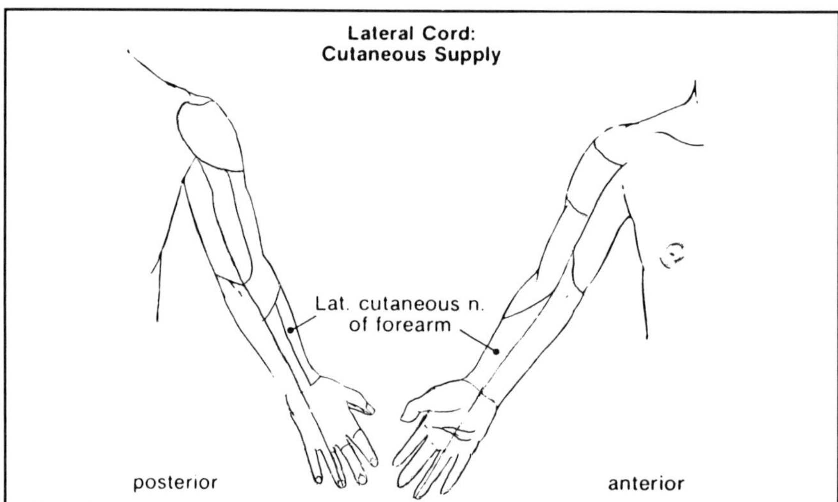

Fig. 6

Reproduced with permission from Malick, M., and Cash, M., ed. *Manual on Management of Specific Hand Problems.* Pittsburgh: American Rehabilitation Network.

The Posterior Cord (Fig. 7) gives rise to five nerves:

- upper subscapular nerve (motor to subscapular muscle).
- lower subscapular nerve (motor nerve to teres major and a branch to subscapularis).
- thoracodorsal nerve (motor to latissimus dorsi).
- axillary nerve (motor to deltoid muscle: sensory to skin overlying deltoid. (Fig. 8)
- radial nerve (motor to extensors of elbow, wrist, and digits; sensory to the lower lateral aspect of arm, central posterior aspect of the arm, central posterior aspect of the forearm, and the dorsal aspect of the radial three and one-half digits to the level of the proximal interphalangeal joints. This cutaneous supply is through the lower lateral cutaneous nerve of the arm, the posterior cutaneous nerve of the arm, posterior cutaneous nerve of the forearm, and the terminal sensory branches. There is considerable overlap with other cutaneous nerves in each of these areas.

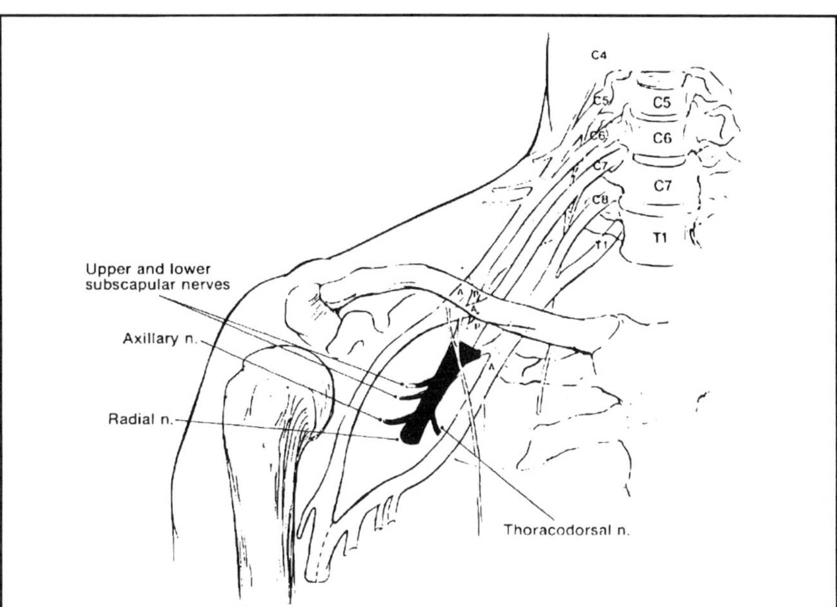

Fig. 7

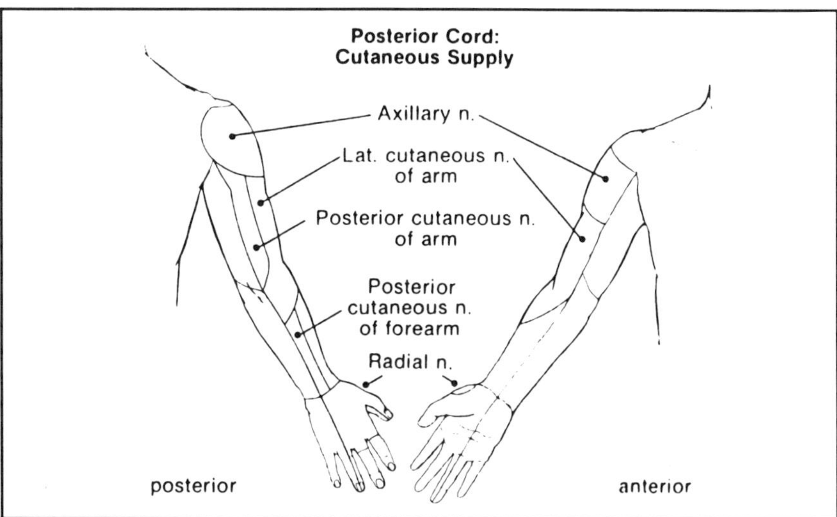

Fig. 8

Reproduced with permission from Malick, M., and Cash, M., ed. *Manual on Management of Specific Hand Problems.* Pittsburgh: American Rehabilitation Network.

The Medial Cord (Fig. 9) gives rise to five nerves:

- medial anterior thoracic nerve (partial innervation to pectoralis minor and major).
- medial cutaneous nerve of arm (sensory to the medial aspect of the arm on both the dorsal and volar surfaces).
- medial cutaneous nerve of forearm (sensory to the medial aspect of the forearm on both dorsal and volar surfaces).
- ulnar nerve (motor to the ulnar wrist and digital flexors and ulnar intrinsic muscles in the hand; sensory to the skin overlying the ulnar half of IV and all of V). Fig. 10
- medial head of the median nerve (motor to intrinsic muscles in the hand; sensory to the skin overlying I, II, III and radial half of IV on the volar surface and distal to the proximal interphalangeal joints on the dorsal surface.

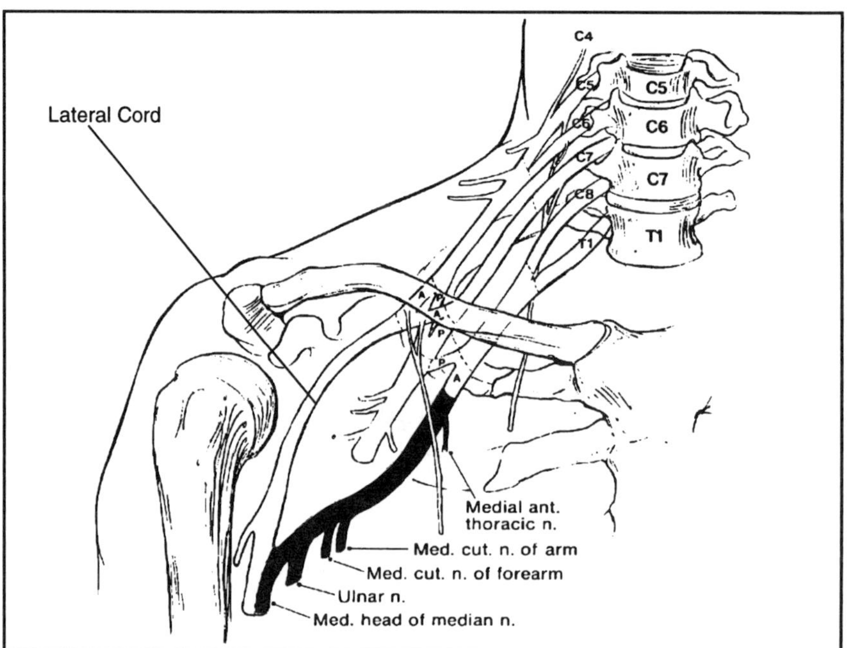

Fig. 9

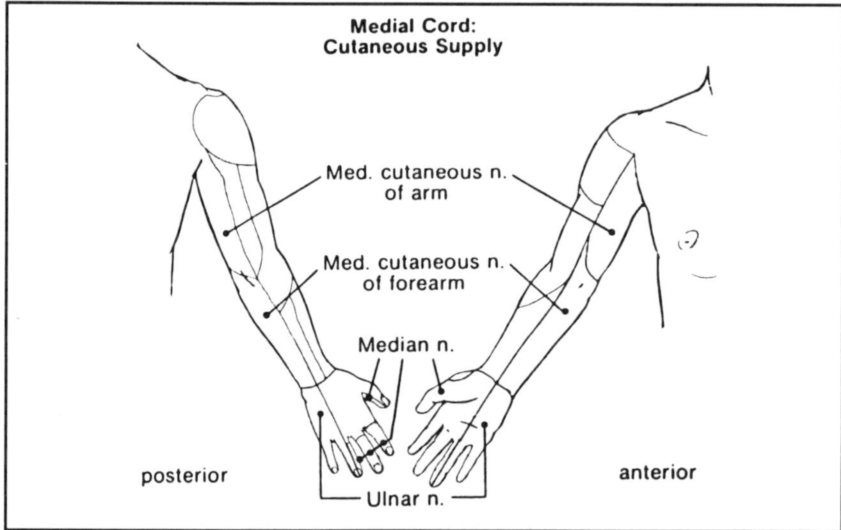

Fig. 10

Reproduced with permission from Malick, M., and Cash, M., ed. *Manual on Management of Specific Hand Problems.* Pittsburgh: American Rehabilitation Network.

INJURIES TO THE BRACHIAL PLEXUS

According to Leffert the majority of injuries affecting the brachial plexus are due to traction in which there is forceful separation of the head and shoulder during a high velocity fall, as in a motorcycle accident. He states that far fewer injuries result from a weight on the shoulder causing compression or a weight on the arm causing traction.

When the injury is above the clavicle, affecting the roots and/or trunks, the motor sensory deficits are segmental in nature. (Fig. 11, 12) In total plexus palsy, according to Haymaker, the sensory deficit may extend proximally to the shoulder girdle, but is more likely to extend proximally to the middle third of the upper arm. At that level it encircles the arm, extending more proximally on the medial side of the arm than on the lateral side.

When the injury is below the clavicle, the cords and/or the nerves to which they give rise are affected. The motor and sensory deficits then follow the distribution of the affected peripheral nerves(s). An injury within the axilla is likely to also affect the axillary artery. Dislocation of the humerus may affect the medial cord, or less frequently, the lateral cord.

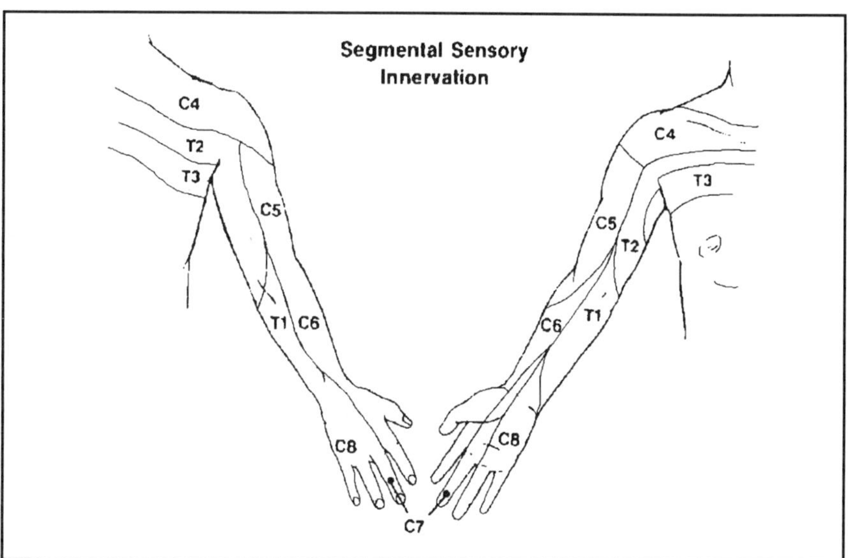

Fig. 11

SEGMENTAL MOTOR SUPPLY TO UPPER EXTREMITY

The asterisks indicate a supply also from the accessory nerve. A line bisecting a segment indicates that the muscle receives minor innervation from that segment (Fig. 12a and Fig. 12b).

Reproduced with permission from Malick, M., and Cash, M., ed. *Manual on Management of Specific Hand Problems.* Pittsburgh: American Rehabilitation Network.

<table>
<tr><th colspan="18">SPINAL SEGMENTS</th></tr>
<tr><th colspan="2">C1</th><th colspan="2">C2</th><th colspan="2">C3</th><th colspan="2">C4</th><th colspan="2">C5</th><th colspan="2">C6</th><th colspan="2">C7</th><th colspan="2">C8</th><th colspan="2">T1</th></tr>
<tr><td colspan="8">Sternomastoid*</td><td></td><td></td><td></td><td></td><td></td><td></td><td></td><td></td><td></td><td></td></tr>
<tr><td></td><td></td><td colspan="6">Trapezius*</td><td></td><td></td><td></td><td></td><td></td><td></td><td></td><td></td><td></td><td></td></tr>
<tr><td></td><td></td><td></td><td></td><td colspan="6">Levator scapulae</td><td></td><td></td><td></td><td></td><td></td><td></td><td></td><td></td></tr>
<tr><td></td><td></td><td></td><td></td><td></td><td></td><td></td><td></td><td colspan="3">Teres minor</td><td></td><td></td><td></td><td></td><td></td><td></td><td></td></tr>
<tr><td></td><td></td><td></td><td></td><td></td><td></td><td></td><td></td><td colspan="3">Supraspinatus</td><td></td><td></td><td></td><td></td><td></td><td></td><td></td></tr>
<tr><td></td><td></td><td></td><td></td><td></td><td></td><td></td><td></td><td colspan="3">Rhomboids</td><td></td><td></td><td></td><td></td><td></td><td></td><td></td></tr>
<tr><td></td><td></td><td></td><td></td><td></td><td></td><td></td><td></td><td colspan="3">Infraspinatus</td><td></td><td></td><td></td><td></td><td></td><td></td><td></td></tr>
<tr><td></td><td></td><td></td><td></td><td></td><td></td><td></td><td></td><td colspan="3">Deltoid</td><td></td><td></td><td></td><td></td><td></td><td></td><td></td></tr>
<tr><td></td><td></td><td></td><td></td><td></td><td></td><td></td><td></td><td colspan="4">Teres major</td><td></td><td></td><td></td><td></td><td></td><td></td></tr>
<tr><td></td><td></td><td></td><td></td><td></td><td></td><td></td><td></td><td colspan="4">Biceps</td><td></td><td></td><td></td><td></td><td></td><td></td></tr>
<tr><td></td><td></td><td></td><td></td><td></td><td></td><td></td><td></td><td colspan="4">Brachialis</td><td></td><td></td><td></td><td></td><td></td><td></td></tr>
<tr><td></td><td></td><td></td><td></td><td></td><td></td><td></td><td></td><td colspan="6">Serratus anterior</td><td></td><td></td><td></td><td></td></tr>
<tr><td></td><td></td><td></td><td></td><td></td><td></td><td></td><td></td><td colspan="8">Subscapularis</td><td></td><td></td></tr>
<tr><td></td><td></td><td></td><td></td><td></td><td></td><td></td><td></td><td colspan="10">Pectoralis major</td></tr>
<tr><td></td><td></td><td></td><td></td><td></td><td></td><td></td><td></td><td></td><td></td><td colspan="8">Pectoralis minor</td></tr>
<tr><td></td><td></td><td></td><td></td><td></td><td></td><td></td><td></td><td></td><td></td><td></td><td colspan="3">Coracobrachialis</td><td></td><td></td><td></td><td></td></tr>
<tr><td></td><td></td><td></td><td></td><td></td><td></td><td></td><td></td><td></td><td></td><td></td><td colspan="5">Latissimus dorsi</td><td></td><td></td></tr>
<tr><td></td><td></td><td></td><td></td><td></td><td></td><td></td><td></td><td></td><td></td><td></td><td></td><td colspan="4">Anconeus</td><td></td><td></td></tr>
<tr><td></td><td></td><td></td><td></td><td></td><td></td><td></td><td></td><td></td><td></td><td></td><td></td><td colspan="5">Triceps</td><td></td></tr>
</table>

Fig. 12a

Reproduced with permission from Malick, M., and Cash, M., ed. *Manual on Management of Specific Hand Problems.* Pittsburgh: American Rehabilitation Network.

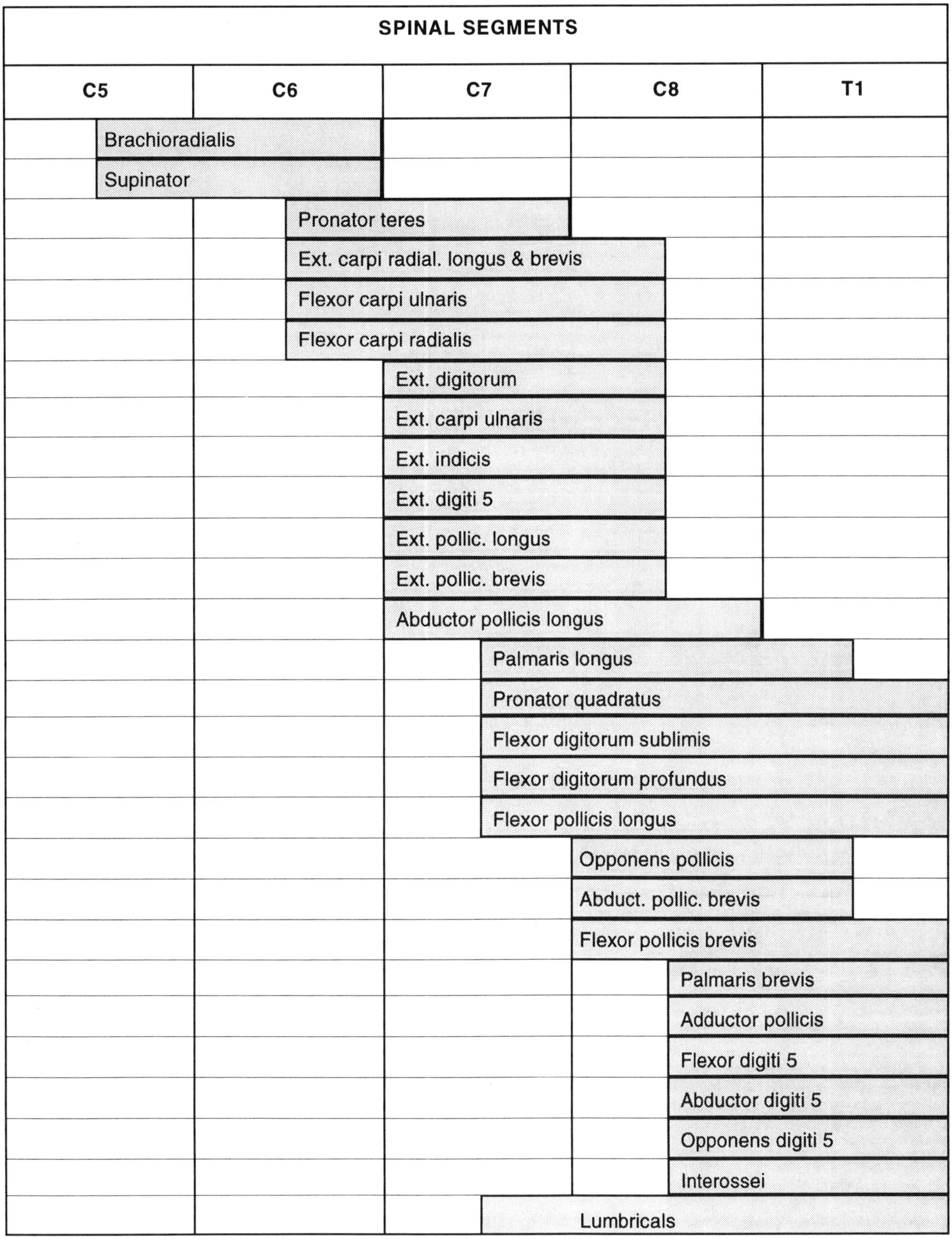

<table>
<tr><th colspan="10">SPINAL SEGMENTS</th></tr>
<tr><th colspan="2">C5</th><th colspan="2">C6</th><th colspan="2">C7</th><th colspan="2">C8</th><th colspan="2">T1</th></tr>
<tr><td></td><td colspan="3">Brachioradialis</td><td></td><td></td><td></td><td></td><td></td><td></td></tr>
<tr><td></td><td colspan="3">Supinator</td><td></td><td></td><td></td><td></td><td></td><td></td></tr>
<tr><td></td><td></td><td></td><td colspan="3">Pronator teres</td><td></td><td></td><td></td><td></td></tr>
<tr><td></td><td></td><td></td><td colspan="4">Ext. carpi radial. longus & brevis</td><td></td><td></td><td></td></tr>
<tr><td></td><td></td><td></td><td colspan="4">Flexor carpi ulnaris</td><td></td><td></td><td></td></tr>
<tr><td></td><td></td><td></td><td colspan="4">Flexor carpi radialis</td><td></td><td></td><td></td></tr>
<tr><td></td><td></td><td></td><td></td><td colspan="3">Ext. digitorum</td><td></td><td></td><td></td></tr>
<tr><td></td><td></td><td></td><td></td><td colspan="3">Ext. carpi ulnaris</td><td></td><td></td><td></td></tr>
<tr><td></td><td></td><td></td><td></td><td colspan="3">Ext. indicis</td><td></td><td></td><td></td></tr>
<tr><td></td><td></td><td></td><td></td><td colspan="3">Ext. digiti 5</td><td></td><td></td><td></td></tr>
<tr><td></td><td></td><td></td><td></td><td colspan="3">Ext. pollic. longus</td><td></td><td></td><td></td></tr>
<tr><td></td><td></td><td></td><td></td><td colspan="3">Ext. pollic. brevis</td><td></td><td></td><td></td></tr>
<tr><td></td><td></td><td></td><td></td><td colspan="4">Abductor pollicis longus</td><td></td><td></td></tr>
<tr><td></td><td></td><td></td><td></td><td></td><td colspan="4">Palmaris longus</td><td></td></tr>
<tr><td></td><td></td><td></td><td></td><td></td><td colspan="5">Pronator quadratus</td></tr>
<tr><td></td><td></td><td></td><td></td><td></td><td colspan="5">Flexor digitorum sublimis</td></tr>
<tr><td></td><td></td><td></td><td></td><td></td><td colspan="5">Flexor digitorum profundus</td></tr>
<tr><td></td><td></td><td></td><td></td><td></td><td colspan="5">Flexor pollicis longus</td></tr>
<tr><td></td><td></td><td></td><td></td><td></td><td></td><td colspan="3">Opponens pollicis</td><td></td></tr>
<tr><td></td><td></td><td></td><td></td><td></td><td></td><td colspan="3">Abduct. pollic. brevis</td><td></td></tr>
<tr><td></td><td></td><td></td><td></td><td></td><td></td><td colspan="4">Flexor pollicis brevis</td></tr>
<tr><td></td><td></td><td></td><td></td><td></td><td></td><td></td><td colspan="3">Palmaris brevis</td></tr>
<tr><td></td><td></td><td></td><td></td><td></td><td></td><td></td><td colspan="3">Adductor pollicis</td></tr>
<tr><td></td><td></td><td></td><td></td><td></td><td></td><td></td><td colspan="3">Flexor digiti 5</td></tr>
<tr><td></td><td></td><td></td><td></td><td></td><td></td><td></td><td colspan="3">Abductor digiti 5</td></tr>
<tr><td></td><td></td><td></td><td></td><td></td><td></td><td></td><td colspan="3">Opponens digiti 5</td></tr>
<tr><td></td><td></td><td></td><td></td><td></td><td></td><td></td><td colspan="3">Interossei</td></tr>
<tr><td></td><td></td><td></td><td></td><td></td><td colspan="5">Lumbricals</td></tr>
</table>

Fig. 12b

MEDIAN NERVE

The median nerve is formed in the uppermost part of the arm by a union of the lateral head derived from the lateral cord and the medial head derived from the medial cord. In the upper half of the arm it lies close to the ulnar nerve. It travels down the medial aspect of the arm with the brachial artery. Fig. 13

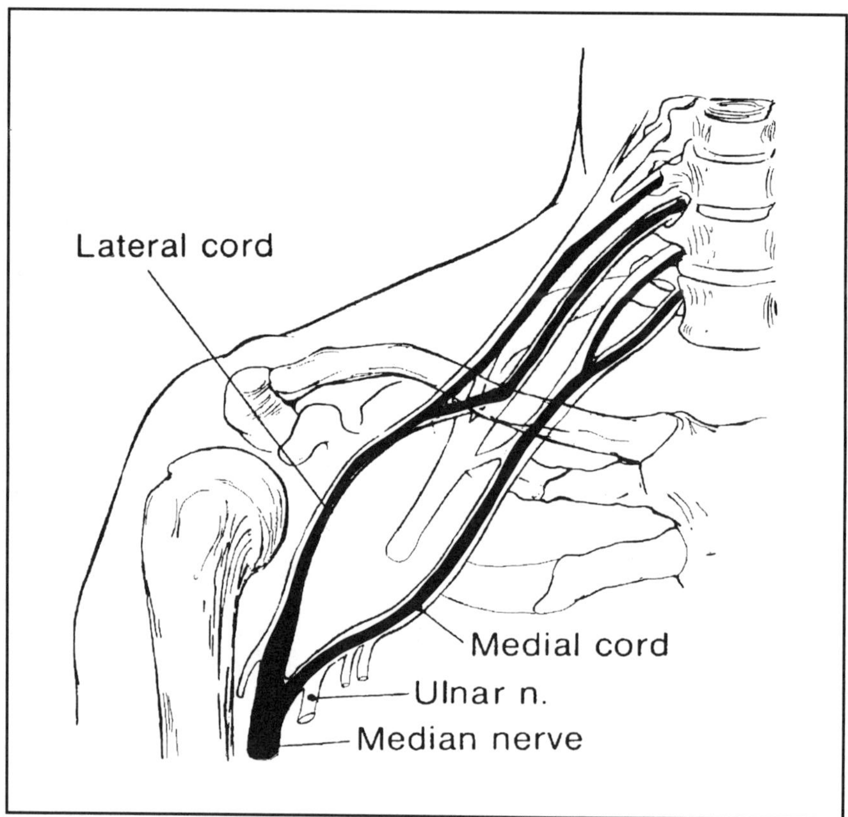

Fig. 13

Reproduced with permission from Malick, M., and Cash, M., ed. *Manual on Management of Specific Hand Problems.* Pittsburgh: American Rehabilitation Network.

At the anterior elbow it lies just medial to the artery which lies just medial to the biceps tendon. It gives off branches to pronator teres and flexor carpi radialis and passes between the two heads of pronator teres. About 5 to 8 cm. distal to the lateral epicondyle it gives off the anterior interosseous branch which innervates the muscles lying just anterior to the interosseous membrane: flexor pollicis longus, flexor digitorum profundus to II and III, and pronator quadratus. The median nerve proper then passes between the superficial and deep flexors, innervating flexor digitorum superficialis and palmaris longus. Approximately 5.5 cm. proximal to the radial styloid it gives off the palmar cutaneous branch which innervates the skin in the proximal palm over the first, second, and third metacarpals. Fig. 14

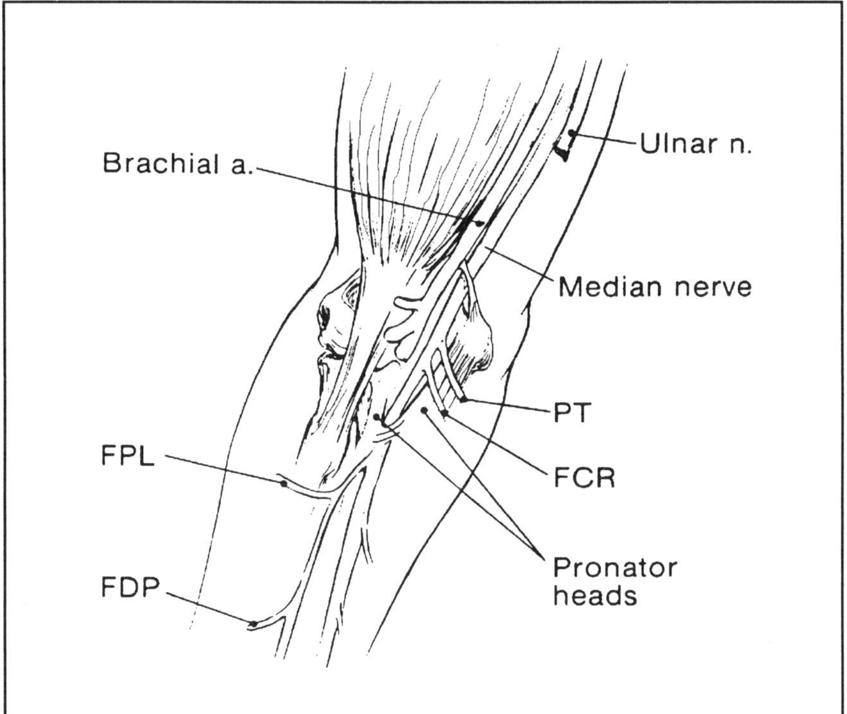

Fig. 14

At the wrist it passes through the carpal tunnel and then gives off a motor branch to the thenar muscles (abductor pollicis brevis, opponens pollicis, and the superficial head of flexor pollicis brevis), terminal motor branches to the radial two lumbricales, and palmar digital nerves to the volar surface of I, II, III, and the radial half of IV, and the dorsal surface of their middle and distal phalanges. Fig. 15

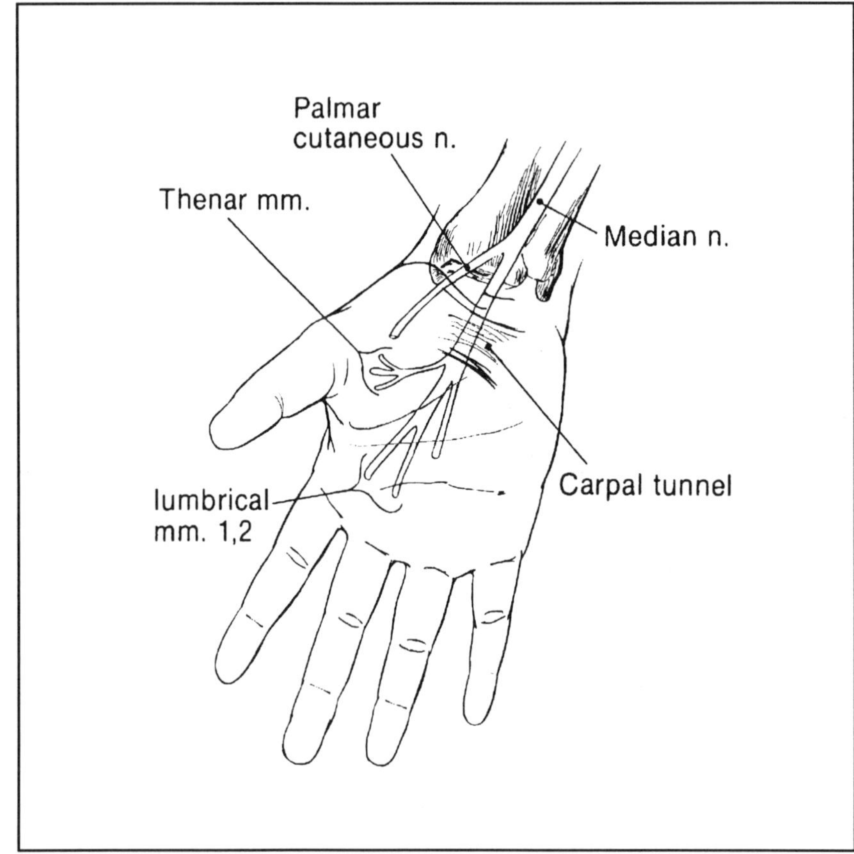

Fig. 15

Reproduced with permission from Malick, M., and Cash, M., ed. *Manual on Management of Specific Hand Problems.* Pittsburgh: American Rehabilitation Network.

Injuries to the Median Nerve

The median nerve is susceptible to injury by fracture of the humerus, dislocation of the elbow, fracture of the distal radius, anterior dislocation of the lunate into the carpal canal and by knife and glass lacerations especially at the wrist. Common compression sites are in the lower arm at the Ligament of Struthers (a ligament bridging a supracondylar process that occurs in 1% of the population and the medial epicondyle), in the proximal forearm (pronator syndrome and anterior interosseous syndrome), and at the wrist (carpal tunnel syndrome).

In a low lesion (wrist level) the functional deficits especially involve precision movements of thumb and index, including: loss of thumb tip to fingertip prehension, loss of pulp to pulp prehension, and loss of protective and discriminative sensibility in I, II, and III, and the radial half of IV.

A lesion of the anterior interosseous nerve results in loss of tip flexion of the thumb and index fingers, making tasks such as writing difficult.

In a lesion at or proximal to the elbow there is the additional loss of wrist flexion strength secondary to involvement of flexor carpi radialis.

ULNAR NERVE

The ulnar nerve emerges from the medial cord in the upper axilla. Fig. 16

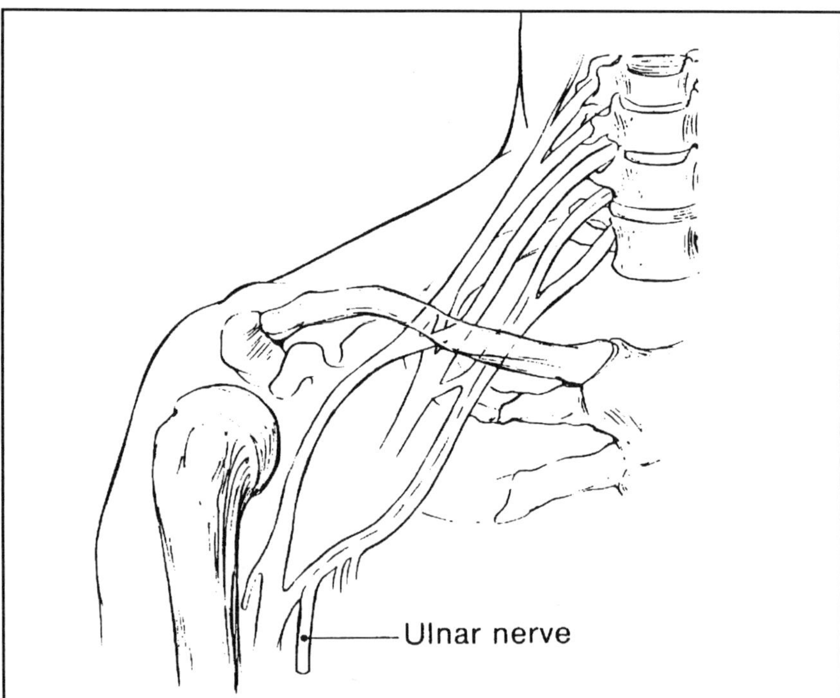

Fig. 16

Reproduced with permission from Malick, M., and Cash, M., ed. *Manual on Management of Specific Hand Problems.* Pittsburgh: American Rehabilitation Network.

It travels down the upper arm closeby and medial to the brachial artery and the median nerve. About halfway down the forearm it descends posteriorly to pass between the medial epicondyle and the olecranon (Fig. 17). In the upper forearm it passes through and innervates the two heads of flexor carpi ulnaris and innervates flexor digitorum profundus to IV and V. It then follows a straight course down the forearm.

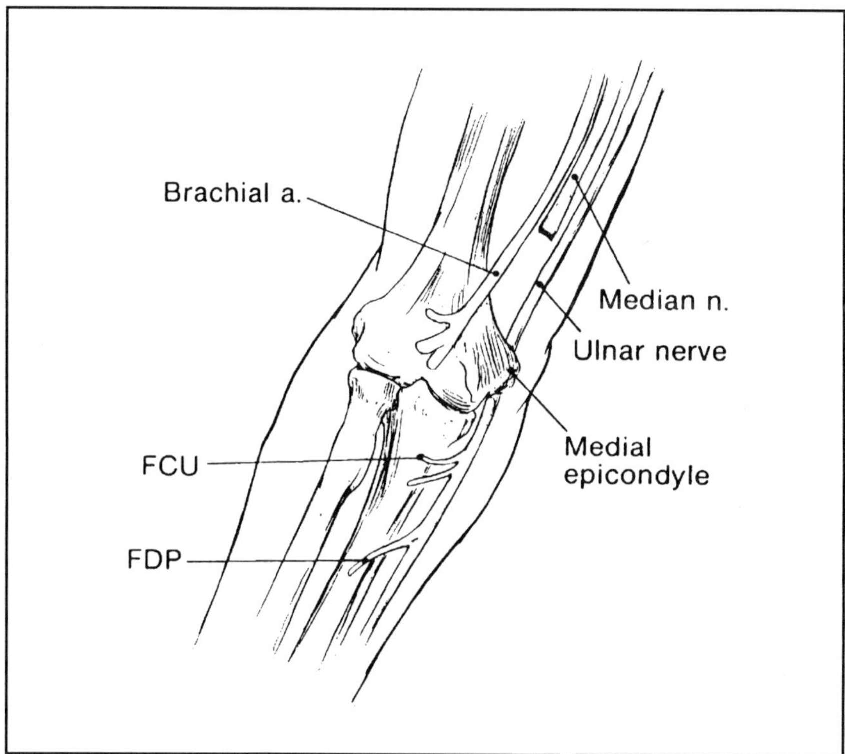

Fig. 17

Reproduced with permission from Malick, M., and Cash, M., ed. *Manual on Management of Specific Hand Problems.* Pittsburgh: American Rehabilitation Network.

Near the wrist it becomes superficial and travels with the ulnar artery. Proximal to the pisiform it gives off a palmar cutaneous branch which innervates the ulnar proximal palm, and it gives off a dorsal cutaneous branch (on the average 6 to 8 cm. proximal to the pisiform) which innervates the ulnar half of the dorsum of the hand including half of IV and all of V. The ulnar nerve proper then passes through Guyon's canal in the wrist where it gives off superficial terminal cutaneous branches to V and half of IV, and a deep motor branch to the hypothenar muscles (abductor digiti quinti, flexor digiti quinti, opponens digiti quinti), the dorsal and volar interossei, the lumbricals to IV and V, adductor pollicis, and the deep head of flexor pollicis brevis. Fig. 18

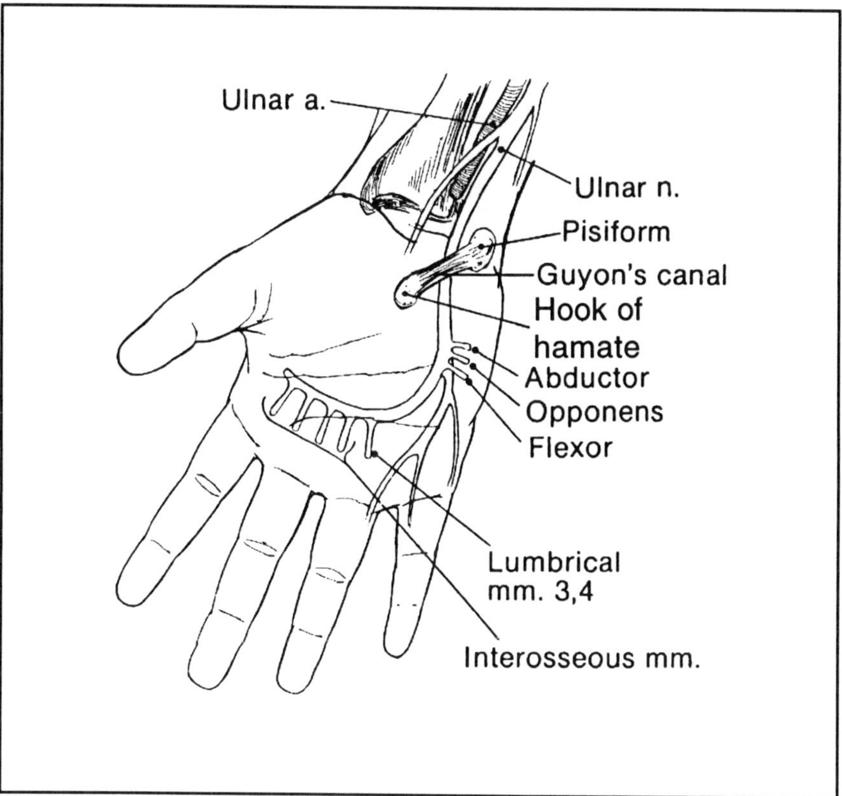

Fig. 18

Reproduced with permission from Malick, M., and Cash, M., ed. *Manual on Management of Specific Hand Problems.* Pittsburgh: American Rehabilitation Network.

Injuries to the Ulnar Nerve

The ulnar nerve is susceptible to injury from fractures of the medial epicondyle of the humerus and olecranon process of the ulna. It is also vulnerable to glass and knife lacerations, especially at the wrist level. Common compression sites are at the cubital tunnel in the forearm and at Guyon's canal in the wrist.

A low lesion of the ulnar nerve (wrist level) results in inability to perform thumb lateral pinch against resistance secondary to loss of adductor pollicis function. Lack of intrinsic function and lumbrical function to IV and V results in:

- decreased grip strength
- inability to fully extend the fingers in preparation for picking up an object ("clawing")
- inability to fully flex the fingers into a cylindrical or spherical grip, limiting grip function to hook grasp.

Moberg has pointed out an additional functional loss: inability to store objects between the flexed fourth and fifth digits and the palm whole carrying out three point pinch activities with the first three digits. All of these deficits are heightened by the loss of protective and discriminative sensibility in the ulnar half of the hand.

In a high lesion there is additional loss of grip strength secondary to paralysis of flexor digitorum profundus to IV and V and there is decreased flexor power to the wrist because of flexor carpi ulnaris involvement.

Reproduced with permission from Malick, M., and Cash, M., ed. *Manual on Management of Specific Hand Problems.* Pittsburgh: American Rehabilitation Network.

RADIAL NERVE

The radial nerve is the major derivative of the posterior cord. It passes through the axilla and innervates the triceps at the lower border of the axilla.

In the upper arm it innervates anconeous and passes via the spiral groove to the radial aspect of the humerus (Fig. 19). Approximately 10-12 cm. proximal to the lateral epicondyle it pierces the intermuscular septum to come into the anterior flexor compartment of the humerus. Here it lies between brachialis and the muscles that arise from the supracondylar ridge: brachioradialis, extensor carpi radialis longus, and extensor carpi radialis brevis. It gives off branches to these muscles.

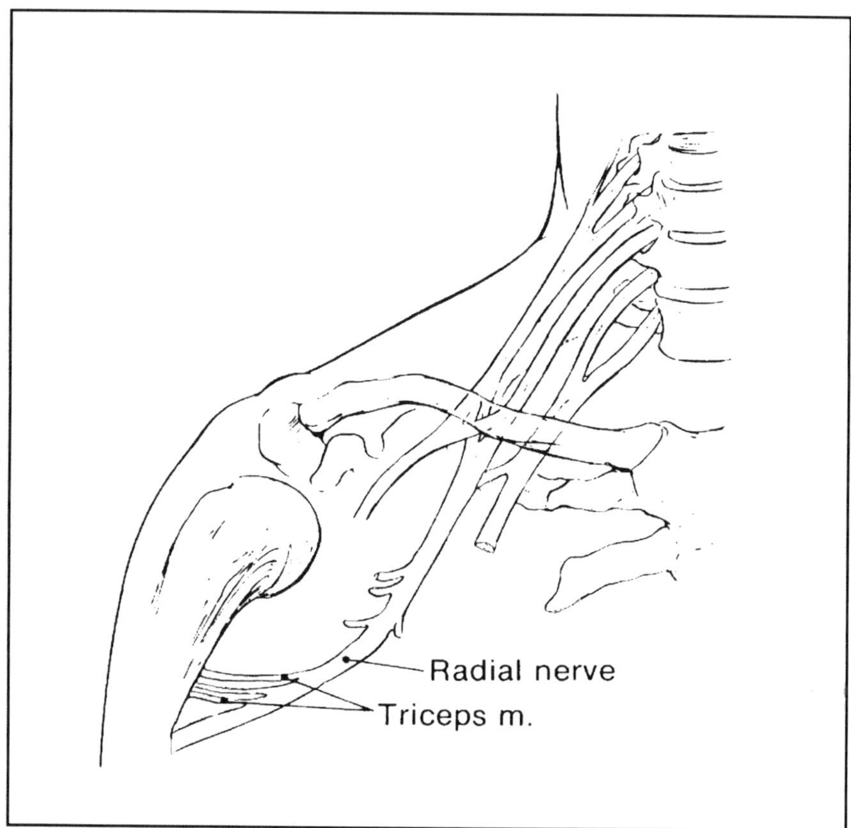

Fig. 19

Reproduced with permission from Malick, M., and Cash, M., ed. *Manual on Management of Specific Hand Problems.* Pittsburgh: American Rehabilitation Network.

At the elbow it divides into a superficial radial sensory branch and a deep posterior interosseous motor branch. The latter nerve immediately innervates extensor carpi radialis brevis, and then passes through the supinator muscle to extend down the forearm along the dorsal surface of the interosseous membrane. As it travels it innervates the supinator, extensor digitorum, extensor digiti minimi, extensor carpi ulnaris, abductor pollicis longus, extensor pollicis longus, extensor pollicis brevis, and extensor indicis proprius. The superficial sensory branch travels down the radial aspect of the forearm, becoming superficial in the distal half of the forearm. Fig. 20

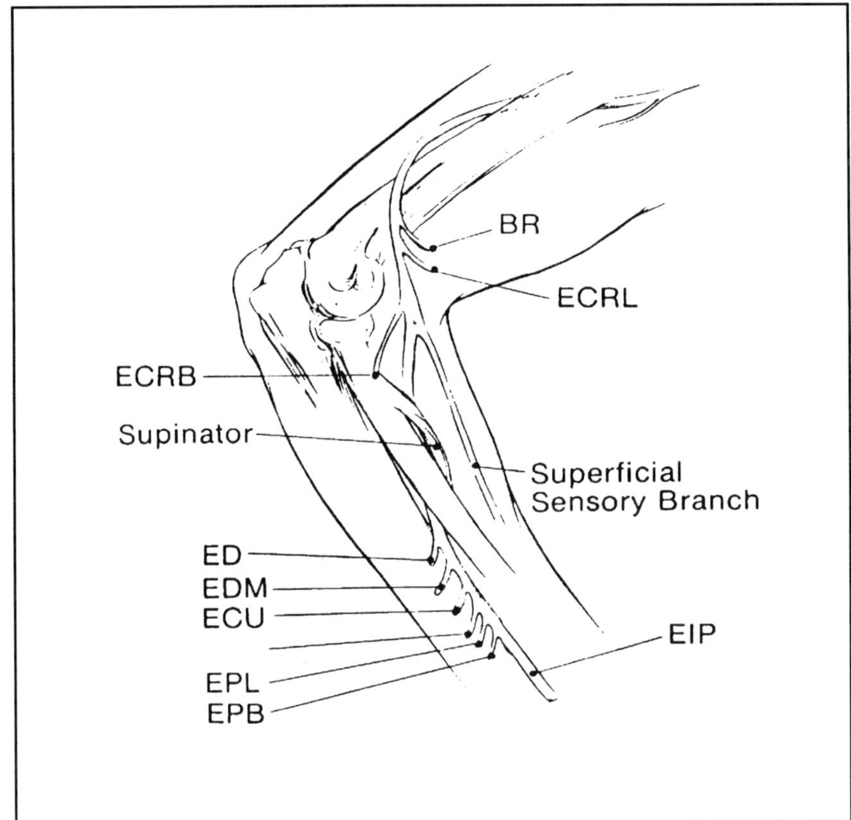

Fig. 20

Reproduced with permission from Malick, M., and Cash, M., ed. *Manual on Management of Specific Hand Problems.* Pittsburgh: American Rehabilitation Network.

At the wrist level, between the radial styloid and Lister's tubercle, its terminal branches provide sensation to the dorsal aspect of the thumb and the dorsum of the second, third, and half of the fourth rays to the level of the proximal interphalangeal joints. Fig. 21

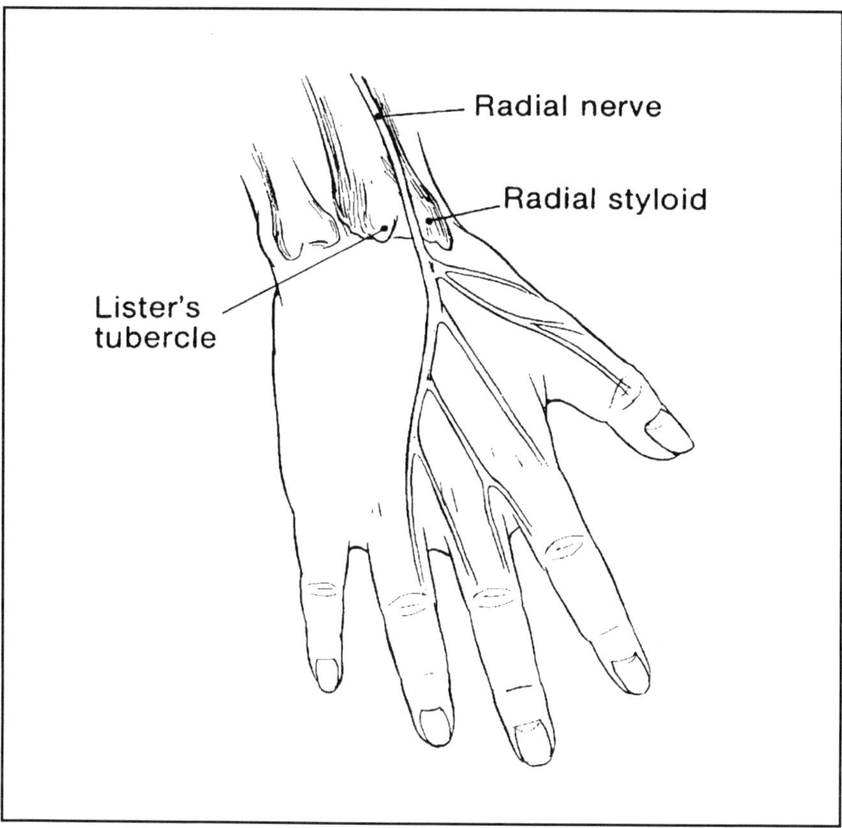

Fig. 21

Reproduced with permission from Malick, M., and Cash, M., ed. *Manual on Management of Specific Hand Problems.* Pittsburgh: American Rehabilitation Network.

Injuries to the Radial Nerve

The radial nerve is the most commonly injured nerve in fractures of the upper extremity, begin particularly susceptible to injury at the mid-humeral level where it travels so close to the bone. At this level it has innervated triceps but has not yet innervated brachioradialis or more distal muscles.

At the elbow level the radial nerve proper and its posterior interosseous branch are subject to injury from dislocation or fracture of the elbow or radius, and from compression at the level of extensor carpi radialis brevis or as the nerve passes through the supinator muscle.

A lesion to the posterior interosseous branch will result in weakness or paralysis of finger and thumb extensors and extensor carpi ulnaris. When a lesion occurs at the mid-humeral level there is added total wrist drop which will significantly decrease grip strength because of loss of wrist stability during grip. A lesion high in the arm adds a loss of elbow extension.

The sensory loss in radial nerve lesions is minimal because of overlap with other nerves, as discussed earlier. The only loss may be over the dorsum of the web between the first and second digits. However, a partial lesion of the radial sensory nerve at the wrist level can be very troublesome to a patient if hypersensitivity occurs. When it does occur it tends to be over the dorsum of the first and second metacarpals and may extend proximally into the forearm on its radial aspect.

LUMBAR PLEXUS

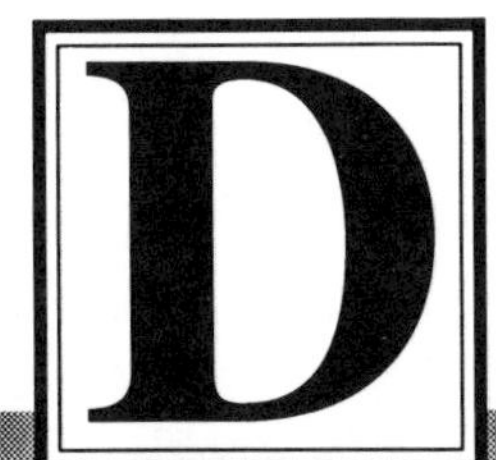

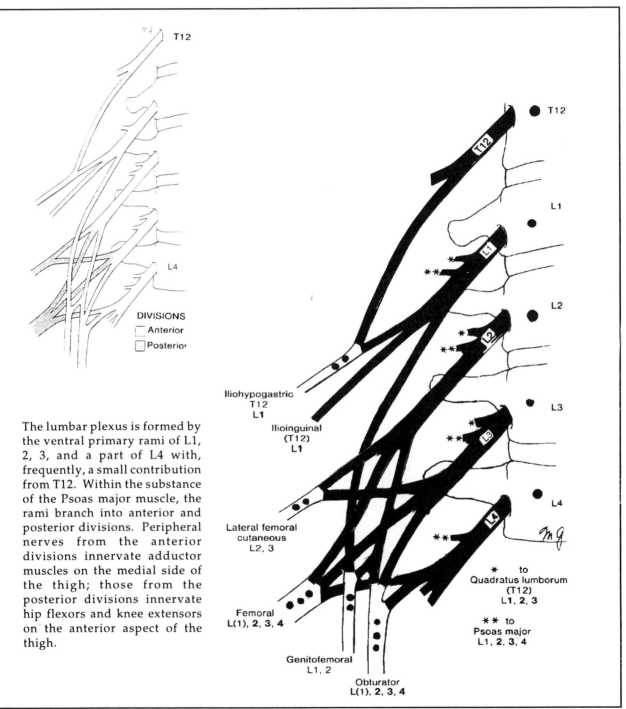

T12
L4
DIVISIONS
Anterior
Posterior

T12
L1
L2
L3
L4
Iliohypogastric
T12
L1
Ilioinguinal
(T12)
L1
Lateral femoral
cutaneous
L2, 3
Femoral
L(1), 2, 3, 4
Genitofemoral
L1, 2
Obturator
L(1), 2, 3, 4
* to
Quadratus lumborum
(T12)
L1, 2, 3
** to
Psoas major
L1, 2, 3, 4

The lumbar plexus is formed by the ventral primary rami of L1, 2, 3, and a part of L4 with, frequently, a small contribution from T12. Within the substance of the Psoas major muscle, the rami branch into anterior and posterior divisions. Peripheral nerves from the anterior divisions innervate adductor muscles on the medial side of the thigh; those from the posterior divisions innervate hip flexors and knee extensors on the anterior aspect of the thigh.

SACRAL PLEXUS

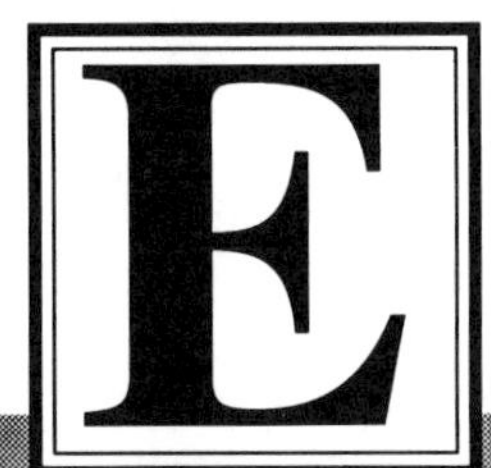

DIVISIONS
Anterior
Posterior

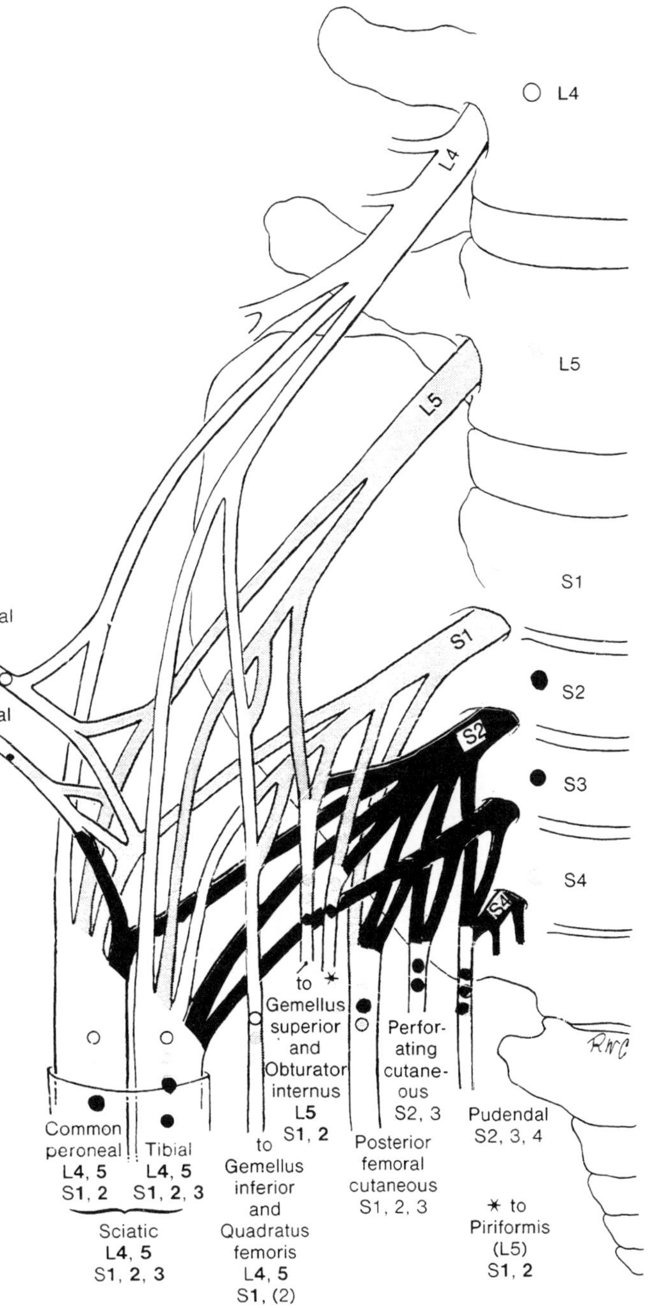

L4
S3

L4
L5
S1
S2
S3
S4

Superior gluteal
L4, 5
S1

Inferior gluteal
L5
S1, 2

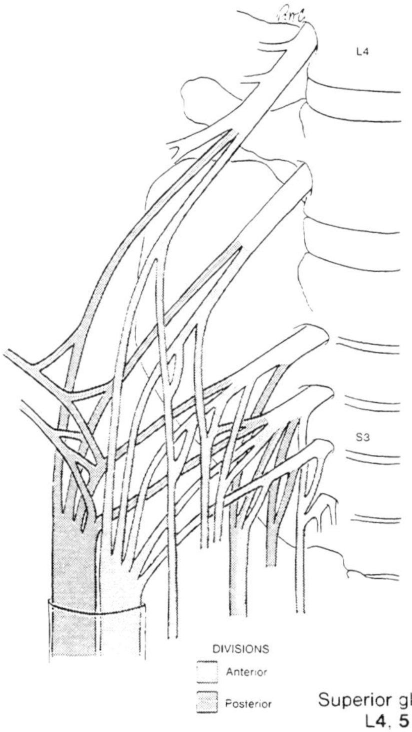

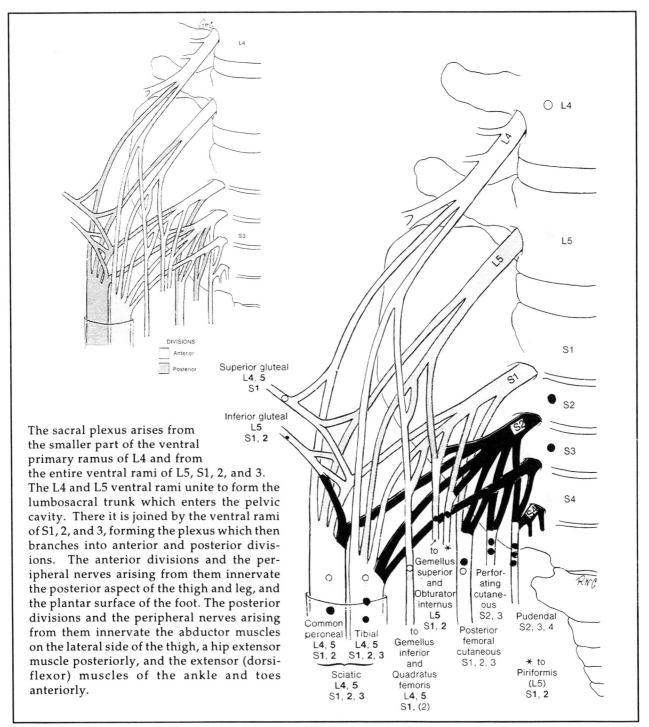

The sacral plexus arises from the smaller part of the ventral primary ramus of L4 and from the entire ventral rami of L5, S1, 2, and 3. The L4 and L5 ventral rami unite to form the lumbosacral trunk which enters the pelvic cavity. There it is joined by the ventral rami of S1, 2, and 3, forming the plexus which then branches into anterior and posterior divisions. The anterior divisions and the peripheral nerves arising from them innervate the posterior aspect of the thigh and leg, and the plantar surface of the foot. The posterior divisions and the peripheral nerves arising from them innervate the abductor muscles on the lateral side of the thigh, a hip extensor muscle posteriorly, and the extensor (dorsiflexor) muscles of the ankle and toes anteriorly.

Common peroneal
L4, 5
S1, 2

Tibial
L4, 5
S1, 2, 3

Sciatic
L4, 5
S1, 2, 3

to Gemellus superior and Obturator internus
L5
S1, 2

to Gemellus inferior and Quadratus femoris
L4, 5
S1, (2)

Perforating cutaneous
S2, 3

Posterior femoral cutaneous
S1, 2, 3

Pudendal
S2, 3, 4

∗ to Piriformis
(L5)
S1, 2

Reproduced with permission from Kendall, F., McCreary, E., and Provance, P. Muscles, Testing and Function, 4th ed. Baltimore: Williams and Wilkins.

QUIZZES ANSWER KEY

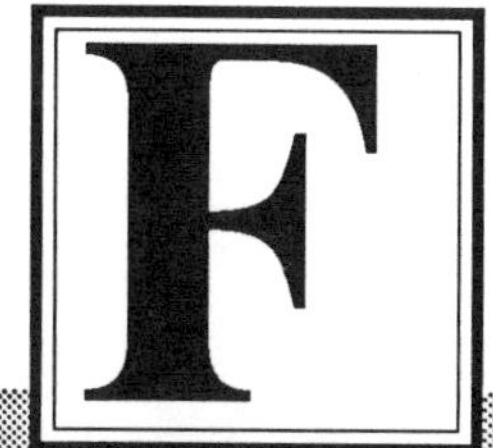

CHAPTER 2
1. False
2. True
3. False
4. True
5. False
6. True
7. True
8. False
9. True
10. False
11. C
12. B
13. B
14. D
15. B
16. A
17. A
18. E
19. C
20. B

CHAPTER 3
Scapula
1. True
2. False
3. False
4. True
5. False
6. False
7. False
8. True
9. True
10. D
11. A
12. E
13. C
14. B
15. C
16. A
17. False
18. True
19. False
20. True

Shoulder
1. True
2. True
3. True
4. False
5. False
6. True
7. True
8. False
9. False
10. True
11. E
12. A
13. D
14. D
15. D
16. C
17. A
18. C
19. B
20. C

CHAPTER 4
1. False
2. True
3. False
4. False
5. True
6. False
7. False
8. True
9. True
10. True
11. C
12. B
13. D
14. B
15. C
16. B
17. E

CHAPTER 5
1. False
2. True
3. True
4. False
5. True
6. True
7. False
8. True
9. False
10. False
11. D
12. A
13. E
14. A
15. C
16. E
17. B
18. C
19. C
20. A

CHAPTER 6
1. True
2. True
3. True
4. False
5. False
6. True
7. True
8. True
9. False
10. True
11. B
12. D
13. C
14. E
15. C
16. A
17. C

CHAPTER 7
1. True
2. True
3. True
4. False
5. True
6. False
7. False
8. True
9. True
10. False
11. A
12. C
13. D
14. A
15. E
16. B
17. C
18. C
19. D
20. B

CHAPTER 8
1. False
2. True
3. True
4. False
5. True
6. True
7. False
8. True
9. False
10. True
11. C
12. B
13. B
14. D
15. A
16. C
17. E
18. B
19. D
20. C

CHAPTER 9
1. False
2. True
3. False
4. False
5. True
6. True
7. False
8. True
9. False
10. True
11. C
12. D
13. A
14. C
15. A
16. E
17. E
18. B
19. A
20. A

CHAPTER 10
1. False
2. True
3. True
4. False
5. False
6. True
7. True
8. A
9. B
10. C

INDEX

I

J

K

L

M

N

O

P

Q